THE UNTOLD
HISTORY
OF HEALING

Also by Wolf D. Storl

Healing Lyme Disease Naturally: History, Analysis, and Treatments

The Herbal Lore of Wise Women and Wortcunners:
The Healing Power of Medicinal Plants

Culture and Horticulture: The Classic Guide to
Biodynamic and Organic Gardening

A Curious History of Vegetables: Aphrodisiacal and
Healing Properties, Folk Tales, Garden Tips, and Recipes

THE UNTOLD
HISTORY
OF HEALING

PLANT LORE AND MEDICINAL MAGIC
FROM THE STONE AGE TO PRESENT

WOLF D. STORL

North Atlantic Books
Berkeley, California

Published by
North Atlantic Books
Berkeley, California

Originally published as *Ur-Medizin* by AT Verlag. Translated from the original German by Annabel Moynihan.

Cover images © iStockphoto.com/duncan1890, iStockphoto.com/mashuk
Cover design by Bill Zindel
Book design by Suzanne Albertson

Printed in the United States of America

The Untold History of Healing: Plant Lore and Medicinal Magic from the Stone Age to Present is sponsored and published by the Society for the Study of Native Arts and Sciences (dba North Atlantic Books), an educational nonprofit based in Berkeley, California, that collaborates with partners to develop cross-cultural perspectives, nurture holistic views of art, science, the humanities, and healing, and seed personal and global transformation by publishing work on the relationship of body, spirit, and nature.

North Atlantic Books' publications are available through most bookstores. For further information, visit our website at www.northatlanticbooks.com or call 800-733-3000.

Library of Congress Cataloging-in-Publication Data

Names: Storl, Wolf-Dieter, author.
Title: The untold history of healing : plant lore and medicinal magic from the stone age to present / Wolf D. Storl.
Other titles: Uz-Medizin. English
Description: Berkeley, California : North Atlantic Books, [2017] | Includes bibliographical references and index.
Identifiers: LCCN 2016048623| ISBN 9781623170936 (paperback) | ISBN 9781623170943 (ebook)
Subjects: | MESH: Medicine, Traditional—history | Herbal Medicine—history | History of Medicine
Classification: LCC R733 | NLM WZ 309 | DDC 610—dc23
LC record available at https://lccn.loc.gov/2016048623

1 2 3 4 5 6 7 8 9 UNITED 22 21 21 20 19 18 17

Printed on recycled paper

TABLE OF CONTENTS

CHAPTER 1

Traditional European Medicine (TEM) 1

The Assumed Origin of Medicine 3
A Modern Myth 8
The Ecological Embedding of Classical Healing Systems 9
European Woodland Culture 12
Great Tradition, Little Tradition 19
Cultural Convergences 21

CHAPTER 2

One Cup of Tea, Three Times a Day 25

The Herbal Tea of the Forest People 26
Chinese Tea Culture 28
Herbal Practices in Other Cultures 31
Fire and Water 35
Rain and Sun 37
From the Beer Mug to the Holy Grail 42
The Daily Cycle 48
The Cross as a Primal Symbol 53

CHAPTER 3

Stone Age Roots, Ice Age Medicine 59

The World of the Paleolithic Big Game Hunters 62
Healing Plants and Diseases of the Old Stone Age 64
The Main Circumpolar Healing Herbs 67
Sweat Lodge and Baking Oven 82
Emetics and Purgatives 91
Shamanism 93

CHAPTER 4

The Healing Lore of Neolithic Farmers 99

The First Farmers 100

Witches, Stags, and Forest People 103

Sedentary Lifestyle and New Diseases 107

Arable Weeds (Segetal Flora) 110

Apophytes 113

Tough Wayside Dwellers 114

CHAPTER 5

Indo-European Roots 121

The Appearance of the Nomads of the Steppes 122

Illness Is a Bad Spell 126

Agents and Causes of Disease 127

Healing Gods 132

Healing Arts 136

Destroying "Worms" 140

The Essence of Healing Herbs 159

Signatures and Signs 162

Roots and Wortcunners 170

CHAPTER 6

The Transitional Period and the Christian Middle Ages 173

Cloister Gardens 176

Religious Legends 180

The Saints and Their Plants 192

The Comeback and Metamorphosis of Heathen Customs 203

Hildegard of Bingen 216

The Turning of the Wheel 219

CHAPTER 7

Alcohol and Burning Pyres 221

Professionalization 222
Heretics 226
Pestilence and Syphilis 227
Arabic Influence in Medical Vocabulary 233

CHAPTER 8

Wise Women and Their Remedies 241

Housewives and Grandmothers 242
Herdsmen and Smiths 252
Midwives 254
Magical and Shamanic Women of the Forest Peoples 258
The Remedies of the Womenfolk 269
Final Words: The Return of Ancestral Wisdom 283

Notes 291

Bibliography 309

Index 317

About the Author 333

CHAPTER 1

Traditional European Medicine (TEM)

The forest is the house of God,
there his powerful breath
labors in and out.

WILHELM MUELLER, JAEGERS LUST (THE HUNTER'S JOY)

They want medicine from overseas, though better medicine
grows in the garden right in front of their houses.

PARACELSUS

Modern mainstream medicine has saved many lives while lessening much suffering. Nevertheless, more and more people are beginning to approach it with skepticism. Despite all of the wondrous chemicals and computer-driven diagnostic techniques, despite the eight to ten percent of Western countries' gross healthcare system budgets spent on treating asthma, arthritis, diabetes, cancer, and Alzheimer's, many chronic degenerative diseases are barely affected, not to mention healed (McTaggart 2013, 26; Coleman 2003, 38). Autoimmune disorders are on the rise; children are at risk from the possible damage of vaccines. It is easy to catch an antibiotic-resistant infection in a hospital, and patients become ill or even die from false diagnoses, unsuccessful treatments, or reactions to regularly prescribed medication.

In the United States, where every year around 40,000 people are killed with guns, there is a higher risk of dying at the hands of a physician than of being killed by a firearm. Professor Juergen Froehlich, director of the Department of Clinical Pharmacology at the Medical University of Hannover, Germany, conducted a comprehensive study in German clinics and found that, in the internal medicine department alone, 58,000 patients die from the consequences of unforeseeable side effects from medicines every year. It is commonly believed that all medicinal procedures that are used today have been scientifically tested, for instance, with randomized, placebo-controlled, double-blind studies and elaborate animal tests. But the magazine *New Scientist* reported that such procedures only take place about twenty percent of the time.

At this point, entire bookcases could be filled with books describing the disastrous situation of our healthcare system.[1] Is it, then, any surprise that people seek out alternative, natural methods of healing, which appeal to them as less invasive and less dangerous? Since the 1980s, ancient, venerable, traditional systems from distant cultures, primarily Indian Ayurveda and Traditional Chinese Medicine (TCM), have attracted many seekers, who try out and practice, with more or less success, Reiki healing therapy from Japan, the Huna teachings from Hawaii, healing massages such as Hawaiian Lomi or Japanese shiatsu, Tibetan medicine, Korean medicine, Indian shamanism, Native American shamanism, pranayama, qi-gong, tai chi, and yoga. Small therapeutic sects have also developed that often contradict each other. Meanwhile, the medical establishment responds with scarcely more than a tired smile for such alternative methods, claiming that they might be entertaining pastimes, but when things get serious, evidence-based, scientific, mainstream medicine is the only one true medicine.

Nevertheless, TCM and Indian Ayurvedic medicine prove effective and are based on thousands of years of experience and tradition. However, they come from cultures that are foreign to us in the West, with basic tenets, healing mechanisms, and particular imaginations often quite alien to us. For example, how can we understand what is meant by "liver-blood"? How does one translate "qi"? Or, for instance, what should one of our experts make of a medical text that states the following?

When the common man rouses away the breath of the soul,
that is: there is too much metal for the wood to accommodate.
When the divine envelops the body of the soul with the breath
  of the soul,
that is: there is too much water for the metal to accommodate.
For the breath of the soul enclosed in the body of the soul
rules those entirely, and makes them wander,
and by wandering the body of the soul flew.

KUAN YIN-TSE OR GUAN JUNZI (IN HEISE 1996, 57)

There are similar questions in regards to Ayurveda, Tibetan folk medicine, and other healing systems. Each medicinal tradition is unique—as are language, religion, and other culturally specific systems of symbols—and has its own personal understanding of the essence of disease and health, their origins and purpose, and the role of the healer and the patient. Each system is closed in on itself, connected within itself, and coherent. Although each has its strong and its weak points, no systems are superior to the others, just as no one can say that there are better and lesser languages. The belief that our model of medicine is universally the best and only way has its roots in our culture—it resembles the assumption that our form of monotheism is the one and only true understanding of God and that there are no other gods; anything else can only be an idol.

In light of this belief, those of European heritage should urgently ask about their own primal medicine. Is there, beyond globalization, beyond international pharmaceutical companies, far removed from complex technology, and independent of today's mainstream medicine, an ancient traditional European lore of healing?

The Assumed Origin of Medicine

In school we learn that so-called Traditional European Medicine (TEM) has its roots in the Middle East. There, about 10,000 years ago, in the region commonly known as the Fertile Crescent, the formerly nomadic,

3

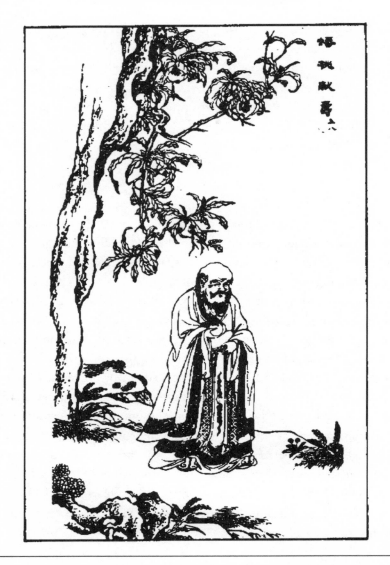

Shou-Hsing, the god of long life and medicine, holding a peach

starving hunters and gatherers settled and began to grow grain and domesticate cattle, pigs, sheep, and goats. Freed from the constant pressures of starvation, humans could now turn to intellectual matters. After the seemingly endless, dull Stone Age, during which people lived from hand to mouth, things began to look up for humanity. The first cities in this region were built, their administration became organized, social hierarchies were established, temples were constructed, and writing was invented. Learned priests replaced the primitive shamans ensnared in magic and superstition. The Near East is, as author James A. Michener (1965) said in his mega best seller, *The Source,* practically the source of all civilization.

In church, we learn that the Garden of Eden, where the evil snake whispered to Eve, was also found in this region. In this region as well, the "one and only true God" revealed himself, the Chosen People lived, and Jesus was born to the Virgin Mary in order to save the world.

In light of all this, we can expect nothing less than to also find the origin of true healing art here in the eastern Mediterranean. Medical historians tell us about the comprehensive medical knowledge of the Ancient Egyptians, for example, the Ebers Papyrus (15 BCE) with around nine hundred recipes; or the Edwin Smith Papyrus with a detailed understanding of wound treatment; or the clay tablets of the Sumerians and the Babylonians with cuneiform writing that already contained rational, empirical aspects although still bound to magical rituals. Then, medical knowledge moved into Greece, to the holy temple of Asclepius, and with the teachings of Hippocrates (479–365 BCE) a rational, empirical method of healing gained the upper hand. The origins of diseases were now less seen as a curse of the gods, bad magic, the anger of the ancestors, or other such things than linked to natural causes, such as a disturbance in the balance of body fluids (humoral pathology) or environmental influences. This movement made its way to imperial Rome where the physician Galen (130–200 CE) turned it into a comprehensive system of medicine.[2] The military physician Dioscorides, a Greek from Asia Minor, wrote the first herbal in the Western world during this time.[3]

But then came the Migration Period. Starving, boozing barbarian hordes, dense berserkers, with little understanding of the subtleties of civilization, overran the Roman provinces. These were primitive people, still caught up in magical and superstitious ideas. Because they did not consider reading and writing powerful, they had also no understanding

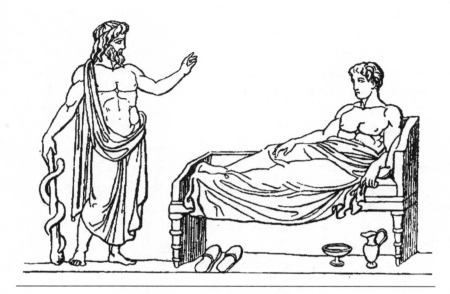

Asclepius with the serpent-entwined staff, which
is still the symbol of medicine

of the value of literary tradition; temples and libraries went up in flames. The recorded knowledge of the wise healers and their recipes were in danger of being lost forever. Fortunately, the monks who cared for this treasure trove of wisdom copied the surviving ancient manuscripts and thus secured them throughout the Dark Ages. In addition, they cultivated gardens of trusted medical plants from the Mediterranean region in their cloisters. After many centuries dominated by the superstitions and idol worship of the heathens, the teachings of Galen finally reemerged by way of monastic medicine.

During the twelfth century, the original ancient texts—mainly Hippocratic aphorisms and the essays of Galen—which had been lost but preserved in Arabic translations, enriched and expanded medical lore. The interest in Islamic sources led to the founding of independent physicians' schools in Spain and southern Italy. Not just alchemy, alcohol tinctures, plant and mineral-based pharmaceuticals, however, enhanced the medical arts; more importantly, diagnostic and practical techniques

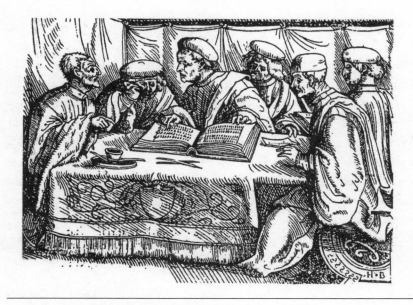

Learned physicians at a disputation, from *Liber theoricae necnon practicae Alsaharavii,* sixteenth century

came to the fore, which were based on scholarship, rational thinking, and clear observation of material reality rather than irrational mystical vision. These were all important steps toward the objective, scientific medicine and modern pharmacy that we enjoy today.

Traditional European Medicine (TEM), which is ever more popular and often endorsed by natural healers as an alternative to "soulless apparatus medicine," also fits into this pattern. It, too, relies on Near Eastern, Greek, and Roman origins, on dietetics, on Galen and his complex Galenic mixtures, and on the teachings of the four fluids (humors)—mucus, blood, yellow bile, black bile—which must be balanced out. It, too, relies on the tradition of dutiful monks and nuns who cured their patients in the name of the Lord with herbal wines, salves and tinctures, bloodletting, compresses and enemas, all with the help of Saint Hildegard, Paracelsus (1493–1541), and whoever or whatever else seemed appropriate—until the theory of bacteria appeared in the nineteenth century.[4]

A Modern Myth

What we read in the books available on the subject of TEM is, from an ethnologist's point of view, no different from a modern, Western myth. Myths, which are expressions and justifications of the images that a society makes of the world and reality, give meaning and order to that world. "Progress" is an integral part of this Western myth, but not every culture assumes that such a thing exists. For example, for the Australian Aboriginals, the world is as it is, and any change would be a distortion of the primordial dream of the ancestors. The indigenous peoples of Central America see the course of things in a decline and believe that only strict ritual behavior and sacrifice can stem the decrease in universal energy.

A further aspect of this European myth is the uncontested assumption that there is only one correct way of thinking and that it has one single source. The drive to convert others, to missionize, and to let others participate in that truth is part and parcel of that worldview. This attitude contributes to the ideological justification for the colonization of less progressive people. The modern version of this worldview can be seen in the "one world" ideology that serves global business and pushes through so-called universally applicable human rights, the McDonald's-ization of culture, the media conformity dictated by a handful of news and entertainment corporations, and, naturally, the medical system dominated by international pharmaceutical corporations—the only system that might be considered valid.

In the post-Christian era, this "one world" advanced to a secular religion, with its main icon the December 1972 photo from Apollo 17 of the planet Earth floating in the atmosphere like a little blue ball. This "Spaceship Earth," as the technocratic visionary Buckminster Fuller explained, needs engineers and technologists (key term: global engineering) as maintenance personnel in order to guide and service it (Storl 2004a, 161). The common citizen shivers in awe, but this image of Earth is, in reality, one of absolute alienation. The moist earth that smells of life in which the plants are rooted, the air that we breathe, the wind that blows through our hair, the whispering breezes of the forests, the revitalizing rain, the blossoming meadows, the trusted landscape, and the people who live here with their own culture and customs—all that recedes into the far distance. We often trust television programs more than our actual surroundings, and Facebook friends are "closer" than the neighbors. Would it not be time to come back to direct experience?[5] And doesn't this also hold true—as it concerns our subject—for medicine?

Research in ethnomedicine has certainly established that each ethnicity, each tribe, and each culture has its own complete medical science, just as each has its own language and unique connection to the spiritual dimension of existence. Each indigenous medical system has grown out of the local natural environment and uses the plants and other healing methods that are available in the region. Everyone grapples with disease and infirmity, which are connected to the local climate, the seasons, the lifestyle, and the nutrition of the people who live in the region. As such, diseases have always been just as much a social and cultural product as is the medicine that fights them (Porter 2003, 13). Consequently, each people and its culture has a tradition that develops within its own context and contains many generations of experiences that go back to the time of the forebears.

This is also the case for the native peoples and tribes in forested central Europe, who possessed an effective medical tradition based on experience. It is this primordial, pre-Christian medicine that we want to explore in this book.

The Ecological Embedding of Classical Healing Systems

Healing systems do not exist in vacuums; they are not merely the result of some professor's abstract theories. Medicine, including that of so-called advanced civilization, is—as far as conceptual models are concerned—embedded in the circumstances of the natural world. The seasons, the latitude and longitude, the local weather and climate, the plants and animals, and the landscape with its mountains, meadows, forests, seas, and rivers not only shape the economic foundation for

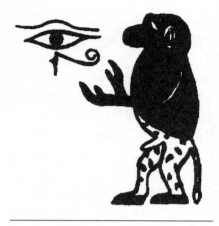

Divine healer Thoth healing the
moon-eye of the Sun God, Re

the society but also influence the conceptual model of the respective medical system (Storl 2010a, 6ff.).

Ancient Egyptian Medicine

Classic Ancient Egyptian medicine would have been inexplicable without the lifeblood of the Nile River, the rising and receding water on the flood plains, the elaborate irrigation system, and the surrounding deserts. According to medical views in the time of the pharaohs, the human microcosm resembled the green Nile Valley. Was human digestion, from mouth to anus, not similar to the life-bringing flow of the great stream? Did blood vessels and veins not resemble the enormous system of canals that regulated and cleaned the water? Did the human pulse not echo the swelling and receding of the river, and were the winds not like human breath? And because the worms and leeches that lived in the canals could make humans sick from infection, it is no wonder that laxatives (castor oil, senna pods, bitter cucumber, figs) or constipating, tannic drugs, vermifuges, enemas, suppositories, diuretics, purgatives, emetics, and bloodletting all played such a significant role in Ancient Egyptian life.

Ayurveda

On the Indian sub-continent, three different seasons provide the basis of Ayurveda, the classical medicine of the Indian high culture:

- the pre-monsoon season with its relentless heat (45 degrees Celsius, 113 degrees Fahrenheit, in the shade);
- the monsoon season with its heavy downpours and high humidity that makes everything moist, slimy, and covered in mildew; and
- autumn and winter with winds and cooler, dryer weather.

Ayurveda describes three conditions (called doshas) that take place in the human microcosm and can be compared to these seasons respectively: Pitta for heat, infections, and inflammation; Kapha for excess fluid and mucous; and Vata for nervous disturbances and anxiety. Medicinal plants and drugs, thus, are prescribed according to the three categories.

Traditional Chinese Medicine (TCM)

The five phases of transformation—water, wood, fire, earth, and metal—of TCM have their roots in the cycle of the seasons: the winter rain (water) lets the new plants sprout in the spring (wood); these are scorched by the heat of the summer (fire), which can lead to forest fires out of which ash (earth) is created and transformed into the soil; from the earth then come metals, such as copper; and on the metallic surface water condenses, closing the cycle (Ody 2011, 38). Everything is bound together and in constant transformation, not unlike the human system with its seasonal rhythms—wind, cold, dampness, heat, and dryness are not only aspects of the weather or change of seasons and not just external forces affecting health, but they also characterize inner conditions affecting organ functions and moods. For example, water is associated with the kidneys, bladder, and bone marrow: it is cold, its time is midnight and winter, and its taste is salty. Obviously, we are dealing with a complicated, highly sophisticated ideational system. All in all, the duty of medicine is to ensure that this transformation runs harmoniously—not too hastily but also not too hesitantly.

Humoral Pathology

Hippocrates's and Galen's teachings of the four humors (called humoral pathology) were based, similar to TCM, on the environment and annual cycles. The warm, moist blood corresponds to the warm, moist springtime of the Mediterranean; the yellow bile, warm and dry, corresponds to summer; black bile to the dry autumn; and mucous to the cold, rainy winter.

The foundation for this classic system of medicine is the vast natural world, the macrocosm. In the human microcosm, the laws work similarly and should be obeyed so that health is assured. Even modern medicine is served by a conceptual model, albeit the machine instead of nature, seasons, and landscapes. During the Enlightenment of the eighteenth century, the clock became the model for the motions of the planets as well as the functions of the body. God, the Creator, was depicted as a cosmic watchmaker who constructed the world and wound it up so that it would tick on its own until the end of time. Humans came to be thought of, as far as the body is concerned, as ticking mechanisms. In the nineteenth century, when the steam engine made its victory march, the idea of a driving mechanical energy was added to the model. And at the end of the twentieth century, the model expanded with the introduction of computers; the human mechanism guides the organism to a highly complicated, cybernetic network of mainframe computers: the brain. Our medical spaceship hovers far above, completely cut off from Earth and from nature. Major Tom has it all under control!

European Woodland Culture

Reference to the native-born people of central Europe in this book should be broadly understood. By no means does the term describe the inhabitants of the national states within today's political borders; the reference is rather to the pre-Christian ethnicities who once settled the vast European forests and worked the land with slash-and-burn agriculture. Mostly, we are talking about the Celts in the west and in the Alps, the Germanic people of the north, the Slavs of the east, and the Baltic people (Latvian, Lithuanian, and Prussian) of northeastern Europe. Even if the languages and individual aspects of any given culture have their differences, these peoples nevertheless have much in common, including their medicine.

These commonalities rest upon these early Europeans' broad forest ecosystem. The forest was the ecological, economical, and spiritual matrix that shaped their way of life. Their farms and towns were found on small, cleared islands within an immense primordial forest, the European rain forest, which grew abundantly thanks to the rain-drenched Atlantic climate. They built their homes from the wood of the forest; the gift of the trees warmed them in the winter and cooked their food; the ashes fertilized their fields; their swine, cattle, and goats fed on foliage in the summer and acorns and beechnuts from the oaks and beeches in the fall; and the bedding for the stalls, leaves, and dried litter came from the surrounding woods.

Under the trees and in the hedges on the edge of the forest grew vitamin-rich wild fruit—sloe berries, hawthorns, blackberries, barberries, serviceberries, raspberries, blueberries, rowanberries, loquats, sea buckthorn, gooseberries, bearberries, lingonberries, whitebeam berries, elderberries, cornel cherries, crab apples, hazelnuts, beechnuts, and so on—which could be dried and stored for winter use. The most potent medicinal herbs also grew in the ecosystem of the hedge, the transitional zone between the forest and the meadows or fields. Precisely these very plants have played a significant role in ethnology, symbolism, and "superstition" for centuries and continue to today.

In the forest, they also encountered nature spirits who had knowledge of the medicinal plants—clever dwarves, magical animals, elves, and gods. Wise, wild Ruebezahl who lives high in the Giant Mountains is a survivor from this enchanted forest world of distant ancestors. Related to him is the Slavic spirit of the forest, the Leschij, who often appears as a small man, but who can also be as big as a fir tree, or as a bird, bear, tree stump, or plant. The bear and the wolf accompany him, and he can whisper softly or howl like the stormy wind. He is partial to magicians and wise women and sometimes inclined to jest and mislead wanderers or mushroom gatherers. Then, there is Rusalka, who lives by forest ponds or in trees and dances naked by the moonlight in the forest. The solitary wanderer might perhaps meet the ancient Forest Goddess transformed into a witch—Baba Yaga (Storl 2014b). The Baltic people also knew about the green-haired "forest mother" who dresses in green clothes, protects the plants and animals, and punishes misdeeds in the forest such as trespassing on the vert (forest vegetation).

Thus, we see that the trees, the blooming wetlands, the cliffs and rivers, the birds, the fish, and other animals of the forest shaped, more than anything else, the spiritual imagination of the primordial inhabitants,

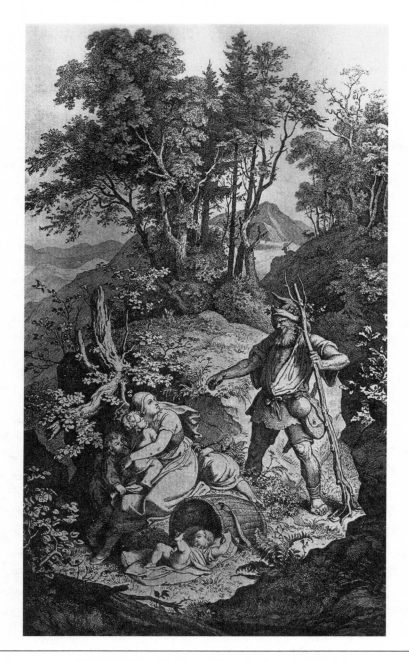

Mountain Spirit, Ruebezahl (Ludwig Richter, 1848)

who in part were the ancestors of modern Europeans and their relatives in America.

Certainly for the Celts, the forest was the embodiment of all that is sacred. Nemetonia is the Forest Goddess of the Gauls, Nemeton the sacred forest, and Drunemeton the oak forest. The Druids, the spiritual leaders of the Celts, were the forest (or tree) wise men (dru = tree; wid = meadow). According to Julius Caesar, the Druid's education lasted twenty years, a span of time during which they lived "like the deer" in the forest and learned its secrets. Merlin, the archetypal Druid, was depicted as a forest dweller in the company of a bear and a stag. For the Celts, wild animals, such as the stag, bear, wild boar, otter, beaver, rabbit, fox, wolf, and so on, embodied the soul of the forest, or were considered manifestations of the gods. The forest symbolized the world itself, the source, the sacred, the eerie Numinosum.

But these forest people knew neither showy temples nor sacred buildings. Why? The forest itself was their temple. "The Germanic peoples, however, do not consider it consistent with the grandeur of the celestial beings to confine the gods within walls, or to liken them to the form of any human countenance. They consecrate woods and groves, and they apply the names of deities to the abstraction that they see only in spiritual worship" (Tacitus, Germania IX). These are the words the Roman historian Tacitus used to describe the Germanic tribes in the first century, a striking resemblance to descriptions of other forest people. The temples that housed the human-like representation of the gods tend to be later developments and can be traced to the influence of the Romans and later that of the Christians.

The beech tree forest was the sacred place of the central European Germanic people. Here in the forest halls, the wise perceived the murmuring of the gods in the rustling of the leaves; here, for the sake of divination, they carved magical runes into twigs cut from the beech trees and painted them with blood or ochre. The runes were then thrown on a white linen cloth in order to decipher the counsel of the gods.[6] The priests also kept sacred horses in these groves, and, as oracles, they interpreted the animals' snorts and hoof beats. Germanic shamans, dedicated to Odin (or Woden, Wotan), the god of magic, experienced their initiation by hanging upside down from the branch of an ash tree for three whole days, without eating or drinking. The shamans undertook this ordeal to loosen the soul from the body, allowing it to fly into transcendental worlds. Their master, Odin, had first practiced the ritual, after having wounded himself with his own spear, when he hung from the Yggrdrasil ash tree for thrice three days and nights.[7] The shamanic god performed this self-sacrifice to acquire the wisdom and power of the runes.

For the Baltic people, the forest served as a gathering place into the nineteenth century, where people brought sacrifices to the gods (Lurker 1991, 811). Still today, important holidays such as summer solstice (also referred to as Midsummer's Eve and Saint John's Eve) are celebrated in these sacred groves. The gods reveal themselves in the trees: Perkunas, the lightning-bearing celestial god in the oak, or Laima, the goddess of fate, who dwells in the linden tree. Even the dead temporarily dwell in the trees of the forest—the men mostly in the oaks, the women in the lindens—until it is time for their journey to continue. They may also roam through the forest as birds or animals until they once again inhabit a human body.

For these people, Adam would not have been modeled out of clay and Eve would not have come from the rib of her husband, as the Bible tells us; the first human couple would have come from trees. Thus, for example, the Nordic myths tell how the three primordial gods, Odin, Hoenir, and Loki (also Lodur), walked along the shores of the primordial sea and came upon the trunks of an ash tree and an elm. Odin breathed the breath of life into them, Hoenir gave them emotions, and Loki bestowed the warmth of life and red blood. The dwarves, who are adept at handicrafts, carved the wood and gave them the shape of a man and a woman.

The Roman legions began to press into the forested land north of the Alps about two thousand years ago. For Publius Cornelius Tacitus, it was *terra aut silvis horrida aut paludibus foeda*—a land covered with horrible forests and dreadful swamps. Although the Mediterranean region was once also covered in hardwood trees, the early urban expansion of civilization—with its intensive clearing for crops, fruit trees, and vine-yards, fuel to heat homes, metal forging, and material for the flotillas and bridge making—eradicated the forests. For the Romans, the forest, which the barbarians honored, was a place of fear, dark and foggy as it was, filled with dangerous wild animals and even more dangerous wild people. In order to break the magic, the Roman general Julius Caesar commanded that a sacred grove, a nemeton, near Marseilles be felled. However, none of his legionnaires dared carry out the orders as "the hands of the bravest were shaking" (Marcus Annaeus Lucanus, Pharsalia III, 399–428). When Caesar saw that even the most hardened veterans stood frozen in fear, he took the ax himself, raised it up high, and cleaved into the two-centuries-old oak whose top was lost in the clouds (Brosse 1990, 156).

The Christian missionaries eagerly followed the Romans in their attempts to destroy the mythical world of the forest dwellers; in order to sow the seeds of "the one and only true faith," they had to vanquish the sacred groves and cult trees. Thus, they let Saint Martin (389–448 CE) fell an ancient spruce tree in Autun, Burgundy, while his student, the Bishop of Angers, had an entire forest, in which the heathens celebrated their "obscene" festivals, burned to the ground. Bishop Amator had a noble spruce, "a blasphemous tree" on which the heads of wild beasts had been hung, chopped down and the stump burned.

The story of the Anglo-Saxon missionary Winfrid (Saint Boniface) is well known, who, under the protection of the armed Frankish soldiers, felled the Donar's Oak (also called Thor's Oak) in Geismar, Germany. (Like other majestic oaks, this sacred oak at Geismar was dedicated to Donar, the Anglo-Saxon Thunar or Nordic Thor, the god of thunder and protector of the yeomen. It represented—much like the sacred oak in Uppsala, Sweden, or the Irminsul of the Saxon tribes[8]—the world tree, the axis mundi, of the Germanic Chatti tribe.) Saint Boniface had a house of prayer built out of this wood and dedicated it to Saint Peter—Peter, as the patron of weather, came to replace the Thunder God Thor (southern Germanic Donar, Anglo-Saxon Thunar), to whom the oak had always been consecrated.

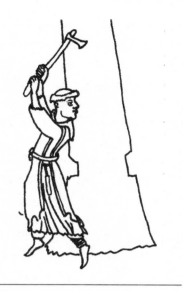

A monk felling an oak tree (French book illustration, ca. 1220 CE)

A few years later, Saint Boniface convened the Synod of Liftinae (743 CE). At this church council, it was officially forbidden to worship trees as well as practice other "heathen" customs, such as worshiping sacred stones (menhirs), collecting bundles of herbs, interpreting bird flights, soothsaying, decorating wells, engaging in festive processions to accompany the dead, and so on.[9]

Charlemagne also supported the desecration of the sacred heathen forest sites—for instance, the Irminsul of the Saxons that was believed to hold up the heavens—and initiated the clearing of the forest. And the zealous Cistercian monks, in particular, made it their mission to drive all of nature far away, the external wilderness as well as the wilderness in the human soul, and to cultivate what was left. Forest and wilderness belonged to the devil and his unredeemed spirits, the wicked wolves and the bears.

The battle of the new state religion, the religion of the sacrificial lamb, against the forest went on for a very long time—the Christian front pushed into the north against the Vikings and into the east against the Baltic people and the Slavs. The bishops and the Grand Masters of the Teutonic Order, over the course of two hundred years of continual religious wars, repeatedly destroyed the sacred groves and trees of the heathen Prussians, Latvians, and Lithuanians. The heathens practiced retribution by slitting open the stomachs of Christian tree defilers, nailing one end of their intestine to the trunk of a damaged oak, and then forcing them to run around the tree as their viscera unwound. To the missionaries, these actions proved the bloodthirsty hate of the godless; to the pagans, these actions demonstrated their high regard for the sacred

18

trees believed to be inhabited by gods (Mannhardt 1875, 29). The Celts, the Germanic peoples, and the Slavs also practiced this sort of punishment on people who sinned against trees.

The battle against heathenism was simultaneously a fight against the forest and the trees, for the indigenous people gained their strength and spiritual inspiration out of the forest.[10]

Great Tradition, Little Tradition

The pagans, of whom we are speaking, were illiterate.[11] They wrote nothing down, and all that concerns the rest of their culture was nearly completely absorbed by the Romans and the Christians, or obliterated. What could we know about their culture under these conditions? What sources do we have? Archeological excavations and the scripts of Greek and Roman writers, such as Tacitus, Caesar, Pliny the Elder, Strabo, or Marcellus Empiricus, are sparse, and the ones that exist are distorted by the worldview of classical antiquity. No wonder cautious empirical historians are quite skeptical about the information concerning the pagans that comes from these classical sources. On the other hand, they also find the gibberish about "channeled" information and the adventurous fantasies of many esotericists and New Agers even more unhelpful. In light of this dilemma, the following question is reasonable: Can one really know anything about the ancient pre-Christian spirituality of the forest people?

The answer is an unambiguous yes, one can. The key lies in the method of comparative ethnology and folklore studies. For example, when one takes certain elements of folk culture, such as the medicinal use of the elder bush, juniper, or hazel bush in the various regions of Europe, and compares them—and, at the same time, takes into consideration the corresponding fairy tales, customs, and superstitions—a larger picture emerges. This can be further expanded by comparing it with similar customs of other cultures, for instance, the Siberians or the Native Americans of the northeastern forests.

During times of cultural transformation, pillaging, and colonizing through alien invasions, the basic understanding of what the world is about collapses—the Irminsul, the pillar that holds up the heavens, breaks. The ancient gods are dethroned, denigrated, and turned into devils, demons, or servants of the new power. The former power elite, the nobles and priests, are disempowered, killed, or turned to be kept as henchmen of the new rulers.

Nevertheless, even if the gods now had new names and new compulsory laws prevailed, the common people stuck to their ancient ways and methods. The farmers continued to rely on their traditional nature calendars as far as sowing and planting, winnowing, and harvesting were concerned. They still knew the nature spirits, the helpful dwarves, the house kobold, or the forest spirit, and tried to keep them kindly inclined toward the humans with prayers, rituals, and acknowledgement. They still observed the behavior of the wild animals and the flight of the birds and knew how to read their messages. And even today holy "Easter water" (once dedicated to the Spring Goddess Ostera) is still drawn from sacred springs in many parts of Europe. Some housewives still sacrifice a bit of milk, bread, or beer under the elder and know how to get rid of pain, sickness, and other injuries by hanging such ailments ritually in the elder branches. Midwives continued to bring children into the world according to trusted and reliable methods. In the evenings by the fire, grandfathers, grandmothers, or aunts still told the old soul-nourishing fairy tales and stories in which the gods and goddesses transformed into magicians, kings' children, hunters, and witches, and live on as such. In particular, ancient, trusted methods for healing and medicine continued. People still knew which herb made one sweat, which one was a diuretic, which one healed a fever, which one eased breathing. The herbs continued to be gathered in the manner as they had always been, at the right time, in the morning dew, at the new moon, at the summer solstice, or whenever it is appropriate for that specific herb. One still knew the magic incantations that drew forth their healing power. The old woman, the grandmother, still knew about the different qualities of the nine woods when it comes to the boiling of a medicinal tea. Children still played their traditional games. And one still spoke the language of the ancestors whose wisdom and knowledge remain inherent in the vocabulary and idioms of today.

In contrast to the "high culture"—the upper classes, the powerful—the "lower culture" of the people remained. The American anthropologist Robert Redfield (1897–1957) discussed the Great Tradition and the Little Tradition (Redfield 1953). He proposed a continuum that starts with the pole of urban civilizations based in written culture and ends at the pole of the illiterate, rural folk culture. On the one side, we have politicians, teachers, priests, and bureaucrats, while on the other side, we have the common people who pass on their knowledge orally from generation to generation and who have a direct relationship to the land and the environment.

Historical writing usually comes from the literary culture of the upper classes. This is the case with the history of Western medicine, which traces its path from the Near East through Greece to Rome and through monastic medicine, incorporating the influence of the alchemists and so on. The oral tradition of folk medicine, however, has found therein little notice, instead actual disdain.

Cultural Convergences

Today, we have distanced ourselves so much from the natural foundation of our existence that we hardly realize how much traditional cultures are embedded in the surrounding nature and landscape. The weather, the rhythms of the seasons, the local flora, the soil conditions, and the fauna have deeper influences on the worldview of a people than arbitrary, abstract ideas do.

In central Europe, as discussed, above all, the deciduous forest has influenced the culture since the Mesolithic. Even the first farmers—who appeared about seven thousand years ago in central Europe, slashed and burned the primordial forest in order to clear the fields, and then moved on when the soil lost its fertility—were, in essence, shaped by the forest.

The European forests stretched from the climate-determining Atlantic Ocean in the west far into the north and to the east, where they turned gradually into boreal conifer forests. In the southeast, they were bordered by the Pannonian and west Asian steppes out of which the waves of the

21

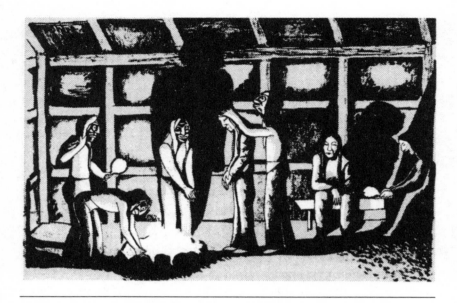

Healing ritual of the Iroquois False Face Society (painting of a Seneca)

Indo-European nomadic shepherds emerged. In the south, they were bordered by the dry Mediterranean. Even if geographical borders cannot be clearly drawn, one can nevertheless confidently speak of a cultural area, cultural complex, or cultural environment of the European forest people just as one can speak ethnologically of the culture complex of the eastern African cattle herders or of the cassava (maniok) growers of the Amazons.[12]

European forest culture can also be compared to the woodland culture complex in the eastern deciduous forests of North America. The indigenous people who lived there spoke derivations of the Iroquois or the Algonquin language families and lived in well-constructed longhouses appropriate for the climate and covered with elm bark. Further north, their wigwams were covered with birch bark. These were also slash-and-burn farmers—they grew corn, squash, beans, sunflowers, tobacco, and various greens. The fields belonged to the women, who also cultivated them. The men were responsible for the hunt and protection against possible enemies. These woodland people could be described as matriarchal,

22

just like the European farmers of the Neolithic era and later the Germanic peoples and the Celts, because of their gendered labor division.[13] Agriculture was supplemented by hunting and fishing, gathering berries and nuts, and, in the spring, tapping maple trees to make syrup. Like the ancient Europeans, they had a shamanic view of the world, and, as animists, they believed everything in nature had a soul and people could communicate with the natural world.

CHAPTER 2

One Cup of Tea,
Three Times a Day

The art of tea,
one must know,
is nothing more than boiling water,
making tea, and drinking it.
 SEN NO RIKYU (1522–1591), JAPANESE TEA MASTER

An ancient German saying goes:
No thing on Earth has such powers and such a rich hoard
 as the stone, herbs, and the word.

Kein dinc hât ûf der erden an kreften alsô rîchen hort,
 sô steine, kriuter unde wort.

In other words: Nothing has as much healing power on Earth as minerals, plants (herbs), and the therapeutic word. In particular, humans have always trusted in the great healing powers of "herbs," the plants that heal. This trust has even been since justified by today's standards. In the meantime, thanks to research on molecular structures, we know that plants are masters of chemical compounds and are living beings that have co-evolved with us and the animals. All over the world, including in folk medicine, herbs, bark, and roots have traditionally played a primary role in the treatment and care of the sick—of both humans and domestic animals.

The Herbal Tea of the Forest People

The possible applications of herbs are many and diverse in every cultural region. The folk medicine of the indigenous forest people includes the following approaches.

Infusion: Hot water is poured over the herbs, one to two teaspoons per cup; it is left to steep for a certain amount of time (three to ten minutes) then strained through a sieve. An infusion is usually what is meant by "herbal tea."

Decoction: First the water is brought to a boil, and then the specified herbs are added; after a brief boil, the pot is removed from the fire, the herbs are left in for a while to steep, and then the tea is poured through a sieve.

Boiling: Barks, roots, and wood, whose essence is harder to extract, are put into cold water (for about a half hour) and then gently boiled for a few moments in a covered cooking pot. Tannin-containing plants (such as oak bark, tormentil, bistort root) only need to be boiled briefly, at most three to four minutes, in order to extract the maximum amount of astringent (contracting, draining) properties. Both the field horsetail (Equisetum arvense) and the rough horsetail (E. hyemale) should boil lightly for about fifteen minutes in order to release the silicic acid. Bearberry is simmered for about twenty minutes in order to extract the arbutin from its coarse, leathery leaves. The standard amount is one to two teaspoons of herbs per cup.

Cold water extraction (maceration): The extraction happens by letting the drug macerate from eight to twelve hours covered in cold water.[1] Herbs with mucilage, such as marshmallow and mallow, are suited for this procedure. A cold water extraction is also recommended for centaury, sweet flag, and goldenrod. Valerian root should be soaked in cold water for ten hours; afterward, it is briefly brought to a boil and left to steep for ten minutes.

Warm water extraction (sun tea): The herbs are put into a pot or a cup with a lid, about one teaspoon per cup. Then, they are placed in the sun or on the warm stove for a few hours where they are delicately heated (to about 85–105 degrees Fahrenheit, 30–40 degrees Celsius).

Plant medicine can also be made by cold and warm extractions in various oils, such as the ruby-red Saint-John's-wort oil (Hypericum perfolatium), or as alcohol tinctures, pills from powdered herbs, salves, herbal beers and wines, compresses and poultices, herbal baths, herbal pillows, and inhalations. We will deal with these in more detail later on, but these additional methods of preparation do not play the same role, by far, in the folk medicine of the European forest people as that of the simple herbal tea—tea was always the first choice in this cultural region. In the Latvian language, it still sounds as it once did: sables, which means "herbs," is the word for medicine in general, and sabler dfert literally means "to drink herbs" but generally means "to take medicine" even if they are pills (Kurtz 1937, 37). The standard is a cup of tea, three times a day, early in the morning about an hour before breakfast, at midday about an hour before lunch, and in the evenings before going to bed. The tea was always taken for a certain amount of time, for example, over a period of about three to six weeks.

Usually, only one kind of plant was used for each tea. For instance, chamomile tea was used for digestive complaints, peppermint for congested gall bladder, coltsfoot for coughs and pneumonia, elder flower for flu and colds, bearberry leaf for bladder infections, skullcap for relaxation, and so on. By using single plants, so-called "simples," one can know the specific effects of the plant better. Of course, plants with similar effects, such as tried and true valerian, hops, and lemon balm for sleeping, or peppermint, milk thistle, and dandelion root for liver or gall bladder ailments, can be used together. In general, folk medicine avoids long recipes, the "composites," such as those the Roman physician Galen used; those found in "theriac," the medieval panacea; the recipes of medieval Arabian medicine; or those found in Chinese or Buddhist medicine.

The simple herbal tea taken three times a day is not a universal but a culture-specific construct of European woodland culture. In other cultures, medicinal plants are administered in many different ways.

Chinese Tea Culture

Herbal teas as medicine are of major importance in Chinese Traditional Medicine. Indeed, even the word tea comes from the southern Chinese word t'e and found its way into European languages in the seventeenth century: French thé, Dutch thee, Spanish té, and so on.[2]

Chinese tea culture is ancient, its origins disappearing in the mists of the Stone Age. Mythology tells that Shennong, in the form of a "divine farmer" and one of the three sublime emperors of primordial times, brought humans agriculture and herbal medicine. He also taught acupuncture and moxibustion, a therapeutic incensing by letting tiny balls of dry, fluffy, smoldering mugwort extinguish on the skin of specific parts of the body. Shennong's Paleolithic roots are recognizable in his iconographic representations, with the horns of a steer on his head and a coat of thick fur. Other gods of the hunters and gatherers of the Old Stone Age, alongside the cave woman, buffalo, and stag deities, were depicted as horned beings as well; thus, the hairy devil with animal hooves and horns is an echo of a buried archaic world.

The legend tells that Shennong tirelessly gathered herbs in order to research their medicinal properties. In one day alone, he was said to have

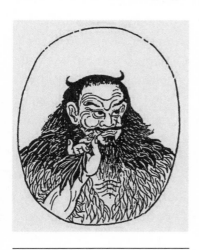

Horned Shennong tests an herb

eaten seventy-two poisonous plants but suffered no ill effects because he knew how to neutralize the poison with herbal tea. One day, after he had once again collected a bunch of herbs, he heated up a kettle filled with fresh water in order to test some plants as tea. (Incidentally, the Chinese symbol for tea means "to test, to try.") As the water began to boil, and without him noticing it, a few leaves from a bouquet of camellia (tea shrub, *Camellia sinensis*) fell into the pot. The water became a beautiful green color, and a lovely, mellow scent wafted into the air. Filled with curiosity, Shennong got a bowl and tasted the brew. He meditated on its effect on the spirit and body and realized that his weariness was gone and his thoughts were clearer than they had ever been. "Certainly," he thought to himself, "heaven has given me these jade green leaves because I am so old and of good heart, so that I might help all living beings" (Gruschke, Schoerner, and Zimmermann 2001, 26).

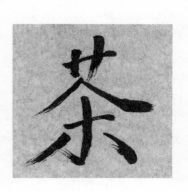 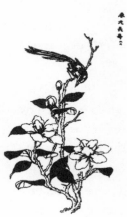

Symbol for *cha* and "leaves of the tea bush"

The Chinese have many different ways of using their healing herbs. Roots, bark, seeds, and twigs macerated and simmered is the most common form of preparation. Blossoms and leaves are added later as an infusion (cha). Cold-water extractions (jian), extractions in oil or alcohol and powder, and pill form are also used (Ploberger 2011, 29–30). The herbs are used as simples (simplicia), but most of the recipes are made with combinations of different plants, making up thousands of medicinal formulas. The main ingredient in the mixture is the "emperor's herb"; "minister herbs" then support the effect of the emperor; "messenger herbs" direct the effects of the other herbs to the appropriate meridians or body parts; and "assistant herbs" weaken any side-effects or alter toxic properties found in the emperor herb. In addition, medicinal plants are categorized according to their five flavors (sour, sweet, bitter, spicy, and salty), the kind of temperature they radiate (hot or cold), their level of toxicity, the four modes of action (rising, sinking, dispersing, and contracting), and their relationship to the major internal organs. This elegant and highly complex system has developed over several millennia.

How is the tea prepared in practice? It looks like this:

1. The tea leaves, as well as the medicinal herbs, are first washed in hot water and then the water is poured off.

2. The tea is then poured into a porcelain or clay pot, and hot water (80–90 degrees Celsius, 175–195 degrees Fahrenheit) is poured over it.

3. The infusion is allowed to steep for about a minute.

4. A cup is placed over the pot in order to hold the aroma; then the cup is rotated a few times around the pot in the direction of the sun; the scent is inhaled to take in the aroma and the delicate essence. Only then is the tea sipped.

5. The same tea leaves are repeatedly used for tea like this over the course of the day.

6. A liter or more of it is drunk over the day. Tea containers, usually thermal cups, are a common sight in Chinese taxis, work sites, offices, or market stands; workers and employers carry them everywhere.

7. An herbal cure with tea continues for three to four months.

Confucius, a Chinese teacher and philosopher, taught that the herbal formulas, with their emperors, ministers, messengers, assistants, and even farmers, mirror a harmoniously functioning society. But, above all, the natural Taoist philosophy is expressed in the cult of cha. Tea symbolizes pure nature; the herbs are natural instead of processed or refined. They are "uncarved blocks of wood" that contain all possibilities within. One drinks the tea over days, not to heal a specific illness, but to calm disease-causing excesses and imbalances, in order to bring the primordial energies (yin and yang) into equilibrium. These primal energies flow through both the human microcosm and the external natural world, and, when they are balanced in the individual, they enable him or her to come back into harmony with the universe, to maintain health. John Blofeld, scholar of Chinese philosophy, wrote, "The spirit of tea is like the spirit of the Tao (Dao): it flows spontaneously, roaming here and there, impatient of restraint" (Blofeld 1997, author's translation).

The Chinese culture of herbal tea has a very specific cultural background that is different—even if there are some similarities—from the central European tea culture.

Herbal Practices in Other Cultures

Herbalism is universal, but, again, the context of the application is culturally specific. Let us have a look at three examples.

Native Americans of the Plains

The Plains Indians, such as the Cheyenne, see plants as powerful beings. Without these "green people," neither humans nor animals can live. Each botanical species is like a tribe, and to be allowed to use the healing power, the healers or medicine people must entrust themselves to the plant and consult the respective chief of the plant's family. When the Native Americans of the Plains say that the medicine people enter "the teepee of the plant spirit," they mean that they step out of everyday consciousness and into the consciousness level of the plants. In this state of consciousness, the healer presents the plant chief with a gift of tobacco, negotiates, and humbly asks to be allowed to take some members of the "green people" in order to heal the sick.

In the same way, hunters go into a trance-like state of consciousness and ask the "chief" of the buffalo, antelope, or any other species of prey to be allowed to kill some of them in order to satisfy their hunger. To simply take without asking would be theft. If the consent is given, a ritual hunt takes place in which the chief plant is circumnavigated four times in the direction of the sun and then in the opposite direction—the direction of death, counterclockwise, that is, against the movement of the sun—and

31

then "stabbed" in the heart with the digging stick (the heart of the plant is understood to be the place at the ground where the root and stem connect). When collecting herbs, the whole plant—root, leaf, and flower—is taken. No iron tools should be used for this task. Collecting herbs is as precisely defined as the way in which animals are to be hunted; they are treated with reverence, placed onto a bed of sacred prairie sage, and then brought into the village.[3]

Although powders, poultices, or salves are sometimes made from medicinal herbs, the herbs are usually boiled for a long time and then drunk as a broth. When I asked a Cheyenne medicine woman why the herbs are boiled for as long as they are (because this causes many essential oils and active ingredients to be lost), she answered, "You need to cook them a long time so that the powerful essence is released. Animal bones also need to be cooked for a long time to extract the mark." The way Plains Indians, therefore, use medicinal herbs cannot be separated from these people's former life as buffalo hunters. The plants are "hunted" and their "flesh and bones" used, as is the case with the animals.

Tibetans

The way Buddhist monks handle medicinal plants is quite different. Tibetan herbalism can only be understood in the context of Mahayana Buddhism. In the sense of "mindfulness," each feature of the plant is precisely considered: color, shape, smell, location, time of year, and astrological aspects. If a plant grows on the cool, shady side of the mountain, then it is ascribed a cooling nature and is used for febrile illnesses. Herbs that grow on the sunny side heal cold diseases. Laxative herbs should be collected in autumn when nature begins to dry, emetics, on the other hand, in the spring, when the plants sprout and flourish. Places where lamas and holy men pray, or in the vicinity of monasteries and temples, enhance the healing power of plants that grow within a certain range.

Prayers, mantras, and deep meditation load the plants with power. On days when the astrological conditions are favorable, and the planetary aspects and the constellations are suited, the medicinal plants are sung

over with mantras—such as the
Medicine Buddha Mantra, or *Om
Mani Padme Hum*—and worked
into salves, ashes, healing butter,
or medicinal oils and incense.

The "jewel pills" are particularly powerful and used in the
treatment of the 84,000 possible
health-related disorders and the
404 possible types of diseases.
They act not only on a physical organic level, the three "life
essences" (wind, bile, phlegm),
but also on a spiritual and soul
level. They act against the three
mental poisons: greed, hatred, and

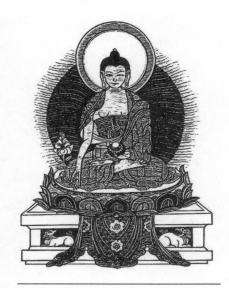

The Medicine Buddha

delusion, which are represented by the pig, the snake, and the rooster.
Karma from the previous life also affects them.

Up to 165 ingredients are used in these pills, which are manufac-
tured on particularly favorable days, such as Buddha's birthday or the
full moon in May *(Vesak)*. The herbs are heaped in the temple and con-
tinuously sung over with mantras by the monks. Crushed gems, all with
high symbolic value, gold and silver, the body wastes of lamas who have
meditated for many years, the crushed bones of deceased monks, and
other valuable things are added to the powdered herbs. The preparation
sometimes takes many days, and the finished pills are then wrapped in
silk or azure-colored silk paper. The blue is the color of the Medicine
Buddha *(Bhaisajyaguru)*. When the "miracle pills" are needed, they are
crushed in hot water and taken at the full or new moon.

South African Bantu

The indigenous peoples of southern Africa are masters of plant medicine. There are around three thousand medicinal plants known to them.
In almost every market, traditional herbalists and herb gatherers, the

inyangas (Zulu for "men of the trees") and *ngakas* (Soto for "herbal healer") are encountered. You can see them with their faces painted white—the color of the spirits—sitting on the dusty ground where they offer their *muthi* medicine spread out on blankets: roots, powder, and dried herbs of all kinds, along with snake skins, bones, claws, offal, pieces of hyena meat and skins, wild cats, and other wild animals. The animal parts are mixed with herbs and cooked with them to give them more "power." The medicinal herbs smell wonderfully aromatic; semi-decayed animal parts on the other hand smell disgusting. The muthi medicine is not only meant for abdominal pains, coughs, or headaches, but also magical purposes, for instance, against the negative influence of otherworldly beings, lovesickness, lightning, or evil spells, or in order to become invisible or invincible, or to win soccer games.

The herbs are taken as a decoction or infusion. They can also be used as incense, smoked, applied as salves or bandages, or used in baths and steam baths. It is especially popular to use the herbs in an enema, as a douche, or flushed through the urethral opening to treat venereal diseases or other disorders of that nature. Eye drops containing medical plant juices are also popular, and a frequently used method of therapy is to "scarify" the skin with razor blades and place plant powders in the scratches.

For the Bantu, diseases have many causes: jealous neighbors, evil spirits, black magic, broken taboos, or unsatisfied ancestral spirits. The disease is always the result of a lack of harmony in social relationships, in which the dead are also included. The most important task of the physician *(sangoma)* is to determine the source of the damage to health by means of a trance or through an oracle, for example, the tossing and interpretation of bones. The patient is not so much diagnosed as the social environment in which he or she lives is. This divination often includes entheogens[4]—that is, consciousness-expanding plant drugs. The *inyanga*, the wortcunner, assists the medicine man with the right herbal medicine.

Though limited and superficially recounted, these examples that have described the cultural contexts in which herbs are applied should be enough to illustrate that medicinal herbalism in one place is not the

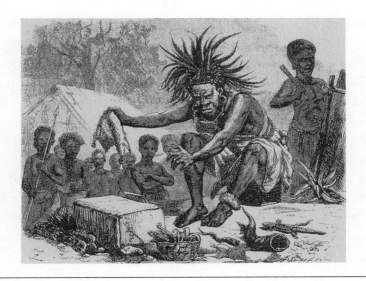

African medicine man (woodcut, J. Leech)

same medicinal herbalism in another, and that tea in one place is not quite the same tea in another. Now let's turn to the tradition of the medicinal plants of the indigenous European forest peoples.

Fire and Water

In German, the word for sick is *krank* which can be traced back to the Old High German word kranc meaning "crooked, bent, or invalid." The English word "cramp" is also related. "Sick" (German *siech*, Dutch *ziek*, Swedish *sjuk*) is an older word for the state of not being healthy. To be healthy is the opposite of sick. Healing (which is related to *hail*, derived from the Germanic *haila, Old English *hæl*) means "healthy, unharmed, whole." It is similar to the Polynesian *mana*, the Arabian *baraka*, or the Iroquois *orenda;* it is a magical force that contains happiness and health.

The word "to heal" is related to the words *holy, whole,* and *health.* "To heal" was reinterpreted by the Christians as a "release from sins," and

---

* It is conventional in historical linguistics to mark the reconstruction of words of prehistoric languages, such as Indo-European, with an asterisk.

the Healer, the Savior, also distinguished himself as a healer of the sick. "Hail" (Old High German *heil wis;* Old English *wes hail* became "wassail," meaning "to celebrate with a toast") was the greeting and toast of the West Germanic peoples. In southern England it is still the custom to "wassail" the trees in the orchards during the twelve days of Christmas, that is, singing and drinking to their health to ensure a good harvest. The common greeting in the English-speaking world "hi" can be traced back to this as well (Grzega 2008, 167).

In order to become healthy and sound (Indo-European **sunto*) again, one must return to the original state of being whole. This return to the origins, to the primal beginnings, is and always was an element of traditional medicine. And in most cultural traditions, fire and water are the origin of things.

In the myths of these forest people, in particular the Germanic and Celtic tribes, the world was created out of the interplay between fire and water or, for the northern Germanic people, between fire and ice. These oppositional forces make up the totality of the world. Thereby, water symbolizes the beginning and fire the end: we are born from the watery uterus, and the funeral pyre releases us again from earthly existence. The virginal goddess of the spring is associated with the cool water that grows the plants; "fire," on the other hand, brings maturity and leads to completion and harvest. In the northern sagas, creation arises out of the ice and ends in the world fire, *Ragnarok* (the twilight of the gods), when the fire giant Surt storms up from the south. Because the Germanic peoples are the ancestors of the original inhabitants of northern Europe, it is worthwhile to take a closer look at their creation mythology.[5]

In their visions, the northern people perceived the glowing hot, fiery home of Muspelheim in the far south, and its very opposite in the far north, icy Nifelheim with its bitter cold. Between these two poles is the "gap of gaps" *(Ginnunga Gap).* The icy cold radiated far into the south; the heat of the seven embers radiated far into the north. And where the primal powers met each other, there it started to steam, sizzle, and simmer, and powerful mountains of clouds formed. These foggy images gradually became denser, then Ymir, the primordial hermaphrodite giant, took form out of them. Audumbla, the primordial cow, also emerged and her milk nourished the giant. The giant had three grandsons, Odin, Villi, and Ve, who slaughtered and dismembered the giant. From his blood came the ocean, from his flesh the earth, from his bones the mountains, from his teeth the cliffs, from his hair the trees and grasses, from his fleas and lice the animals of the forest, from the intestinal parasites the clever, small dwarves, from his eye the sun, from his skull the sky, and from his brain the clouds. Essentially, his body is identical to the world tree.[6] For these peoples, their familiar world was a sacrifice of the gods and as such, sacred. In the depths, deep under the two opposite poles, is the effulgent spring Hvergelmir, the cauldron of chaos, the cauldron of the threefold goddess (Grimm 2012, 467).

Thus, at the beginning of all things, was water (or frozen water) and fire. And also a cauldron.

Rain and Sun

We will see how the forest people always used words and roots (worts), in other words, incantations and healing plants, for healing. Most of the incantations have been lost to us; however, some have lasted until current times. When a small child falls down and gets hurt, has a stomachache, or has been stung by a bee, often the dear old grandmother, in northern Europe, will speak these words:

> Holy, holy blessing,
> Tomorrow it will rain,
> The day after, the sun will shine,
> And then my baby laughs,
> And everything is good again.
>
> (*Heile, heile Segen; Morgen kommt Regen; Uebermorgen Sonnenschein; Dann wird das Weh vorueber sein!*)

An Irish equivalent:

In the name of Dagda, Bridget, and Diancecht. The wound was red, the cut was deep, and the flesh was sore; but there will be no more blood, and no more pain, till the Gods come down to Earth again.

While speaking the words, the abrasion is cleaned or the grandmother rubs a little spit on the wound, and soon the child is feeling much better. Archaic cultural lore is in this treatment, as there often is in traditional children's culture: hopping games have roots in ancient cult dances, counting rhymes are remnants of magical charms, bows and arrows, as well as cowboys and Indians, are based upon primal cultural recollections as far back as the Stone Age from the times in which the people still spoke with animals. In the healing charm or song that I used as an example, the primal elements of water (rain) and fire (sunshine) are called out (Pfleiderer 2009, 21). In the north and west of Germany, the charm goes "heal, heal gosling . . ." Such primordial images are called up by the flying wild geese who live in harmony with the year's rhythms and have been an image of the free soul for the Celts, Germans, Slavs, and Baltic for a long time. Shamans, as we will see, also fly in the form of geese out into the otherworld.

Cold Snow and Warm Blood

The ancient fairy tale from northwestern Germany called *Machhandelboom*—which means juniper tree and is one of the most sacred and ancient medicinal plants of the forest people—tells the story of a rich man and his beautiful, virtuous wife; they loved each other very much but they had no children. One day in winter, the woman was peeling an apple underneath the juniper tree that grew in front of the house. She cut her finger, and blood dropped onto the snow. Then, she sighed and said, "If only I had a child as red as blood and as white as snow!" And as she went back to the house, she became happy because she realized that she felt a baby nestled under her heart. Other fairy tales, such as Snow *White and the Seven Dwarves,* bear this same theme. The white, cold snow and the red, warm blood represent the oppositional forces out of which something new can be created, a new universe, or a child.[7] The Christian symbol of the red rose that blossoms in the middle of the ice-cold winter and signifies the birth of the Savior echoes this primordial, mythical theme.

Juniper *(Juniperus communis)*

"This happened a long time ago, around two thousand years ago." With these words, the fairy tale of *Machhandelboom* begins. The story contains heathen elements that reach back more than two thousand years into ancient times and tells of a small boy who is cut into pieces and cannibalized; his crying sister collects his bones and puts them under the juniper whereby the bush begins to burn and shake. A peewit bird then miraculously appears out of the rising smoke and begins to sing. With this dismemberment and transformation of the dead boy into a bird, we find the ancient theme of shamanic initiation whereby the shamanic apprentice is hunted by demons and eaten, a bird mother collects all of his bones, dresses him in new flesh, and brings the initiate to her nest on the shamanic tree where he matures as a shaman and attains the ability to fly.

That it is a juniper under which his bones are placed is no accident. During historical periods in which the forest people cremated their dead, juniper was the preferred wood for the funeral pyre. The conifer's aromatic-smelling smoke accompanied the departed one's soul and offered it protection. Juniper is called, in the Bavarian and Austrian dialect, *Kranewitt* (Old High German *krane* = crane, *witu* = wood). The European indigenous peoples also considered the crane to be a bird of the soul, a messenger of the Mother Goddess, the Goddess of Death, the Celtic Caillech (Botheroyd and Botheroyd 1995, 352).

Juniper is used as incense and for ceremonies everywhere it grows in the northern hemisphere from Europe to North America, from Siberia to Tibet. Juniper is believed to cast out "snakes" (not just empirical snakes, but spirit-snakes, or snake-like, worm-like meta-physical beings) and ghosts, and in Estonia it is said that with a juniper branch one can even scare away the devil. Juniper smoke protects against "contagion" as a German saying goes, "drive it away with juniper" *(Etwas muss mit Wachoder vertrieben werden)*. Juniper, as well as mugwort (or in the United States, prairie sage), Saint-John's-wort, and, due to Christian influence, possibly also frankincense, were part of the blend used to incense the house and barn in the nights of winter solstice. Sick rooms and dining rooms were also smudged with the dry twigs of the bouquet. Today, the Bonpo shamans honor the mountain deities with juniper smoke and use it as incense during their shamanic séances.

Before treating the sick, the Cheyenne medicine people cleanse themselves with smoke from juniper, sweetgrass *(Hierochloe oderata),* bitterroot *(Lewisia revidiva),* and an undetermined species of dried mushroom. The shamans put the herbs on the glowing wood coals and, using their palms, swirl the incense and heat into the face. During the healing ritual, they put their hands back into the smoke periodically then hold them high up to the sun and down to the earth before turning back to the patient.

In the regions in central Europe where the Alemannic people live, juniper is called *Reckholder,* and, according to folk etymology, it is linked to the German word rauchen (smoke) and *raeuchern* (incense); in Moenchengladbach, Germany, the plant is called Roekkrut (incense herb). The Prussian name *Kaddig* is related to the Lithuanian *kadagys* and the Latvian *kadikis (kaditi* = incense) and comes from the Indo-European root *ked* (smoke, smudge).

Juniper is used as medicine throughout the northern circumpolar region in similar ways. In Siberia and Russia, a decoction of the berries is used as a diuretic, while branches and bark are used for women's health, tuberculosis, fever, and stomach and bowel problems. The same indications—as a diuretic for kidney and bladder issues, a tuberculosis medicine, a treatment for fevers, rheumatism, and women's health—are also known to the North American native

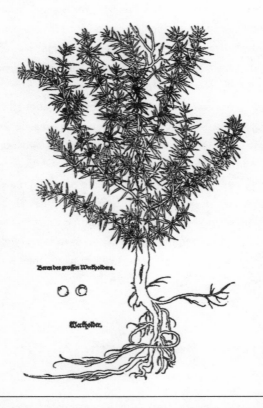

Juniper (woodcut, Hans Weiditz, sixteenth century)

people. The Cheyenne and other tribes use juniper in their sweat lodges by placing them on the glowing hot stones, in particular for a feverish cold. Given the wide geographical spread of the juniper and its similar medical and ritual use, ethnobotanists conclude that this conifer played an important part in the ancient circumpolar Paleolithic culture stretching from the Atlantic coast via Siberia all the way to the New World. This light-loving plant, growing in the steppes where the mammoth elephants roamed, is part of our oldest heritage of shaman- ism and healing.

Like the elder bush, juniper was considered a threshold to the otherworld. In central Europe, mothers placed wool and bread under the juniper when their children were sick and chanted, "Dear Hollen and Hollinnen, I bring to you something to spin and something to eat, so that you might forget my small child and leave him in peace."[8] This Swiss saying shows us how much this bush is honored: "One should tip the hat for elder and bow down for juniper."

Dwarves are clever, and, of course, they know about the healing power of all plants. The following old folk tale is revealing. Once during a plague in Obersimmental, Switzerland, farmers went out to catch dwarves in order to demand that they reveal an effective medicine. The farmers poured some sweet wine into a hole in the cliffs and waited for the curious spirits to get drunk on it. Despite their tipsiness, though, all the swift little folk escaped except for one. From behind a bush, however, the others called to their fallen comrade, "No matter what they try to get out of you, don't tell the secret of the juniper bush!"

From the Beer Mug to the Holy Grail

Fire and water are also the main elements of the Celts, the primordial people who descended from Indo-European nomadic herders and indigenous Bronze Age farmers of the central European forests, and are seen as the father and mother of existence. The warm radiance of the sun fertilizes the water in the kettle of the Great Goddess and in this way brings forth the visible creation. The sun, with its form-giving fire power, is considered the masculine pole of existence; the vessel, the container, with its sensitive, fertile water, is the feminine pole. The fertile cauldron and the fertilizing spear of light are a leitmotif in Celtic mythology and remain so today.

Clay pots and jugs, in which grain was stored and beer was brewed, were already being used in the early Stone Age or Neolithic period. The brewing of strong beer, often with the addition of psychoactive herbs, was an early discovery. Probably, as is still done with the chicha beer of South America, the grain was chewed by the women and spit into the pot, whereby the enzymes of the spit trigger fermentation; another possibility is that the fermentation process was left to free-floating yeast spores already in the air.

Intoxication brought the gods and spirits closer, or, in other words, whenever they approach the otherworld, humans lose their mundane consciousness and become somewhat ecstatic. Most traditional peoples know rituals and ceremonies that open the door to dreamtime, allowing humans to dance and become euphoric. In the springtime, when the Virgin of Light, the White Goddess, appeared once again and fresh sap and power shot through the trees, the late Stone Age hunters and gatherers tapped the birch trees and caught the sap in buckets made from birch bark. After a short while, the slightly sweet liquid began to ferment and became alcoholic. It was probably one of the first intoxicating drinks of the Stone Age until the Neolithic farmers replaced it with beer made from fermented barley juice.

Baking and Brewing

It was not because of a loss of food that the people in the Occident gradually settled, but because they found in the fermented grain to which herbs have been added a drink that lifted their spirits[9]—at least this is the well-founded thesis of evolutionary biologist Josef H. Reichholf (2008). Stone Age hunters and gatherers regularly came together—probably at the time of the full moon—and celebrated festivals in specific places where they also erected centers of worship. Evidently, such centers, for example, Gobekli Tepe in southern Anatolia around 12,000 years ago, existed even before the first permanently inhabited towns had been built. Similar ceremonial places are known, built far away from settlements, in other cultural areas as well (for example, those built by the Mayan people).

In order to protect the seeds of the wild grains, as well as the treasured brew made out of them, humans began to make jugs and pots out of clay. For hunters, however, it was practically impossible to carry heavy pottery around as it would limit their mobility, so some of their tribe members had to stay behind. In addition, the places where the wild cereal grains grew—the first "fields"—needed to be protected from pests and foraging animals. Incidentally, baking bread was a later development than brewing beer. The words *bread, brew,* and *to brew* have roots in the Germanic root word **brauda,* and, in turn, these go back to the Indo-European word **bhreu* (to brew, to ferment, based on water and fire).

Along with grain cultivation, harvest, and breadmaking, brewing was usually the domain of women—thus, the cauldron and the oven both belong to them. Both are analogous to the fertile, life-giving feminine womb. For the Latin people, Ceres (Greek Demeter) was the goddess of grain, agriculture, and plant growth in general. She was represented with a crown of grain on her head and a basket full of poppy blossoms. As Ovid writes in *The Metamorphoses,* "Ceres first turned the soil with curving plough, first gave the crops and the produce as gifts to the land" (Ovid, Metamorphōseōn libri V, 341). (Implied in this verse is that Ceres gave the earth fruits and mild, wholesome, vegetarian foods. Some translations speak of "un-bloody" food.) We find her name again in the word *cereal* (Latin *ceralis* = grain) as well as in the Spanish word for beer, *cerveza* (Latin cervesia).

Ceres is related to the Celtic Mother Goddess Cerridwen. The etymological roots of her name come from the Indo-European *ker* (to grow). In the medieval Welsh saga, she is no longer a goddess but a clever magician. It is told that she gave life to two children: a daughter who is the most beautiful girl in the world, and a son, the ugliest boy in the world. But she knew how to help her son have good standing in society despite his unsightly appearance—for this, she had her witch's cauldron that had to simmer for a year and a day without being disturbed, during which time she picked medicinal plants each day when the stars were aligned just right, murmured a magical spell over them, and stirred them into the brew. In this way, she was able to extract the three drops that held the essence of wisdom meant for her son. But as the young servant, Gwion Bach, stirred the brew just one more time before it was finished, three drops spilled onto his hand. After he licked the burning liquid from his hand, he became enlightened and instantly turned into Taliesin, the greatest bard that ever came out of Wales (Scheffer, Mechthild, and Storl 2012, 46–47).

In European folklore, such cauldrons, as well as brooms, cats, owls, and magical herbs, continue to be connected with witches and their work. The old Mother Holle (also known in English as Mother Hulda or Mother Goose)—including her medieval incarnation as the devil's grandmother—is also often depicted with a steaming cauldron.

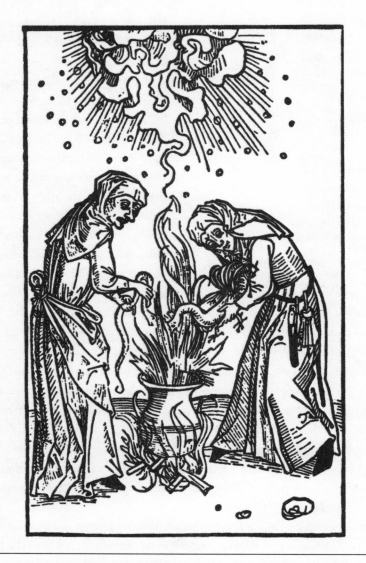

Witches' cauldron (wood cut from the book *De laniis et phitonicis mulieribus,* by Ulricus Molitor, 1491, Strasbourg)

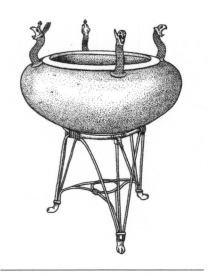

Celtic cauldron made of bronze (from a prince's burial mound, "La Garenne," near Sainte-Colombe, France)

The Celtic gods who emulated the Great Goddess Cerridwen also had cauldrons, including Dagda, the benevolent Sky God, and the Lover of Dana (Dea Ana), the Earth Goddess, who had a cauldron "that would never empty and go dry." The Raven God, Bran, dipped his fallen warriors in his cauldron and thereby brought them back to life. Of particular interest regarding this theme is the simmering cauldron of Diancecht, the divine healer and physician, which contained 365 medicinal plants. He was able to heal the sick and wounded and bring the dead back to life with this herbal brew while chanting spells. Because the cauldron is a symbol of power, the Celtic chieftains made a point of having one themselves as well. They boiled meat or brewed intoxicating mead in it in order to keep their warriors and allies in good spirits and to observe the laws of hospitality.

Springs and wells, swamps and moors are considered the Great Goddess's "cauldrons" and entryways to her realm, thresholds to the otherworld. This theme is shown, for instance, in the fairy tale *Mother Hulda* (Holle) in which a girl—who symbolizes the human soul itself—falls into a well and lands on the other side in a green meadow (Storl 2014b 54–55). Incidentally, contact with the otherworld is always a requirement for healing, for only in this way is a true metamorphosis, a transformation, possible.

An Irish saga tells of a magical spring that is surrounded by nine hazel bushes. Every once in a while, the fiery red hazelnuts fall into the cool, clear water, whereby bubbles of inspiration rise up. Salmon eat the nuts and thereby get their brilliant red color. Similarly, a central European myth tells of the hazel snake or hazel worm—a white snake with a golden crown that lives under the roots of very old hazel trees. Such old hazel trees often have mistletoes growing on them. Whoever captures such a snake and eats of its flesh will have magical powers, attain wisdom, understand the language of animals, and know the healing virtues of herbs (Storl 2009, 201). Sylvia and Paul Botheroyd comment, "this is an obvious image and explanation of the Indo-European concept of fire-in-water, of the divine, fiery spark that makes the water fecund" (Botheroyd and Botheroyd 1995, 274).

The heathen Europeans of long ago considered hot springs and thermal pools especially medicinally powerful, with the primal elements of fire and water at play. The Celts believed that the sun heated the chthonic water during its journey below the earth during the night. Such water contains the power of the sun. One of the most sacred Celtic thermal springs was Aquae Granni on the northern edge of the Eifel mountain range. The Romans consecrated these hot baths to Apollo Grannus, who was the Hyperborean Sun God;[10] Grannus (Grian in Irish) is one of the many Celtic names for the sun. For the Celts, the Sun God, a mighty warrior, was the protector of the Great Goddess's womb (the cauldron). Today the city of Aachen, Germany, lies here, where the Sun God drove his fire power into the depths of the Great Goddess. It was in this place of power that the Frankish king, Charlemagne, had his main castle and cathedral built.

The Celtic primordial image of the sacred cauldron and the fertilizing, warming, protecting spirit of the Sun God still lives on today, despite the conversion, in the legends of the Grail Knights. Here the cauldron has mutated into the chalice for the Christian Eucharist, and the spear became the Lance of Longinus, which was jabbed into the side of the Savior when he hung on the cross.[11] The medieval Legend of the Grail tells that, when the goblet and the spear are separated, the land becomes dreary and dark, while pestilence and infertility abound. But healing is generated when the goblet and spear, springs and sunbeams, fire and water, are joined together again. We also see that the vessel with the hot, healing herbal tea is in full harmony with this cultural theme.

The common people, carriers of the Little Tradition, have not forgotten this. Despite the orders of the *Indiculus superstitionum et paganiarum* (the index of superstitions and paganism) from the time of Charlemagne (eighth century) in which false cults in the forests and the worshiping of trees, stones, and springs were forbidden, the people held firmly to their sacred springs. On days of celebration, or saint's days, these locations continued to be frequented and decorated with leaves and flowers. People also continued to collect holy water in the form of Easter water before sunrise on Easter. It is still said today that this water stays fresh year-round and not only heals diseases but also bestows beauty.

With the flower remedies of the Welsh physician Edward Bach, Celtic medicinal knowledge has celebrated a resurrection. In order to produce this medicine, the flower of a medicinal plant is placed in a bowl with pure spring water and set out in the sun on a bright day. The energy of the sun transmits the "information" of the flower into the receptive water. Next to the "sun potentiation," Dr. Bach also used the "cooking method"— above all with tree flower essences—whereby the heating occurs over fire. Fire from natural heat sources such as wood is, of course, nothing other than the sun's light from years past. The flower essences work less on coarse physical levels, but flood the soul with positive, harmonizing information (Scheffer, Mechthild, and Storl 2012, 67–68).

The Celtic cauldron also lives on in popular culture. In the Asterix and Obelix comics popular among French schoolchildren since the 1960s, the bearded Druid Miraculix diligently stirs his cauldron in which the secret, invincible-making "energy drink" simmers.

The Daily Cycle

The question arises: Why is the herbal tea drunk three times a day, morning, noon, and evening?

Three is an absolutely sacred number for the Indo-Europeans, as well as for the Siberians. The universe is divided in three: upper world, middle world, and lower world. The world tree has three times three branches and as many roots. A magical spell or charm must be spoken three times in order for it to work. Even the gods appear as a trinity. The primordial goddess (i.e., the three Celtic matrons, the Nordic Norns, the Greek Parcae, the Indian Devi) appears, for instance, in a three-part formula: as a white virgin, as a red bearer of life, and as a black elder. In the fourth century, even the Church had to capitulate before the power of this ancient presence—the monolithic God of the Bible became the Holy Trinity.

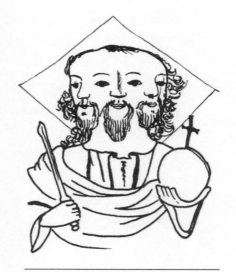

The trinity (a peasant panel from Tyrol, around 1600)

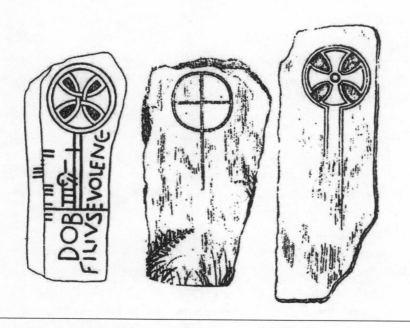

Representations of the sun wheel in Wales

49

But four was also significant. For the forest people, time was like a rolling wheel with four main spokes, which represented the four times of day:

dawn, when the sun comes up;

midday, when the sun stands at its zenith and the shadows are shortest;

twilight, when the sun disappears below the horizon; and

midnight, when the sun is at its nadir and has reached its lowest point.

Thus, abstract mental constructions are not at play here, but celestial phenomena.

Morning

The brief occurrence of the dawn, when the bats disappear, the swallows appear, and the sun nears the horizon, is a blessed time. The tender light disperses the nocturnal spirits. Now the nighttime demons, the oppressive nightmare that rides the sweating, sick person, flees. With the golden morning light, new power floods the land. The birds are taken up in this wave and twitter and sing joyously for the day star, the sun. Dew glistens on the meadows and refreshes the plants. The blossoms of the daisy, the chicory, and other flowers open to the light from the east. The human soul also opens to the divine power at the dawning of the day. "Early to bed, early to rise, makes a man healthy, wealthy, and wise"—dawn is filled with medicinal power. This is the time to, like the sun, "rise and shine" and to rinse one's hands and face with refreshing, cold water. The cows will soon be mooing into the barn and will want to be milked and fed.

The herbalists went out in this morning twilight to collect healing plants or healing water from a spring. They went silently, in a meditative state and unseen; in other words, they took care that nobody talked with them. They paid attention to the signs and which animals they encountered. They went with uncovered, unbraided hair and barefooted; in heathen times, they went naked to gather herbs. In folk customs, it was considered a bad sign to encounter a nun or a priest, who frightened off the helpful nature spirits. With their gaze directed to the east, while speaking a charm or prayer, the herbalists collected dewy herbs. Dew is considered pure, newly created matter. For the Celts, dew was a gift from the in-between world; it came neither from the earth, nor did it fall as rain from the clouds. The in-between world is a magical place, where nothing is yet fixed, but everything is possible—it is the in-between space in which healing can also take place.

The morning hour is also the time in which—an hour before breakfast—the first cup of hot, healing herbal tea is sipped.

Noon

Twelve o'clock midday is the next magical time. Now the sun is at the zenith of its daily path. It is the transition point, the moment when the sun hovers between its rising and setting. For the ancient Europeans, the midday hour, when the shadows are the shortest, represented a break in time in which the sun remains still for a bit. This still standing of the sun was a magical moment, another in-between time, in which the otherworld came closer. This space outside the influence of time was considered by the Germanic people and the Celts a moment of truth, when it was beneficial to conduct a divine judgment (trial by ordeal) and a way to determine right from wrong, guilt from innocence. It was high noon—we still know about this from the North American mystery plays, the traditional westerns, when two men are in a duel and the invisible hand of the gods (or God) guides the hand of the true hero.[12]

It is a very natural phenomenon, part of the overall bio-rhythm, that people rest, take a break, eat a noontime meal, and become a bit drowsy in the middle of the day. Work done at this time brings little success at most and at worst downright bad luck. During the harvest, farmers often took a nap after a big meal and dreamed of the midday spirits, of the Lady Midday or the Noon Witch who asked them riddles. The West Slavic people have a midday spirit called Poludnitsa, who threatens the sleeping with her scythe and causes them to awake with a headache. Sometimes the midday spirit is a grain maiden who glides over the grain fields, or one hears (in the Swiss French dialect) the grain spirit *(le pleurat)* crying. People can have visions during the midday hour at crossroads and enchanted places. And it is also said that herbs picked at this hour on St. John's Day are particularly potent.

Naturally, one drinks a second cup of the healing tea during this magical time a bit before the noon meal.

Evening

The breaking of the evening twilight brings the promise of rest and the end of the workday. It is the third sacred station of the day. The birds sing their evening song, the ravens fly in pairs to their nests, the dairy cows return home to their barn, as it once was, and after the milking all work comes to a pause. The whole family sits down to eat dinner.

With the coming of the darkness, the bats and the moths fly out, and the dwarves and the night spirits get to work. For the people close to the earth, this is no idle fantasy. Without the distraction of the internet or television, one can recognize these beings with ease. The Christians mark this sacred pause, like the other cardinal points of the daily cycle, with bells. It is the right time to turn away from mundane reality and with meditation prepare for the night journey into the spiritual dimension—into the realm of Mother Holle.

Naturally, it is the evening hour that is also the right time to drink the third cup of healing tea.[13]

Midnight

There is also a fourth cardinal point, and that is the middle of the night, when the sun has reached its lowest point. There is no healing tea drunk then, for it is the hour of ghosts, the restless dead; nightmares and strange spiritual beings are underway. This is the best time, protected in a warm featherbed, to stay with Mother Hulda, or, as a Christian, to put your trust into the protection of the angels. Midnight is the suitable hour for witches to fly and shamans to practice their work, undisturbed by the stressful tumult of the day. But in the still of the midnight hour, black magic can also be concentrated on the soul (astral body) of the sleeping in order to wield power over them. Those who are aware, even today, may feel, in the deep of the night, attacks of dark, pessimistic, fear-filled, and negative thoughts. Since pre-Christian times, people have sought protection against these attacks by, for instance, hanging mugwort or Saint-John's-wort in the sleeping area.

In the indigenous Occidental cultures, these four main times of day were halved, so that the cycle of the day was divided into eight spaces of time. This division was retained in the Christian cultures as the time for prayers and bells. These additional in-between times, however, played a subordinate role and were usually used for small snacks, for example, a ten o'clock break or tea time around four o'clock.

The Cross as a Primal Symbol

Like the day, so the year. The ancient Europeans also saw the year as a circle, with four cardinal points determined by their annual path of the sun: spring equinox, summer solstice (midsummer), fall equinox, and winter solstice (midwinter). These four seasons were symbolized by a wheel with a cross.

This sun-cross—also called a Celtic cross, Slavic cross, wheel cross, or sun wheel—could be called the medicine wheel of the European forest people. It represents the path of the sun through the twelve horoscopes, the four cardinal directions (north, east, south, west), the seasons (winter, spring, summer, fall), the four ages of life (childhood, adulthood, old age, death), and much more. This cross is at the same time a glyph of the world tree. The vertical axis of the cross reaches up into the nine upper worlds and at the same time down into the nine levels of the underworld, deep into the earth. The horizontal axis of the cross, in contrast, is the middle world (Midgard); it is the ground level upon which we ourselves walk during our normal day, on which the animals move about and the plants grow. And where these two axes cross is the center: the middle of being, the gate to the highest mystery, the heart—our own heart and also the heart of the universe.

This cross symbolism is much older than the cross of the Christian church.[14] The Ice Age hunters of the European Magdalenian cultures already knew this motif. We also find it in the Mesolithic age, when humans were still hunters and gatherers, and above all in the New Stone Age megalithic culture. In the spring, the first farmers carried the cross decorated with a crown of fresh green branches (today it is called a *Questenkreuz* in Germany, from the medieval word for a *wreath of leaves carried on a pole*) in the direction of the sun, that is, clockwise, around the fields in order to bless them with growth and prosperity. This green wheel cross still survives in the palm processions on Palm Sunday (Storl 2014b 24), which is a remarkable cultural continuity!

Like the cross symbolizing the daily cycle, the cross of the year was quartered once again at some point during the megalithic period so that there were eight spaces of time to the circle, each developed into a particularly powerful, magical transitional day. These so-called cross quarter days were originally connected to the full moon and fell during the months exactly between the four cardinal points of the solar year.

> **February:** Candlemas, Imbolc, Lupercalia, or Groundhog Day is celebrated when the pre-spring moon announces that winter is losing its strength and the "sun buck jumps." It is the celebration of the virginal White Goddess, Bridget, who transforms ice into flowing water, awakens the plants from their deep winter sleep, and encourages the sap to rise in the trees.

> **May (Beltane):** The full moon in the merry month of May, when the migratory birds have returned, is the feast of the marriage between the flower-decorated Vegetation Goddess and the young Sun God. The May pole or May tree is, still today in wide parts of Europe, erected in the villages as a symbol of their union and love. Dancing around the May pole and crowning the queen of May is part of the festival.

> **August (Lughnasadh or Lammas):** On this full moon, the feast of the fire and harvest gods and the revered matrons are celebrated. It is the beginning of the harvest season and the time of

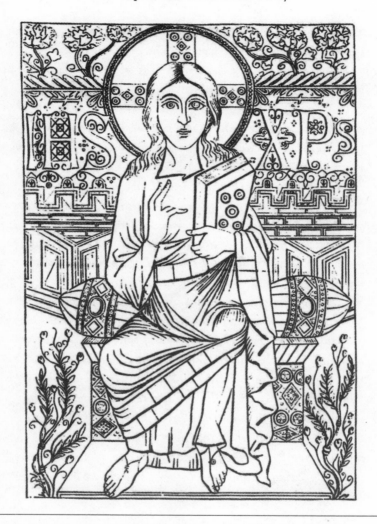

The wheel cross as Christ's halo, from the Godescalc Gospels commissioned by Charlemagne (ca. 782 CE)

herb gathering. The Great Goddess now pours her cornucopia of cereal grain, healing herbs, and fruits over the land.

November (Samhain): This moon, to which the ghosts are headed, marks the end of the year and the beginning of the rest period. It is a festival honoring the dead.

In this way, the wheel of the year developed eight spokes—four primary spokes and four intermediary spokes.

Like the cross of the day, the cross of the year was important in the herbal medicine of the forest people:

- *Around the spring equinox women collect "blood-cleansing" green herbs, which disperse scurvy and connect humans to the spirit of the new cycle of life. In German-speaking countries, the Czech Republic, Slovakia, and Hungary, people still eat a "green Thursday soup" on Maudy Thursday; the "Frankfurt green sauce" is an echo of this former cult food. In the American Midwest, a friend's great-grandmother made a spring soup of burdock leaves, dandelion leaves, and nettles and called it "a mess of greens."*
- *Midsummer, summer solstice or Saint John's Eve, is the next high point of the medicinal calendar. At this time, summer herbs such as Saint-John's-wort, which are full of the power of the light and warmth of the sun, are gathered and blessed at the time of the summer solstice fire. Herbs such as linden or elder flowers, which bestow warmth and are diaphoretic (as modern phytotherapy now tells us) and which strengthen the immune system, have played an important role since the megalithic times. Yarrow, bracken fern, fennel, mallows, vervaine, and arnica were included in what used to be called the "medicinal herbs of Saint John" and were gathered at this sacred time.*
- *The August herbal blessing is the next important time for herbalists. The hottest month of the year brings out the herbs' essential oils and active ingredients, the most powerful medicine of the plants. It is the fiery blaze of the gods Lugh, Loki, or other fire gods that brings the herbs to maturity and ripeness. These powerful herbs belong to the cornucopia of the Great Goddess.[15] Ever since the Virgin Mary took over her role, the herbal festival is celebrated in Christian culture on Mary's Assumption Day on*

August 15th. The message is, although Mary is leaving the earth, she leaves her blessings behind in the form of medicinal plants.

- *In the foggy, dreary days of November, when the songbirds and swallows fly south and the spirits of the dead are roaming, the herbs have no power, for they are then taboo, or, like the Celts say, they are* pucca—*meant for the spirits, for the pucks or phookas.*

This brief glimpse into the cultural history and symbolic background of the simple tradition of drinking one cup of tea three times a day for health demonstrates neither a universal custom nor something randomly invented; rather, it is a culturally specific form of medicine. It is typical of the circumpolar forest people and has its roots with the farmers of the megalithic culture. But the roots of European folk medicine go much deeper than what was inherited from the megalithic farmers. These roots go back to the big-game hunters of the Ice Age.

CHAPTER 3

Stone Age Roots, Ice Age Medicine

For Indians medicine and religion are closely bound and
*   interwoven.*
The one is a substantial part of the other; one can't work
*   without the other.*
It is nearly impossible to determine where the practical medi-
cine starts and the ceremonial healing begins.
<small>JOSEPH MEDICINE CROW, ABSAROKEE CHIEF AND</small>
<small>MEDICINE MAN</small>

Shamans can heal; this I know. And their healing is enduring.
<small>BEATRIX PFLEIDERER, ETHNOMEDIZIN</small>

Medicine, in particular the use of healing herbs, was not discovered at some certain time. No primordial Einstein experimented doggedly with plants and came to rational conclusions, such as that this herb is poisonous, a different one strengthens the liver, and yet another soothes back pain. The discovery of healing herbs is lost in the mists of primal times. Nevertheless, behavioral biologists have confirmed that animals use precisely sought-out healing plants when they are sick or injured. "Instinct" and "innate abilities"—this is the bewildered explanation for this behavior that is difficult to understand rationally. For example, wounded chamois goat antelope roll around in alpine plantain, which is styptic, a vulnerary, and slightly bacteriostatic; wolves eat nettles for their indigestion and then vomit; heavily pregnant elephant cows eat the bark of the red seringa tree to induce labor; South American sheep find the leaves of the Boldo bush, whose essential oil kills liver parasites and alkaloid stimulates the liver; bears eat laxative herbs after their hibernation to get their bowel movements back into swing; tiny red ants plant broad-leaved thyme on their mounds, which protects against mold and bacterial attacks.

Chimpanzee researchers have discovered that the great apes have a veritable herbal apothecary; for example, during the rainy season, when intestinal parasites become a problem, they seek out a bitter herb as a vermifuge (Storl 2011, 34). Pollen analysis of plant remains that were found during the excavation of prehistoric people (Homo erectus) who lived during the interglacial period nearly 400,000 years ago in central Germany (Bilzingsleben) has shown that they also had a well-developed healing plant knowledge (Wolters 1999, 80). With the Neanderthals, it is even clearer. In Kurdish Iraq, for example, a Neanderthal was found that had been laid to rest on a bed of flowering healing herbs (also revealed through pollen analysis) that were all plants still used in phytotherapy today (Pabst 2013, 210). That was 60,000 years ago—a long time ago if one considers that humans only became settled around 10,000 years ago or that the "eternal" Roman Empire was founded 2,500 years ago.

The Stone Age people were intimately connected to nature. Civilized humans can scarcely imagine anymore how intertwined with their natural environment and the rhythm of the seasons early people lived. Collecting edible roots, herbs, fruits, berries, and nuts, and also hunting animals, took place in a state of undivided attention. These traditional hunting and gathering people did not make nature into an external object that could be analyzed. They achieved their knowledge through unconditional attunement, through being one with the plants and animals. They were very quiet, thereby putting aside the distracting noise of unnecessary thoughts. That is what I experienced again and again as an anthropologist with indigenous people that included the Cheyenne medicine men, herbalists in Kerala and other places in India, and some with the Xhosa in South Africa. Priority was given to immediate perception, conscious

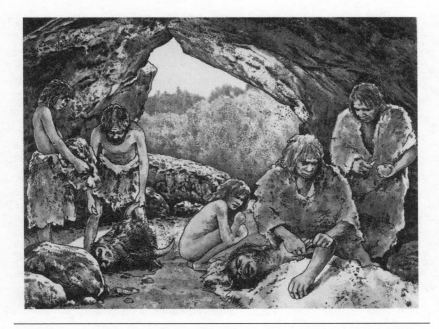

Neanderthals caring for a sick family member (from U. Creutz, *Rund um die Steinzeit,* illustration by Stephan Koehler, Kinderbuchverlag, Berlin, 1990)

being-here. When one is thinking, one is distracted and not connected to the here and now. This, of course, does not mean that natives are not able to think. They have fantastic intellectual abilities, but they only use them at the appropriate time.

The natural person slips into nature and lets all of the senses resonate with it. It is not a case of observations directed out at the world, measuring, weighing, and diagnosing, as we have learned to do after many years of training within the four walls of a school or a school laboratory. But it is an interior perception, a looking into "the mirror of the soul." With the soul, one perceives the soul of nature, the plants and the animals, just as our "energetic body" (etheric body) perceives the energies in nature. As one looks at nature in this way, inner images can arise. The group soul of the wolf or the raven can appear in some form and speak with people in a language they can understand. In this way, the stone can convey its wisdom in the form of a gnome. There, one can make out the illness as a "worm" that avoids the light of day. There, the plant deva, when it is benevolent, can tell the medicine people which healing power healing plants have.

Humans do not have a highly sensitive nose such as most animals possess; they cannot decidedly distinguish poison or medicine like many animals can. Their instincts have shrunk to a certain degree; nevertheless, they have the ability of true sight or "vision." Some people are naturally more gifted in this area than others, and are therefore obliged to support their tribe as a healer. These abilities can be strengthened with shamanic techniques and spirit-moving plant drugs (entheogens).

Anthropologists and scholars of pre-history can confirm that shamanism has deep roots. It was as much a part of the life of Paleolithic big-game hunters in the Ice Age tundra as it was of the foragers of the post–Ice Age forest. And this actually brings us to the European ancestors where we shall see that a considerable part of medicinal knowledge and herbal tradition can be traced back to them.

The World of the Paleolithic Big Game Hunters

About 18,000–24,000 years ago, the last ice age reached its peak. The glaciers advanced so that much of northern Eurasia and North America were covered by a thick sheet of ice. So much water was frozen that the sea level was 400 to 425 feet (120 to 130 meters) lower around the entire world than it is today. Relatively dry and cold grass steppes formed on the edge of the immense ice sheets, which made an ideal habitat for large herds of herbivorous mammals: woolly mammoth, reindeer, woolly rhinoceros, Przewalski's horse, musk ox, red deer (wapiti), bison, saiga antelope, and others. With the help of their dogs, the people in these latitudes followed the big game.[1] They lived in a way similar to that the Plains Indians lived up until three hundred years ago (who mainly hunted bison). The flesh of large mammals nourished them; the leather and skins dressed them; the fat fed their lamps; animal stomachs and bladders were used as containers, bones and horns as tools, tendons as thread; and even dwellings, when there were no willow or birch branches, were often built from mammoth bones spanned with animal skins. In summer, these people lived in teepee-like, portable, small tents; in winter, they lived in earth lodges or semi-subterranean houses (also called pit houses) that were partially dug into the ground.

Because the sea level was so low due to the water bound in the ice, the herds as well as the hunters could easily roam from eastern Siberia to North America. The Bering Strait that now separates Kamchatka, Russia, from Alaska, was a dry, rich grassland filled with game during the period between 24,000 and 14,000 BCE. In addition, a wide-open track, a corridor, in Canada existed between two gigantic ice-sheets that led into the warmer south;[2] the herds used this corridor, and the Ice Age hunters followed them.

Scholars of pre-history paint us a picture of Stone Age big-game hunting culture that is similar in almost all aspects from Europe to North America. This is not only the case in material culture, such as housing (teepees and pit houses dug halfway into the earth), clothing, and hunting weapons, but it also applies to the spiritual culture. To the latter belong the stories about the mighty bear, the wolf, the deer, and the mischievous fox or the wise raven; included was the vision of the world tree as the world axis and the threefold structure of the universe, as well as the idea of the sky's arc as a huge tent (the "firmament") with holes in the fabric that let the light shine through as stars. To this came the belief that animals have spirit guardians specific to their species, and that one must first have their permission to hunt them. In addition, the archaic circumpolar worldview included the belief that trees and plants have their own spirit guardians and that the grandmother of all souls lives deep under the ground, that the world is animated and responsive, that shamans have the ability to travel to other dimensions, and much more (Schlesier 1985, 69ff.). The shamanic healing techniques, the sweat lodge (*banjas* and saunas), and, that which is of particular interest to us, the knowledge of healing plants of Stone Age ancestors continue to be effective today as part of indigenous folk medicine.

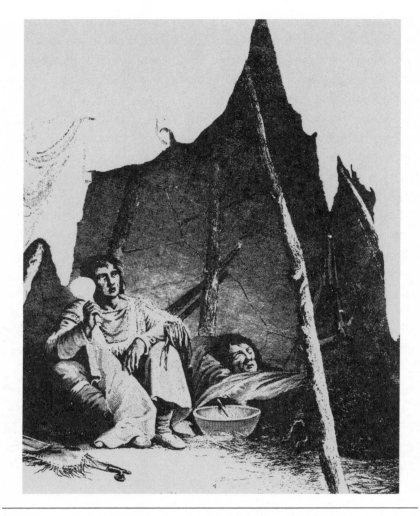

Dakota healer (Henry Schoolcraft, nineteenth century)

Healing Plants and Diseases of the Old Stone Age

The Stone Age hunters and gatherers of the Holarctic tundra, steppes, and taiga plains lived in a healthy environment. The water and the air were clean. There were fewer parasites and pathogenic microorganisms in the cold air than in the tropics. The low population density also contributed to the lack of infectious diseases. Their way of life provided the physical activity necessary to keep heart and blood circulation active and healthy, and body cells well supplied with oxygen. Their protein-rich diet based on wild game, supplemented by wild herbs, roots, nuts, berries, bird eggs, mushrooms, and possibly beetle larvae, kept people healthy. Deficiencies and bone and tooth damage were scarcely found, unlike later settled farmers who ate a carbohydrate-filled diet of mainly cereals (and dairy products).[3]

With the receding of the Ice Age and the rapid warming of the climate about 12,000 years ago, the large herds of steppe animals lost their basis for existence. They either died out or moved farther away to the northeast, and the last of the big-game hunters followed them. Forests—birch, willow, pine, hazel bushes—began to cover the once wide-open spaces. The remaining game hunters now hunted smaller game, such as deer and wild boar, and collected more nuts, acorns, and grass seed, such as the floating sweet-grass *(Glycera fluitans),* as well as all kinds of roots and shellfish. They also fished. They lived in a healthy environment and did not yet suffer infectious diseases, which would later plague the sedentary farmers.

What illnesses and ailments did these Stone Age people have to endure? The main complaints were:

- **kidney** and **bladder** disorders and **rheumatism,** due to lying on animal skins directly on the earth in the cold, earthen homes or the huts spanned with animal skins, including even on permafrost during the Ice Age;
- **diarrhea** and **gastrointestinal** disorders, in part because of spoiled food stocks;
- **skin diseases,** probably due to poor hygiene;
- **respiratory** diseases, possibly caused by smoke-filled dwellings;
- **wounds** and **bleeding,** and **fractures,** which among others things happened during hunting accidents; and
- **gynecological complications** during childbirth.

A circumpolar flora of healing herbs, bark, and roots that grew across Eurasia and extended to North America held a store of healing plants ready to help alleviate all of these problems. To this day, the indigenous North American and eastern Siberian healing lore consists of further development of this Ice Age medicine, without much influence from other cultural traditions (Wolters 2000, 6ff.).

Although the land-bridge between Alaska and Kamchatka was already flooded by 11,000 years ago, and the old world was separated from the new from that time forward, Russian and Siberian folk medicine as well as Native American healing lore continued to use the same medicinal plants that were used during the Ice Age (Kay 1996). This is also true among the European forest peoples, although to a lesser extent due to the additional influence coming from the Mediterranean and the western Orient. Despite pressure from the Byzantine Empire, the Oriental influence had less of an impact on folk medicine in Russia than in the rest of Europe.

About 32,000 species of native vascular plants (plants that have a vascular system for transporting water and nutrients) can be found in North America (Moerman 1999, 11). As the Paleo-American hunters moved ever farther south, their medicinal lore expanded. Of the plant species of the Western Hemisphere, North American Indians used—and to a degree still use—more than 2,800 medicinal plants. A disproportionately large share of these medicinal plants are circumpolar species, which means that the Paleo-Indians brought their healing knowledge with them to the New World and continued to use the medicinal plants they knew from the Old World. If the specific plants were not available, they used closely related, similar-looking species that would have the same effect. For example, common mugwort *(Artemisia vulgaris)*, which grows from Europe to China, replaced with an American species, such as prairie sage *(Artemisia* spp.), is used almost identically.

But the Paleo-Siberian immigrants, who became the Paleo-Americans, brought an entire cultural system across the Bering Strait that is integrated with their medicine; this included a shamanic worldview, the use of a drum to induce a trance, archaic techniques of soul travel and vision quests, animals as helping spirits, emetic and purgative agents for the purpose of "purification," sweat-lodge rituals and herbal steam baths, the sucking out of magic arrows and "worms" (disease-causing spirits), the entheogenic use of fly agaric *(Amanita muscaria)*, and more. They probably even introduced some of their important healing plants to the Americas, such as the stinging nettle, tarragon *(Artemisia dracunculus)*, sweet flag *(Acorus calamus)*, or chamomile *(Matricaria discoidea)*.

The Main Circumpolar Healing Herbs

Let us now select a few of the most important healing plants that are used similarly and have been important since the Upper Paleolithic period (the Late Stone Age) in European, Russian, Siberian, and North American indigenous medicine.

Yarrow (Achillea millefolium)

Though chamomile is the medicinal herb most commonly used by central Europeans, the Chinese prefer angelica, and the North American indigenous peoples favor yarrow. It is the most important hemostatic and vulnerary medicine plant and is used in a bath or as a cover for a wound. A tea is also drunk for gastrointestinal imbalance, liver problems, gynecological problems, and fever (flu, cold) (Moerman 1999, 42–43). An almost identical application can be found in Russia, Siberia, and Europe.

Bog Rosemary (Andromeda polifolia)

The small bog shrub with pink flowers, which is related to marsh rosemary and Labrador tea (Rhododendron spp.), is toxic and contains andromedotoxins that can lead to a dangerous decrease in heart rate and respiratory paralysis. Nevertheless, knowledgeable herbal healers in Baltic countries and in Russia as well as in North America made an infusion or decoction of the leaves; its diaphoretic properties are used to treat rheumatism and tuberculosis (Demitsch 1889, 164).

Angelica (Angelica archangelica, A. sylvestris;
A. atropurpurea, A. sinensis)

The roots of the angelica plant are what is usually used as a medicinal remedy. Many different closely related species of angelica grow in the circumpolar region. The primary use of angelica is to treat colic, gastrointestinal complaints, and catarrh problems. In addition, it is used as a support for the immune system against contagious diseases such as colds, typhoid, or cholera. They say everywhere, including among North American indigenous people, that this plant has a good spirit; the North American indigenous people of the forest consider it a bringer of good luck and a banisher of evil spirits. The young shoots are cooked as a vegetable from Lapland to Canada.

Bearberry (Arctostaphylos uva-ursi)

For the Germanic tribes, Celts, Siberians, and North American indigenous peoples, the bearberry plant was seen as a bear plant. Not only because bears, as well as humans, like to eat the red berries, but because humans were convinced that the bear is a master of healing plants. Decoctions of the leaves are universally drunk for inflammation of the urinary tract, cystitis, and gonorrhea. North American indigenous peoples smoke it as part of the herbal mixture in their medicine pipes—the pipes should be understood to be portable altars, where the smoke rises to the gods.

Fringed Sagebrush (Artemisia frigida)[4]

This delicate but tough species of mugwort likes cold and dry places. It grows in a wide swath from northern Europe to North America. For the tribes of the Plains, such as the Arapaho, Cheyenne, Dakota, Omaha, Pawnee, and others, it is "woman's sage," which is used as a gynecological remedy, to bring on menstruation, for example. For Cheyenne people, this plant is absolutely taboo for men; they may neither look at it nor even mention it. Otherwise, this herb that tastes similar to wormwood—as bitter as bile—is also used in small doses to treat gastritis and indigestion.

Birch (Betula spp.)

The birch was one of the colonizers of the tundra after the glaciers retreated. A light-loving companion and friend to the people who have lived in the circumpolar area since the Ice Age, the birch tree helped them survive. Its innermost bark could be cooked and eaten as a "vegetable" when food was scarce. In the spring, tapped birch sap is refreshing and cleansing. Eastern Woodland Indians, such as the Iroquois and Algonquin, used the small, hollow elderberry branches to tap the birch sap and then mixed it with sweeter maple sap. Native Americans in Canada and Inuits in Alaska smoked fish and raw meat over slow-burning birch wood and its smoldering leaves—it may well be that the Stone Age people in Europe and northern Asia cured in a similar way. The Paleolithic hunters used birch tar distilled from birch bark to "glue" their stone blades to the spear shafts. Recent studies indicate that more than 80,000 years ago this complicated method of pitch preparation was known and developed by the Neanderthals of the interglacial period.

Before there was earthenware, the Stone Age people in the Old as well as the New World made watertight containers and pots out of birch bark. Cooking was done by placing glowing stones into pots filled with water, meat, roots, or greens. In this way, the soup was cooked from within. Even the Later Stone Age man Oetzi, who was discovered in the melting glaciers of the Oetztal Alps after more than 5,000 years lying encased in ice, was carrying two birch bark containers with him.

Because birch bark contains many essential oils, it is suited for lighting fires, even in the rain. For Stone Age people of the Old and the New World, for Siberians and Native Americans, the birch was and is a veritable pharmacy. The parts used include buds, root powder, and bark as a decoction for stomachache, diarrhea, hemorrhoids, and indigestion; ointments made from the bark are used for skin fungus, rashes, and wound healing. Teas from bark or leaves are drunk for colds and lung diseases. Crushed twigs are placed on the red-hot stones in the saunas to cleanse the lungs. Teas help with kidney and bladder stones. In general, the tea from the bark

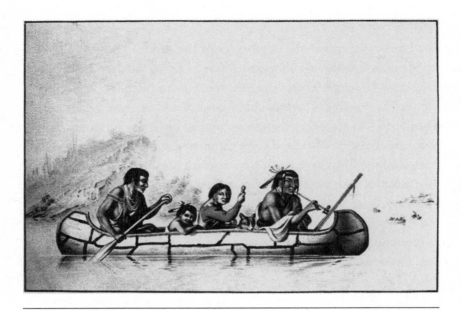

Ojibwa family in a birch bark canoe, by Peter Rindisbacher (1806–1834)

and leaves has analgesic, antipyretic (fever-reducing), expectorant, diuretic, blood-cleansing, disinfecting, gout-mitigating effects, and is a vermifuge (Ruoff 2014, 46).[5] It is known that northern Germanic people wrapped broken arms or legs in fresh birch bark, which then hardened upon drying and served as a "plaster" cast.

The birch is a symbol of light everywhere that it grows. It is the tree of the White Goddess, the goddess of spring, the Celtic Brigit as well as the Indian Sarasvati, the goddess of inspiration and of the true word. The Vedas, the oldest sacred texts of the Hindus, were at first written on birch bark. Like the young goddess herself, birch symbolizes purification and a new beginning. With a broom made of birch twigs, one sweeps rooms and sacred places; during the Alemannic carnival, the archaic, colorful festival at which many costumed and masked people parade as various "spirits" in February, the witches still carry a birch broom, occasionally "riding" it and symbolically swooshing it around to cleanse the atmosphere. The role of the witches is usually played by men because it is believed that women are more receptive in nature and more likely to be possessed by the spirits represented on the masks.

The Ojibwa, a people of hunters and wild rice collectors from Lake Superior, not only lived in birch bark wigwams, but they also built canoes from this bark, boiled their food in birch pots, healed with the bark and leaves, and buried their dead in birch bark. Wrapped in this bark, the dead would find protection, just as their culture bringer Manabozho, who found protection from the thunderbirds in a birch tree.

Fungi That Grow on Birch Trees

In the Stone Age, the different types of fungi that grow on and around the birch were already important for humans. To begin with, the birch polypore, or birch bracket mushroom *(Piptoporus betulinus)*, only grows on birch. At the time, it was an important part of a first aid kit because it is anti-inflammatory, antibacterial, and hemostatic and thus suited to treat various injuries and wounds. Oetzi, the Ice Man, also carried a few pieces of dried birch polypore along. Intestinal examinations revealed that Oetzi suffered from a parasitic whipworm infestation. Perhaps he was using the fungus internally to kill the worm's larvae. Birch polypore is edible when it is in a very young stage of growth but has a rather bitter taste. The birch polypore also grows in North America and was used medicinally by the Okangan and other tribes of the Pacific Northwest.

Oetzi also had some tinder polypore *(Fomes fomentarius;* also known as tinder conk) among his belongings. The dried tinder conk has been used, as its name suggests, as a fire starter since the Stone Age. In the Old and in the New World, the fungus is also used as a sponge for wounds and for cauterizing festering wounds. The felt-like *trama* (the inner "fleshy" portion of the fruiting body of the shelf mushroom) is pounded out until it is flat and soft, heated until it is smoldering, and then placed on the injury. The native people of North America used the tinder conk in this way, as did the Siberians and the ancient Europeans. The tinder polypore that infects decaying birches and beech trees was also lit up and brought to a glimmer in order to serve as a substrate upon which fragrant herbs—such as mugwort, juniper, and others—could be burned to make aromatic smoke in circumpolar ceremonies (Grienke et al. 2014, 564).

Chaga, or clinker polypore *(Inonotus obliquus),* is another mushroom associated with birch. It grows as a bulbous, black, brittle parasite on the trunks of old birch trees. The fungus has been making a splash in the alternative medicine scene under the name *chaga.* In fact, chaga is a giant when it comes to its healing powers. The tea or decoction is used internally in Russia, the Baltic countries, as well as in China to treat gastrointestinal inflammation, tuberculosis, malignant tumors, and other ailments with its detoxifying, anti-inflammatory, antiviral, and antioxidant properties; and it is used externally for its fast and effective wound healing. The name chaga comes from the language of the Khanty people (formerly called Ostyaks), a small tribe of reindeer herders on the west Siberian taiga. They use the tea that has been boiled a few minutes to detoxify the liver, get rid of intestinal parasites and stomach ailments, and more. The Ainu, the indigenous inhabitants of northern Japan, as well as several indigenous Canadian tribes, such as the Micmac, Cree, or Gitxsan, drank a decoction of chaga and also made an incense with the fungus.

The lovely, red fly agaric *(Amanita muscaria)* lives in symbiosis with birch and spruce. People have used this circumpolar mushroom to communicate with dwarves, gods, and ancestors in Eurasia as well as in North America since at least the Upper Paleolithic period, especially during the dark nights of the winter solstice time. The fungus seems to shine the sunlight caught by the birch directly into the depths of the soul, even into its darkest corners. Fly agaric is sympatholytic, meaning it relaxes the sympathetic nervous system so that one is completely relaxed after ingestion, the motor functions are inhibited, and the saliva flows. Bright light is disturbing because in this state one perceives the light of the otherworld.

First, shamans travel through the world of dwarves—thereby basically becoming dwarves themselves. When the trance is deep

72

enough, they come into the world of the ancestors; they themselves become one of the dead and learn their knowledge, wisdom, and instructions. In this profound state of immersion, the shaman becomes witness to the midwinter rebirth of the light—the shaman is conscious of the birth of the sun child in the womb of Mother Earth. The winter solstice is therefore the right time for such communion. Ingesting the fly agaric is never done alone as an individual hedonistic "trip," but always within the framework of a cultural, ritual context. The shaman experiences the nearly complete loss of motoric skills during the session, which can obviously be very dangerous and is never undertaken alone. Anthropologists such as Christian Raetsch believe that Santa Claus, with his red coat trimmed with white fur, is a personification of the fly agaric with its white-speckled red cap. In Germany and also in western Slavic countries, small imitations of fly agaric made from marzipan (sweetened almond paste) are still part of the celebration of the twelve holy days from Christmas to New Year's and Three Kings' Day (January 6th). They connote good luck, as do figurines of chimney sweeps (who clean the chimney, the ghosts' entryway), little marzipan pigs (which are reminiscent of the gold-bristled boar Freyr who pushes the wheel of the year to get it rolling again), and the Celtic cross in the shape of a green shamrock.

According to Germanic lore, the magic mushroom sprang up from the earth where foam had dripped from the nostrils of Odin's eight-legged horse. The Slavic people have a similar myth in which the saliva of Swantowit's horse produces the fungus. Odin's horse, with its eight legs, is a metaphorical image of the (funeral) bier—a fitting image, because the shaman is "dead" while in a deep trance induced by mushrooms and while his soul travels. Like their cousins in Siberia, Algonquin sorcerers inhabiting the birch forests of the Great Lakes region knew "red thunder mushroom" and used it in shamanic practices, especially to contact the dead.

For the Germanic people, the Slavs, and the Paleo-Siberian tribes—less so for the Celts, who were rather mycophobic (feared toadstools)—*Amanita muscaria* was the main entheogen. For several participants, seven to nine dried mushroom caps were taken together with reindeer milk, often with cranberry or crowberry juice, or tea made of the narrow-leaved willow herb (*Epilobium angustifolium,* or fireweed, as it is called in the United States) (Rosenbohm 1991, 143). In the tundra of the far north, where this mushroom does not grow, its value was such that it was exchanged for sable and fox pelts or even reindeer. Since the active ingredient, the muscimol, remains unchanged in urine, the northern Siberian people collected the urine of the shaman. Some other members of the tribe then drank it so that they could "travel."

The missionaries with their new ideas about "the one and only faith" condemned fly agaric, and it was banned. The men of God had a different kind of Holy Communion in mind, and the legend that the mushroom is fatally poisonous can be traced back to this time. However, the fungus has less to do with "poisoning flies" than with "flying" in the sense of shamanic flight. More relaxed about the fungus than Europeans, Russian, Siberian, and Japanese people macerate the toadstool so that the water-soluble toxins (ibotenic acid) are soaked out and then use it in various mushroom dishes. In Russia and Siberia, the fungus is referred to as *mukhomor* and considered a useful cancer remedy, particularly for gastric cancer; it was also used in the same way in Rhineland folk medicine.

The fly agaric trance requires the absolute silence of the winter night. Every sound can end the trance. In today's world, where a mobile phone suddenly rings, the refrigerator automatically starts to hum, or an aircraft flies over, such a state is hardly possible. In addition, the shaman should be called upon by the ancestors and gods before such an attempt. Would-be shamans who hold onto their egos will likely end up on a kind of horror trip.

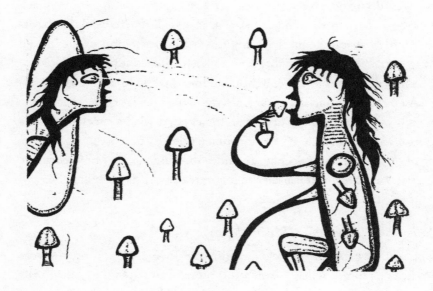

Bogbean, Bitter Clover (Menyanthes trifoliata)

The bogbean is a marsh plant that roots in shallow waters. Despite its trifoliate leaves, it is not a real clover but is a member of the buckbean family. Throughout the circumpolar region, the root, like gentian, is used as a bitter agent for upset stomach, constipation, and "internal diseases." In times of need, the indigenous people eat the roots.

Common Clubmoss (Lycopodium clavatum)

This herbal fossil, also called stag's horn clubmoss, ground pine, and wolf's claw, is of carboniferous origin (it existed before the coal period). One finds the mossy forest plant all around the globe. In the taiga, they form large, closed ground covers. Stone Age peoples used, and Siberians and Native Americans all across the continent still use, the abundant yellow spore as wound powder and baby powder; it is also powdered on the navel of the newborn in order to promote healing. Throwing the greasy, aluminum-containing spore into the fire results in a terrific, fiery explosion. Shamans, and later stage actors, used this pyrotechnic effect for their dramatic representations. In Russia, the spores are drunk mixed in kvass (a fermented bread drink) as a laxative. Decoctions of the shoots are diuretic or can be used as a mouthwash. Farmers in Europe hung a twig of the plant on the stable door to keep witches at bay.

Closely related to the common clubmoss is the fir clubmoss (*Lyco-podium selago; Huperzia selago*), also known as devil's claw. This *selago*, which was sacred to the druids and harvested with a special ritual, is poisonous. In Polish, it is called "women's death" because it was used as an abortifacient. As a decoction, under the guidance of knowledgeable herbal practitioners, it is used as a purgative as well as for killing lice and other pests.

Elder (Sambucus nigra, S. canadensis)

The natural habitat of the elder, a nitrogen-loving bush, is open spaces in the taiga forest, where mammoths, buffalo, and other large mammals gathered to rest for the night (Hempel 2009, 132). Certainly, the purple juice of the berries that ripen in autumn were an important source of vitamins for the Paleolithic hunters. The berries contain large amounts of vitamin C (18 milligrams per 100 grams), along with vitamins A, B12, and B2, potassium, carotenoids, and other nutrients. We now know that elderberry juice or even the dried berries strengthen the immune system as the weather begins to get colder. The juice stimulates peristalsis and cleanses the colon, which is an important organ of the immune system. Modern phytotherapy demonstrates that the juice is effective with viral infections and neuralgia. It is also recommended for shingles (herpes zoster), a viral disease.

Wherever it grows, the white flowers that blossom at midsummer are used as a diaphoretic for feverish diseases. An infusion of the flowers has a strong diaphoretic and diuretic effect and stimulates the immune system. Certainly, this application was already known by the people of the Upper Paleolithic period as elder flower tea is used by Native Americans, wherever the shrub grows. Eastern Europeans have it as a beverage during the sweat house ritual or the banja. Today, in Europe, one still makes hot elder flower tea, combined with a hot bath to prevent the onset of a cold or flu. The scraped bark (phloem, the inner, living bark) was known to the hunters and gatherers on both sides of the Bering Strait, and in Eurasian folk medicine as well as that of the Native Americans, such as the Winnebago, Menominee, and the Iroquois, as a strong purgative, sweat-inducing, emetic, diuretic, and mucus-producing material. The leaves can be used for bruises, contusions, frostbite, burns, tumors, and rough, raw skin; for this purpose, they are preferably macerated in ointments such as boar, bear, marmot, or badger fat.

By the end of the Upper Paleolithic period (the Magdalenian era), the reindeer hunters developed a drilling technique to perforate antlers, wood, or even stone. They used hollow elder twigs that they spun between their palms or put into motion with a bow drill; wet flint pebbles served as emery. Ethnobotanist Bruno Wolters was able to show that the varied applications of the elder among Native American indigenous peoples and the people of the Old World are shared at a rate of more than seventy-five percent (Wolters 2000, 15).

Field Horsetail (Equisetum arvense) and Rough Horsetail (E. hyemale)

Native Americans, such as the Blackfoot, Chippewa, Okanagan, Potawatomi, and many others, use horsetail as well as rough horsetail primarily in a tea or decoction as a diuretic and cleansing remedy. It is used for kidney pain, uterine bleeding, blood in the urine, urinary retention, and is also used by women who drink the tea during childbirth. It is a dermatological agent and is used for washing and hemostasis of abrasions, and to heal skin diseases (Moerman 1999, 213–216). In the spring, the pale beige shoots are eaten as a vegetable, and the tubers are cooked like potatoes. The tubers are difficult to harvest because they are very deep in the earth, so some North American indigenous peoples raided and gathered them from the nests of lemmings and other rodents. Rough horsetail is also used as an astringent skin medicine and as a diuretic.

With its signature of a jointed stem, it is used for pain in the spine. The siliceous shoots—the ash contains almost ninety percent silica—served as abrasive paper and were used for scouring soapstone pipe bowls, bone tools, arrow shafts, and bows. In Eurasia, horsetail is used in exactly the same way. While the western Europeans do not use the rough horsetail as a healing plant, in Russia and Siberia it is applied exactly as in North America, which points to a common Paleolithic heritage. The idea that the siliceous horsetail decoction can also be effectively used to treat tuberculosis can be traced back to the herbalist Father Kneipp, who cured himself of pulmonary consumption with the plant. The understanding that drinking the decoction makes broken bones heal faster seems to have come at a later time.

Fireweed or Willowherb (Epilobium angustifolium)

These delightfully rosy and lovely flowers are in the primrose family. They grow up to six feet (two meters) high by mid-August, at which time the womenfolk collect their healing herbs and consecrate them to Mother Mary.[6] Where a forest fire has raged, the plant quickly covers all scorched surfaces, which is why it is called fireweed in American English. In fact, its relationship to fire is its signature—the circumpolar willowherb is used to heal burns. It is a good tannin and is a remedy for inflammation, diarrhea, and uterine and urinary-tract infections; as a gargle, it cures gingivitis and tonsillitis. It is also used in Russia to treat both leucorrhea and epilepsy. Wherever it grew, the Native Americans roasted the root and crushed it to make a hot poultice for boils and ulcers. The young spring shoots are enjoyed everywhere as a vegetable, and in Russia the dried grass-like leaves are drunk as a pleasant tea that tastes similar to black tea. In Siberia, as already mentioned, the tea is part of the shamanic fly agaric ritual. The woolly white seed hairs were also used for stuffing clothes and pillows.

Juniper (Juniperus communis, and other Juniperus species)

The juniper was, along with mugwort, dwarf birch, crowberry, bearberry, buckthorn, and other light-loving, cold-resistant tundra vegetation, among the first colonizers of the cold steppes as the glaciers receded. In other words, the small tenacious conifer was well known to the Ice Age hunters, who brought the branches into their dwellings and sweat lodges to use as incense. A tea or a decoction of the berries works as a strong diuretic. The blue berries contain germicidal, aromatic, fat-soluble oil. When boiled in bear lard, they produce an ointment for joint pain and rheumatism; chewed, they help with heartburn and gastrointestinal disturbances. When simmered, the twigs release expectorant and antiseptic scents that help with mucus and pneumonia.

Knotweed Species (Polygonum spp.)

The various circumpolar knotweed species include the annual common knotweed *(Polygonum aviculare)*, water pepper *(P. hydropiper)* and bistort (P. bistorta). All three contain astringent tannins and are used to treat diarrhea, bleeding, and wounds. The young leaves and shoots of the knotweed are edible. Water pepper is spicy-hot in taste and applied externally as a poultice, works as a rubefacient, reddens the skin, and increases subcutaneous blood circulation; thus, it helps with swelling and inflammation, similar to a mustard plaster. The bistort roots are also eaten but must first be soaked in water overnight.

Marsh Labrador Tea (Ledum palustre, syn. Rhododendron palustre, R. tomentosum)

This resinous moor plant grows where birch and pine thrive. The Canadian and Alaskan indigenous peoples and the Inuit of Greenland drink the aromatic, mucolytic tea for colds and coughs. The Russians cook the flowers in butter and make a salve for skin diseases and rheumatism. In wide areas of Siberia, the dried leaves were mixed with shamanic, trance-inducing intoxicants. In northern Europe, marsh Labrador tea was used as a beer additive in the heady *gruit-ale* (an unhopped beer with herbs) long before the use of hops came about. The Tanana people in Alaska use the branches as bathing brushes in their sweat lodges.

Marsh Marigold (Caltha palustris)

This circumpolar flower from the buttercup family grows in wet areas. The roots, the young leaves, and the buds can be eaten in the spring. They must be well cooked, and the water must be discarded; otherwise, they

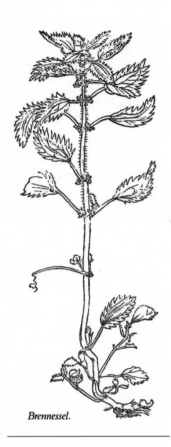

Brennessel.

Stinging nettle (Otto Brunfels, *Herbarium Vivae et Eicones,* Strasbourg, 1530)

will cause a severe irritation to the mucous membranes. Heat, however, destroys the protoanemonine responsible for the discomfort. The vegetable is eaten from Finland to North America, with a preference for pairing it with greasy meat. The root of the plant is drunk as a laxative, diuretic, and diaphoretic. The Iroquois used the tea as an emetic if they wanted to purge unwanted love spells. The impressive, greasy, shiny, golden-yellow flowers are used in cult and ritual ceremonies.

Nettle (Urtica dioica)

An herb that can sting so severely is obviously a plant of power with which one can practice magic. The applications as a healing and magical plant among the circumpolar peoples are correspondingly varied. Among Native Americans, such as the Abenaki, and Russians, it was considered a most effective styptic. The roots and leaves were grated into a powder and sprinkled on fresh wounds; the fresh juice of the leaves is used to stop internal bleeding, such as in the lungs, or hematuria. The plant is also considered a vermifuge. For rheumatism and arthritis, affected body parts are brushed with the fresh shoots. It is also an effective diuretic and was used as such throughout Eurasia and by the Algonquin. A tea of the whole plant without the roots is drunk for dropsy (edema), urinary semolina, bad skin (pimples and rashes), and "to improve the blood."

Since the Stone Age, rope, nets (for fishing and carrying), textiles, and snares have been prepared from nettle fibers. The etymology of the connection between nettles and words such as *net, naehen* (in German "to sew"), and *needle* has been well researched by linguists; all of these words can be traced back to the common Indo-European root word **ne*. The Native Americans—the Algonquin, Iroquois, and even the ancient Hopewell, the mound builders who settled in Ohio some 2,000 years ago—sewed with nettle fibers, using porcupine quills as sewing needles. The Jesuit missionary Father Hennepin reports in 1698 that the Iroquois fashioned nets from nettle fibers and the bast fibers of the linden or basswood tree that were up to fifty yards (three thousand meters) long and spanned the Saint Lawrence River such that up to four hundred whitefish and some great sturgeons were thus collected (Erichsen-Brown 1989, 444).

Wherever nettles grow, the shoots are eaten like spinach and seeds are gathered in the autumn as a food supplement. The plant is invigorating and healthy; in England, there is still a saying: "three nettles in May keep diseases away."

Water Avens (Geum rivale)

This plant of the rose family is found growing on the banks of streams. It has a drooping reddish flower head that looks like a congealed drop of blood, which was taken as an indication the plant could stop bleeding. Throughout Eurasia and North America, the root is boiled and used internally for diarrhea, dysentery, and spitting up of blood and externally to treat wounds. In fact, it is an excellent tannin drug that justifies such applications.

Winter Green, Pipsissewa (Chimaphila umbellata, syn. Pyrola umbellata)

This pretty little herb of the heath family (specifically of the subfamily of wintergreen plants or *Pyrolacae*) grows in sandy pine forests. It has always been used, similarly to the bearberry leaves, as a decoction to treat cystitis, prostate problems, and rheumatism. It is also used externally for washing lichens and rashes. American herbalists use the Algonquin word *pipsissewa* for this plant.

Sweat Lodge and Baking Oven

Another legacy of Paleolithic big game hunter culture is the steam bath. It is a place where physical and spiritual healing and renewal can take place by encountering spirits and magical animals. In the Native American sweat lodge, such as the Lakota inipi rite or Cheyenne *emaom* (little sweat lodge), the archaic sweat lodge has been preserved in its purest form. The Russian steam bath *(banja);* the Scandinavian and Finnish sauna; the Baltic sweat house *(pirts);* the hot Japanese baths; the Turkish bath *(hammam),* probably brought by the Turkic tribes from their original home in the central Asian Altai region; the sweat house of the Aztecs *(temazcal);* and the Celtic sweat lodge *(allus bothan)* in ancient Ireland are further developments of the simple Paleolithic sweat lodge. And the portable sweat lodge yurts in the central Asian steppes should also be included. The Scythians, the wild nomadic horsemen of the eastern European steppe, used teepee-like tents covered with felt mats for performing initiation and funeral rites. According to reports by the Greek historian Herodotus (440 BCE), hemp *(Cannabis)* was sprinkled onto glowing stones in these tents. The inhalation of cannabis smoke helped the participants put everyday consciousness aside and accompany the deceased on their path to the otherworld for a stretch.[7]

For the Plains Indians, the sweat lodge represents the belly of a bison;[8] this in turn embodies the ancient Earth Mother, the Grandmother, the guardian of animals and plants. To build the framework of the low, dome-shaped hut, materials such as flexible willow branches are driven into the earth and in a circle and tied together in the center, in a north-south axis. The curved branches represent the ribs of buffalo (the Earth Mother), and the axis is her spine. The framework used to be completely covered with buffalo skins (today with blankets).[9]

Generally, the narrow opening is in the east—regarded as the vulva of the Earth Goddess—because from this direction comes light and life.[10] In front of the entrance is a fire in which round boulders are heated up until they glow then carried with sticks or moose antlers into the pit in the middle of the sweat lodge. Participants crawl through the low

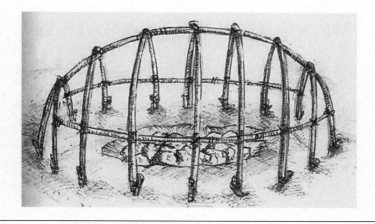

The structure of a typical sweat lodge
(from Christiane van Schie, *Im Schoss der Erdmutter*)

entrance—so to speak, through the vagina—into the belly of the Earth Mother where, in total darkness, as naked as embryos, the people squat and sweat. Water is poured repeatedly onto the hot, glowing stones, forming swaths of dense steam. The heat, which can become almost unbearable, catapults participants out of their ordinary state of consciousness so that they can perceive the gods and animal spirits and communicate with them. During the sweat-lodge ritual, which can sometimes take a night or a day and a night, all sense of time is lost so that one finds oneself beyond normal time, in dreamtime. Prayers are said and medicine songs are sung, and possibly the medicine pipe is smoked. Four times the participants leave the hut to jump into the icy river or pond or to roll in the snow or in the fresh dew, and then to sweat again.

When the sweat-lodge ritual is over, each participant feels like a new person. Mother Earth has taken them in her hot lap, incubated them, cleansed and released them back with full force into existence. The Cheyenne tell that even the dead have been revived in a sweat-lodge ceremony. The ritual is thus a return to the womb of the Great Mother. It is she who receives the souls of animals as well as the seeds of plants, guards them, and dismisses them again into the external world. It follows that the Central American sweat lodge *(temazcal)* has also been designed as the belly of the Great Goddess. The Russian banja has also been traditionally associated with "moist Mother Earth," the second mother *(vtoroi mat)* of humans; in pre-Christian times, it was the goddess Mokosh. For the Latvians, the "mother of the sweat house" *(Pirts Māte)* is seen as an aspect of the Earth Goddess *(Zemes Māte).* The sweat bath itself is her womb.

In this context, it also follows that the sweat lodge of many peoples is the privileged place where births take place. In Finland, pregnant women may still prefer the sauna room to give birth. Even in rural regions of Latvia, as well as in Russia, children are still being brought into the world in the steam bath house. It was also the case in ancient Ireland. The custom can certainly be traced back to the mammoth steppes of the retreating Ice Age. Where else could a woman giving birth in a cold, windy climate find more security and protection than in the warm sweat lodge, scented with aromatic herb mugwort (McKee 2007, 1)?

Although deviations among the many different ethnic groups in the execution of the sweat lodge abound, there is nevertheless a basic pattern that shows the common cultural origin.

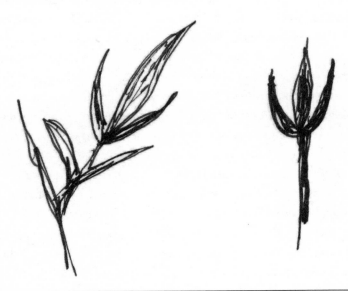

The tip of a mugwort leaf, which is similar to a Shiva trident

- Water is poured on heated stones to produce steam. Here we meet again the theme of the two contradictory primary elements: fire and water.

- To cool down, the sweating is either interrupted or brought to a close, and the participants jump into a cold lake, pond, or river, or roll in the snow or the dew-fresh grass.

- The body of the sweating person might be gently brushed during the ritual with bundles of specific aromatic herbs or twigs. Birch twigs are generally preferred as a brush or tuft; sometimes, the brush is made out of branches from a juniper species, for example, in Latvia, from the fragrant bog myrtle *(Myrica gale)*. Often mugwort shoots *(Artemisia* spp.) are added to the brush. For aching, swollen limbs, arthritis, and rheumatism, the Russians like to use bunches of wormwood twigs *(Artemisia absinthium)*. To be brushed down with wormwood is supposed to clarify the spirit. For the same purpose, the Athabaskan people use a tuft of Tilesius' wormwood *(Artemisia tilesii)*, and the Aleut people turn to Kamchatka wormwood *(A. vulgaris var. kamtschatica)*.

- Herbs with essential oils and healing properties are scattered onto the glowing stones or into an infusion. Ethnobotanist Bruno Wolters writes that Native Americans know at least 164 species that are suitable for the sweat lodge (Wolters 2000, 22). Fifty-five percent of them belong to genera from northeast Asia that are found in the circumpolar regions and have been known since the Upper Paleolithic period. Among them are the following: mugwort, yarrow, tarragon, fringed sage *(Artemisia frigida)*, wintergreen, juniper, mint, self-heal, ferns, elder, nettle, pine, spruce, angelica, cherry, oats, sweet gale, and calamus.

- To help induce sweating, large amounts of a tea made out of diaphoretic herbs are drunk in advance. The Native Americans of the Rocky Mountains, for example, the Cheyenne, drink an infusion of bee balm (bergamot, *Monarda fistulosa*), which grows there and is used similarly as the elder flower is used among the

Iroquois and other eastern woodland indigenous peoples; people in Russia use elder flower in a similar way as well.

Meanwhile, physicians have recognized that these sweat cures indeed have a strong impact on one's health.

- The intense sweating washes toxins and metabolic slags from the body tissues.
- The heating (hyperthermia) acts like an artificial fever. A fever is, as we now know, a natural immunological defense reaction: It activates the lymphocytes and inhibits bacteria, viruses, and fungi.
- The alternate sweating and cooling cleanses the skin, opens the pores, and stimulates blood circulation so that the tissues and muscles are better supplied with oxygen (Storl 2010a, 160ff.).

These observations are natural, rational, and empirical and correspond to our worldview. For the Native Americans, eastern Siberians, and probably also Paleolithic peoples, such healing is regarded as a gift from the spirit beings present during the sweat-lodge ritual.

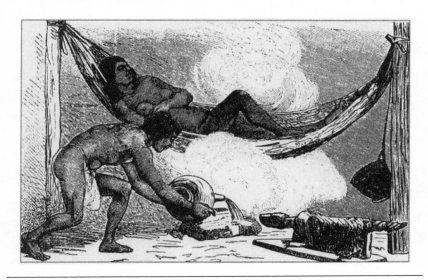

Sweat bath of the Rouquouyennes (by Creveaux, 1881)

Mugwort *(Artemisia spp.)*

Like juniper, mugwort is one of the first pioneer plants that grew after the glaciers receded. The mammoth and reindeer hunters at the edge of the glaciers knew the grayish-colored, aromatic herb very well. They will have used mugwort in the same way everyone still does today throughout the northern hemisphere. They surely burned mugwort incense in order to drive away unpleasant spirits and negative influences; it was used in midwifery and as a medicinal plant for women's health, and they decorated their cult places with it.

In the Alps, mugwort is part of the mixture used to incense the house and barn during the sacred nights of winter solstice. The Plains Indians use an incense mixture for sacred ceremonies and séances that includes sweetgrass *(Hierochloe odorata),* red cedar *(Juniperus virginiana* or *Thuja plicata),* and steppe sagebrush *(Artemisia tridentata, A. ludoviciana,* and other *Artemesia* species). The Native Americans west of the Mississippi say sagebrush creates a sacred space, the "cedar" protects them, and the sweet-smelling grass attracts good spirits. Similar use can be found with Tibetan Bonpo shamans and Nepalese Jhankries. The latter recognize the trident of the shaman god Shiva Mahadeva in the three points of the mugwort leaf; Shiva has many characteristics rooted in the Stone Age, such as when he appears as a dancing shaman, or the Lord of the Animals (Pashupati), or the master of ecstasy (Storl 2012, 42–43). The trident is a symbol of the shaman not only in India but also throughout all of Siberia.

Everywhere, mugwort is known as a dispeller of evil spirits. Its use in Traditional Chinese Medicine as a moxa plant, in which tiny balls or cones of the plant are burned directly on the skin (on certain meridians), originally chased bad spirits from the body. Indigenous peoples in what is now Canada put mugwort *(A. vulgaris, A. arguii, A. douglasiana)* under the pillow to further lucid dreams; in China, mugwort is stuffed into the pillow to ensure good, quiet sleep. In Europe, people did the same thing as an aid against bad dreams. And Plains Indians depend on it to keep ghosts at bay. Even today, mugwort is one of the main plants used by midwives.[11]

The petite, strong, fringed sagebrush *(A. frigida)* that contains camphor is preferred in eastern Siberia and North America to regulate fertility and menstruation. Women drink decoctions of this and other sagebrush species during certain stages of labor to facilitate the birth or to help the placenta detach. As a gynecological herb, mugwort, and especially *Artemisia vulgaris,* is used universally for leucorrhea, vaginitis, irregularities of the menses, and for increasing fertility. The *Macer Floridus* (eighth to ninth century), the standard work of medieval herbal medicine, praises the action of wormwood for preventing miscarriages. With the help of mugwort, midwives once knew how to turn a fetus that was in an awkward position and at risk of a breech birth (Madejsky 2008, 60). It is considered highly likely that this herb was used in these ways already in Paleolithic times. In the rural population in China and eastern Asia, women would squat over a mugwort steam bath while in labor. The sacred herb was most likely used in the sweat lodge during birth since the old Stone Age. The Plains Indians still cover the floor of ceremonial teepees with sagebrush today.

In the famous Anglo-Saxon Nine Herbs Charm, a testimony of ancient Germanic herbalism, the mugwort is mentioned as the very first plant. It is called the *yldost wyrta,* "the oldest wort" (healing plant). Her name is Una—this is a deliberate reverse spelling of Anu, a so-called anagram (an ancient practice to ensure magical protection by which the letters are reversed), and grants magical protection. Anu or Ana is the ancestor, the primordial goddess, and is identical to Mother Holle and the Earth Mother. She is also the Dea Ana of the Indo-Europeans, the mother of the Celtic divine race of the Danu.[12] She also represents the Roman mistress of animals and wildlife, Diana. As nourisher, this goddess appears as Annapurna in India and, with the Latin-speaking Indo-European tribes in Italy, as the ever-recurring Anna Perenna, a former Etruscan earth goddess who once saved the people from starvation. As Saint Anna, the mother of the "Mother of God," she is cloaked in a Christian guise. This primordial goddess was dedicated to mugwort. The name Artemisia is based on Artemis, the Greek goddess of the wilderness and of childbirth. She was considered the first midwife because she was born before her twin brother, the Sun God Apollo, and immediately helped to bring him to the world.

In German, the common name is Beifuss, which means something like "at the foot," and generally one thinks that the name is related to the practice of tying the herb to the foot so as not to be tired while walking. However, this is not the case. This German plant name— Hildegard of Bingen called it *biboz*—comes from the Middle High German bozen (to pound, hit, or smite) and is related to the German word for anvil, *Amboss,* upon which the smith's hammer smites. Thus, it is the "pounding herb," with several possible significances.

- It is an herb that is pounded or crushed with a pestle.
- Because the plant is connected to sexuality and fertility, it is an indication of coital "thrusts."
- The herb wards off poltergeists, that is, spirits that make bumping and thudding noises in the night, such as the Swabian *Butz* or the *puck* of Nordic folklore.

Mugwort is undoubtedly one of the oldest shaman herbs. The camphor-like fragrance of the pulverized dry flowers alone, or when placed on incense coals, opens the soul and sharpens mental perception. In eastern Asia, from Tibet to Mongolia, mugwort was used by shamanic healers for moxibustion, presumably to drive the spirits of disease out of the body. Moxibustion with *Artemisia* has been incorporated into Traditional Chinese Medicine and, over the span of millennia, was refined utilizing needles that conduct the heat of the burning mugwort into specific acupuncture points. The Indo-European shamans, as well as the shamanic seers of Nordic peoples, the *Voelvas* and *Veledas,* consecrated themselves with the herb on certain days before flying "as wild geese" out to the worlds beyond. Mugwort also played a role in the holy days of the solstices. People danced around or jumped over the midsummer solstice fire with a belt made of braided mugwort and then offered it up in the flames, which symbolized the casting away of the past year.

There is little doubt that the indigenous peoples of central Europe also once used sweat lodges. From the Neolithic and Bronze Age, round, beehive-shaped stone huts were partly set in the earth; their function puzzles archeologists. Were they for grain storage, or were they places of worship? Closer examination of these structures showed an accumulation of stones that were splintered by fire, and pollen analyses of the soil revealed mugwort and other aromatic herbs (McKee 2007, 1–2). Similar archeological finds exist in Mecklenburg, Germany. In Kilkenny County, Ireland, prehistorians discovered the outlines and charred remains of a Bronze Age sweat lodge. This cabin had been, like other Stone Age sweat lodges, built from hazel branches (Van Schie 2010, 36), although generally such Irish sweat lodges were built with stone and resembled grave chambers. They were heated with peat and served the purpose of sweating out of diseases.

Through contact with the Roman civilization, the relatively simple steam baths were replaced with sophisticated bathhouses in much of Europe. From the twelfth century on, though, baths with stone ovens and benches similar to the sauna in which herbs were placed to vaporize on the stove again appeared. Menstrual complaints and pain were treated in these bathhouses with tansy, feverfew, and mullein (McKee 2007, 9). Henbane was also placed on the stove, which caused merriment and brought about hallucinogenic states—thus, the otherworld found its way once again into the bathhouse. When the black plague came and later syphilis raged—after Columbus had brought it back with him from the New World—the bath houses everywhere were closed and the bathing culture came to a virtual standstill.

Nevertheless, people continued to sweat as a therapeutic treatment at home for "fever" (including rheumatism and neuralgia), other pains, rashes, warts, or infestations. After the bread loaves were taken out of the baking oven, patients stretched out inside as it slowly cooled. Sometimes the patient lay in the oven for a while bedded in hot sand, ash, salt, or, as in Russia, clay.[13] Ailing infants were taken here to "re-bake," and changelings were ritually returned and exchanged.[14] In Hungary, as she ritually put a bogus changeling in the oven, the midwife said: "Here, take the little Devil, and give me back my own child." After this, the child would be free of the evil spirit.

The oven symbolized a womb in the view of the farmers—similar to the sweat lodge of even older cultures. Taking the freshly baked bread from the hot oven resembled birth; the fresh, warm loaf is not unlike the small body of a swaddling child (Storl 2014b 57). Children cursed by a witch (enchanted) could be disenchanted here. The oven was a mystical place where ancestral spirits or the friendly house gremlin and the dwarves hung around. On occasion, even the dead were put into it to dry them a bit, before being given a proper burial (Baechtold-Staeubli and Hoffmann-Krayer 1987, Vol. 1, 783). The oven, like a fireplace or a forging place, is a site of transformation—even the witch's oven in the story of *Hansel and Gretel* points to this significance. The Church regarded this as superstition and, thus, forbade such uses of ovens.

Emetics and Purgatives

Another legacy of the circumpolar ice age medicine is the use of purgatives and emetics. Today, we would call these "cleansing or detoxifying therapies," but for the indigenous people, it meant more than merely the sudden emptying of the colon and the stomach contents to get rid of toxins or pollutants. Often, this cleansing was carried out before a healing session with a shaman to remove pernicious disease spirits or magical poisons (intrusions) that had been perceived in a clairvoyant state or shamanic trance (Storl 2011, 133–134). Occasionally, the healers prepared not only their patients but also themselves in this way for the healing ceremony. Vomiting and purging were also often part of initiation rituals for youths. The Seminole people in Florida practiced ritual vomiting before their council meetings. Nothing should weigh on the participants; they should not carry bad spirits into the council; words and ethos should be clear and true.

Native Americans knew about two hundred plants that were emetic and around 150 that served as laxatives. Many emetics, such as puke weed (Indian tobacco, *Lobelia inflata*) are species endemic to North America.

However, many other laxatives and purgatives are native to both the New and the Old World.

One of the most important medicinal plants of the forest natives of North America, the Siberians, the Russians, and the western Europeans, as we have seen, is the elder bush *(Sambucus nigra, S. canadensis)*. In circumpolar regions, the inner bark (phloem or bast) is used as a purgative and laxative. And Russians, Siberians, ancient Prussians, Upper Bavarians, Celts, and even the polymath Albertus Magnus (twelfth century) in the text *Vegetabilis* have stated something similar: If the inner bark of a young tree is scraped upward, then the decoction causes vomiting; if it is scraped downward, then it causes diarrhea. The North American woodland tribes, such as the Winnebago, Menominee, and Iroquois, tell that this scraping upward or downward has been transmitted in their healing methods. In Romanian folk medicine, "worms" are either expelled through the mouth or through the anus in this way. The fact that these similarities in this "sympathetic magic" did not happen by chance, but are a cultural practice that has its roots in the Upper Paleolithic period, is obvious.

The Celtic-Gallic term for the elder is *skobiém* with the linguistic root sco, which is related to "rasps" or "scraping." The names for elder derived from Slavic and found in Silesian or Upper Saxon dialects, *Schibbeke, Schibchen,* or *Zibke,* also allude to the scraping of the bark. In European folk medicine, the bark is best scraped during the new moon in early spring or in late fall. As the Gaul Marcellus Empiricus (turn of the fourth and fifth centuries) wrote, a piece of bark roughly the size of a hazelnut is cooked and consumed in the morning on an empty stomach (Hoefler 1911, 24).

Our question in this regard is: Does it work? Is vomiting really brought on when the bark is scraped upward? Is the result a vigorous bowel movement when it is scraped downward? Or is this pure superstition? The answer is, for at least 15,000 years, an unequivocal, "Yes, it works." Since the elder bark, as well as the leaves, is mildly toxic due to cyanogenic glycoside sambunigrin, which the body flushes out as quickly as it can, sweat and urination occur accompanied with vomiting or diarrhea if the dose is too strong. The therapeutic word of the healer triggers the reaction—the way the plant has been harvested signals the patient's psyche to which elimination process is appropriate: down through the intestines or up to cause vomiting.

Shamanism

Quite a few elements of shamanism, which dates back at least until the Upper Paleolithic period, are also still part of our folk medicine. The limestone cave paintings, etchings, and drawings, colored with yellow and red ocher, black charcoal, and white chalk, which were discovered in the Franco-Cantabrian region, leave no doubt that shamans already existed. In addition to the animals vital to survival—buffalo, reindeer, aurochs, mammoths, horses, and others—strange human figures are also depicted. In the cave of Lascaux, for example, one sees a bird-headed little man, who apparently finds himself in a trance (Illustration 25a); in the cave of Espelugues, the "Wizard of Lourdes" carries deer antlers and has an animal tail similar to the Tungus shaman (Illustration 25b); the cave complex of Trois-Frères (Illustration 25c) displays dancing "sorcerers," with stag's antlers, wolf ears, and bear paws, as well as a dancing figure with a buffalo mask (Illustration 25d); in Dodogne, Abri Mège, a horned ibex dancer is carved into bone (Illustration 25e).

There are many interpretations of this cave art. For cultural anthropologists such as Hans-Peter Duerr, caves are entrances to the otherworld and regarded as the womb of the Earth Goddess, the mother of the animals. Here, deep in the earth, in her belly, animal souls mature until the goddess releases them into the external world. The shamans, the mediators between the worlds, enter these dark depths to negotiate with the goddess, perhaps even to sleep with her and fertilize her in order to secure the population of the wild game (Duerr 1990).

So this is what constitutes shamans: they are not simply conjurors of spirits. Shamans have the ability, and have mastered the technique, to leave the body and travel afar. They are, as defined by Mircea Eliade, masters of ecstasy.[15] Ecstasy (Greek *éksta-sis*) means "to emerge out of

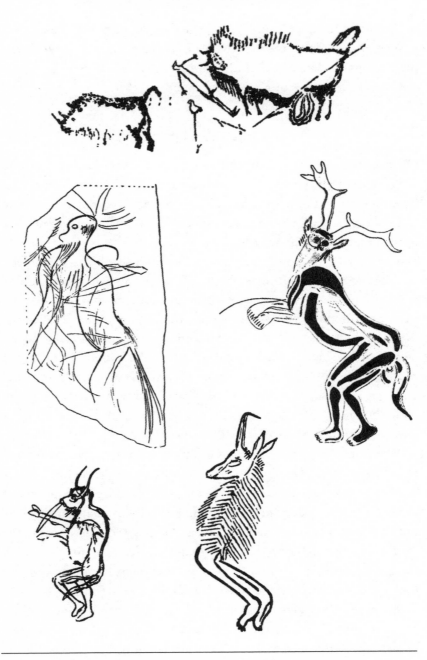

Shaman representations from the Upper Paleolithic period

oneself," to send one's soul in conscious astral travel to the "inside" of nature, into the other dimensions of existence, to the worlds of ghosts, gods, and demons. Unlike representatives of spiritualist séances or the African voodoo tradition, shamans are not possessed by spirits or deities.

That there is this metaphysical plane of existence, this world of spirit beings, was never questioned—that is, other than in our current materialistic, rationally oriented culture. We mostly interpret these worlds as psychological projections. This is not true for traditional peoples—for them, the otherworld is a fact. Nor is it merely a religious matter of faith, but it is truly experienced. It is neither of subjective fantasy nor imagination but affects and influences our everyday existence and being.

So what do shamans do in the tribal society? They use their skills to make things happen on the meta-level, in the world of spirits, to provide order in the otherworld before these things condense into concrete material reality. They are active not only on the horizontal axis of everyday reality, but move also on the vertical axis, which connects us with the upper and the lower nine worlds. They fly or climb up the branches of the world tree or down to its deep roots. Shamans know how to deal with the spirits, and they use their abilities to:

- cure diseases;
- retrieve and bring back souls and soul parts that have been lost in the astral world or have been stolen by spirits;
- find out where the herds and big game are and ask permission to take some animals;
- ask the plants about their healing powers and ask for their help;
- escort the dead into the spirit world;
- find out the truth; and
- avert impending disaster before it manifests in the material world.

What is, in terms of the healing process, the difference between a modern doctor and a shaman?

The physician's diagnosis is based on the most precise, empirical investigation according to the latest scientific study by using techniques such as ultrasound, X-ray, magnetic resonance imaging (MRI), endoscopy, and an entire battalion of physiological, biochemical, and microscopic tests. The treatment is rational and contains scientifically tested pharmaceutical drugs, surgery, and the like.

While shamans do not have such impressive technical means, they observe the appearance of the sick person for fever, pain, excretions, skin color, and so on. But they do not stop there. They embark to the "inside" of the phenomenon, while in a trance. They see the essence—the "worm," the disease spirit or the magic arrow, the magical intrusion that has affected the sick person. With the strength and assistance of their animal allies and helping spirits, with the power of words and song charms, they are able to then overcome these fiends and render them harmless. They can draw out, drum out, smoke out, suck out disease-causing "magical intrusions," "worms," or "snakes" and then discard them. All this is done on the meta-level, in the dimension of becoming, where everything is still in flux and not in the dimension of what has become.

If a seasoned physician who doesn't believe in ghosts observes a patient who is still feverish and lying helpless and debilitated after a successful shamanic healing session, he or she is likely to say that nothing has happened; the patient is still in critical condition. The shaman, however, says, to the contrary, "No, the patient is on the road to recovery, because the worm is out!" And then, to advance the healing, the patient is given suitable herbal teas, decoctions, or ointments and possibly some protective amulets.

As we will see, European forest peoples continued to use this kind of shamanic healing for a long time. The speaking and singing for the sick, the expelling of "worms," "elves," spirits of disease, magic arrows, and the like were a component of rural folk medicine until the early part of the twentieth century. The evil spirits that were perceived on various levels were transferred from the patients onto beetles, birds, and trees—particularly the elder near the house (where the bush prefers to grow)—and so "disposed of."

Before conversion to Christianity, the culture of the forest peoples was marked by shamanism. For the Germanic peoples—from the

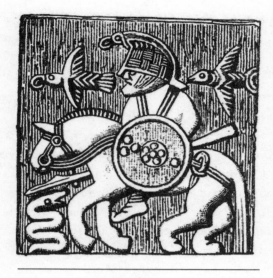

Odin/Wodan

Scandinavians in the north to the Lombards in northern Italy, from the
Anglo-Saxons in the west to the Rus *(Varangians)* on the Volga—the
main deity was a shaman. It was Odin (German Wotan, southern German Wodan, Anglo-Saxon Woden, Alemannic Woutis, Langobardian
Godan). Only much later did the Scandinavian nobility stylize the one-
eyed god *(Aesir)* into a god of war. But he was first and foremost a magician. Wolves and ravens—typical shaman animals—were his companions.
He knew the healing songs and was a master of the medicinal plants, as
we know from the Merseburg Healing Incantations and the Anglo-Saxon
Nine Herbs Charm, or Nine Worts Galdor. Hanging on the world tree,
he experienced his shamanic initiation and could thus bring the wisdom of
the runes to awareness. Odin was a magician, a shape shifter, a wanderer
between worlds, a companion of the dead, a rescuer of the cauldron with
the mead of inspiration, a master of trance and ecstasy. His name refers
to "rage" within the meaning of shamanic frenzy and goes back to the
Indo-European **uat* (blow, breathe, inspiration). The Latin name *vates*
(seer) and the Old Irish word *faith* (seer, soothsayer) are also etymologically related.

Some cultural researchers believe that Odin, or Wodan, was an immigrant deity from Siberia, but it is probably because the common Paleolithic shamanic roots make it appear that way. Incidentally, it is said that Odin learned his magic from Freya, goddess of love, life, and joy. Freya comes from the family of the Vanir, the even older gods. Thus, Odin's knowledge of magic is rooted in the female primal ground.

The shamanic knowledge, which was supported by the myth of Odin and Freya, stood in the way of the declaration of the "true faith in the one God" by Christian missionaries. Shamans, with their direct access to the world of spirits and gods, were and are the rivals of the priests and their book religion. Nevertheless, many shamanic elements have been retained in simple folk medicine. The carriers of this medicine were later brutally persecuted during the time of the Inquisition and witch hunts in the fifteenth and sixteenth centuries (Mueller-Ebeling, 2010), and the Enlightenment tried to make a clean sweep to completely wipe out the remnants of shamanic consciousness.

CHAPTER 4

The Healing Lore
of Neolithic Farmers

*People of the Middle Stone Age gathered and stored hazel-
nuts for the winter. Today people work in order to buy hazelnuts. In the time in between then and now, they have created
cultivated landscapes.*

WERNER HEMPEL, BOTANIST

The glaciers were receding. The tundra disappeared and, with it, the great
herds of the plains and northern steppes. Grasses and shrubs such as
buckthorn, willow, and juniper began to populate the landscape, followed
by birch, pine, hazel, and other trees. And then, during the Climatic
Optimum (the Holocene Thermal Maximum or HTM) eight thousand
years ago, the annual temperature rose—to as much as two degrees higher
than it is today—so that the countryside was soon covered with dense
oak, elm, and linden forests. The hunters and gatherers in central Europe
adapted; they collected more vegetable foods, hunted smaller game and
birds with bows and arrows, fished with fishhooks and harpoons and
with nets made from nettle fiber, expanded the use of dugout boats,
widened their knowledge of rope-making from willow bast fiber, and
fashioned water-proof containers from birch bark. They began to live
year-round in huts made of wood and reeds.

The First Farmers

While people continued to live off fishing, shellfish harvesting, and hunting in the northern coastal regions of the North and Baltic Seas, around 5000 BCE the first farmers appeared in the south along the upper reaches of the Danube River. They are referred to as the Linear Pottery culture for the type of decorations on their ceramics. With time, these farmers spread into the Rhineland and to the east into Ukraine. Archeologists long believed that these Neolithic farmers were solely immigrants, but now we know that they emerged largely from the indigenous Mesolithic population who took on the new economic and agricultural practices coming out of the south (Korn 2006, 37).

These Neolithic farmers settled mainly on fertile, loessial soil where a mixture of oaks and hornbeams grew. With polished stone axes and torches, they cleared the land and planted wheat, one-grained wheat, spelt, peas, lentils, millet, field beans, and flax, and made pastures for their cattle, pigs, sheep, and goats. In the midst of clearings, made by slash-and-burn techniques, they built small hamlets with longhouses where matrilineal extended families lived.[1] The thatched or reed houses—65 to 150 feet (20–45 meters) long and 16 to 25 feet (5–8 meters) wide—contained bedrooms and living rooms, workshops and storage, and a fireplace and an oven for bread baking in the middle area.[2]

The traditional division of labor established that the women, as daughters of the Earth Goddess and owners of the land, tilled the fields, sowed, hoed, and harvested. The women themselves were seen as similar to the Earth Goddess as they could also receive a seed and bring forth life. Already during the Paleolithic era, it was mainly groups of women—young and old women, mothers with their children, and babies—who gathered roots, wild fruit, and other food plants as well as healing plants while the men hunted. Consequently, it was the women who took care of the crops during the Neolithic era. In addition to the garden and field work, they put up food stores, milled the grain, baked flatbread, and cooked porridge—with added greens and herbs, and vegetables such as celery, leeks, and fennel (later poppy and hemp seeds were added). They spun and wove textiles, made pottery, healed the sick and injured, and brought up the children. The men cleared the land, built the houses, made the stone tools, and took care of the cattle. This division of labor was maintained, more or less, until the early twentieth century.

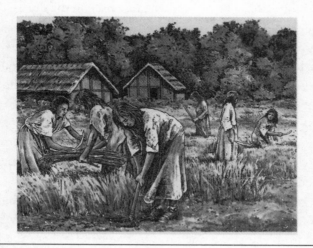

Women farmers of the Linear Pottery culture during the harvest

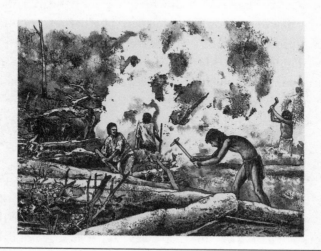

Men of the Linear Pottery culture using slash-and-burn methods to clear the forest (illustrations by Stephan Koebler, in Creutz, Ulrich. 1990. *Rund um die Steinzeit*. Berlin: Kinderbuchverlag)

So that a field might recover after the harvest, they left it to lie fallow and turned their cattle on it. Over time, soil fertility decreased, and the weeds increased. This is probably the main reason the farmers moved on to clear a new patch of forest after one generation, approximately a quarter of a century later. The forest then grew back in the deserted places.

Although these farmers supplemented what they reaped in agriculture with hunting and gathering herbs and edible wild plants, their activity had a much stronger effect on nature compared to the previous hunters and gatherers. Not only did their fields and pastures tear holes in the forest canopy, but they also used timber and large amounts of firewood for heating, baking, and pottery making. They cut branches to use as leaf forage fodder for their animals and drove their pigs into the forest in the fall to fatten them with roots, beechnuts, and acorns. And as they altered the environment, their worldview also changed.

There, where forests and grasslands meet, a distinct habitat with a unique botanical community forms. A dense hedge develops where cattle and goats nibble at the branches. On one hand, where the livestock browse, the branches produce many side shoots; on the other, the browsing encourages the survival of thorny and prickly bushes and shrubs (blackberry, hawthorn, dog rose, sloe berry, barberries, sea buckthorn) as well as poisonous shrubs (spindle tree, black haw, clematis, privet, Scotch broom, honeysuckle). Thus, for these farmers, in contrast to the previous hunters and gatherers, the world became divided into two parts. Outside in the wilderness lurked wild animals—bears, wolves, aurochs—and unpredictable forest spirits. Inside the hedge, the neat farmland, green pastures, and fields with the farmstead in the middle were an island of peace.

Of course, not everyone in central Europe was a farmer or shepherd at that time. Hunters and gatherers continued to survive in the vast forests. They did not see a contrast between nature and culture like the Neolithic farmers did; for them, the forest was neither strange nor dangerous, but an extension of "home" (Descola 2014, 59). The idea of Midgard—a peaceful world, with a garden in the middle protected by the gods, surrounded by a perilous, external wild world (Utgard)—is based on this late

Stone Age ideology. (And Asgard, the home of the gods, was the other of these three worlds of Nordic mythology.)

Witches, Stags, and Forest People

Ecological transition zones, such as hedges and forest edges, have a great abundance of botanical species. Not only are many kinds of woody plants represented, but a variety of herbs also grow there: hedge nettle, germander, groundsel, oregano, veronica, nettle, hemp nettle, cranesbill, and dozens of other species. Among the early farmers, it was probably the old, white-haired women, the aunts and grandmothers whose children had grown and who no longer toiled in the field, who tended to the hearth and healing.[3] They were wise because they had been through and experienced much in their lives. And since they were no longer involved in the active daily work, they could surrender themselves to contemplation and deepen their spiritual life in quiet meditation.

The hearth was the heart and center (Latin *focus* = focal point, stove) of the home and the clan. Fire has been sacred since it arrived more than one and a half million years ago to the early humans *(Homo erectus)*, making them truly human. Not only does it cook food, provide warmth, aid in healing, and bring light into the darkness of the night, it also connects humans with the gods and ancestors. The old clan mother is the fire guardian, who would sit at the fire place and let her soul fly out with the smoke through the flue opening on the gable, much like the Ice Age shaman once did who flew through the smoke hole of the tent (yurt or teepee) into the spirit world. The spirits came and went through this smoke hole, this "wind eye" (hence, "window"). Upon encountering them, the clan mother received visions that could be used when needed. Even the medieval image of the witch flying on her broom out through the chimney to some lonely hilltop (such as the Brocken, the mountain of the gods, or the Puy de Dome) to unite with the horned god (the devil) has its cultural historical roots in the Ice Age.

Often, old women could be seen collecting medicinal herbs and brushwood in the hedge, in the thorny, wild habitat of the intermediate region between field and forest, between this world and the other. This was the place where the best medicinal herbs as well as "nine" kinds of wood were found with which humans and farm animals could be kept in good health.

The nine different kinds of wood the women collected were later often associated with witchcraft and sorcery. However, behind this is the knowledge that each wood has a different quality, a different smell, a different color and strength, and of course each emits its own type of heat. This heat can actually even be measured with thermometers and recorded on a numbered scale. But that is very elementary because it only says something about the amount, or quantity, of the heat and not about the quality. As my teacher, the forest homesteader Arthur Hermes, once said, the healing of an herbal decoction or infusion can be strengthened or otherwise influenced by using this or that type of wood. Healers knew this from experience and tradition.

The Stag

The image of the wise elder who hangs around the hedge survived to our time in the English word *hag,* as well as in the German word *Hexe* which means "witch" (from Old High German, *hagzissa,* meaning "hedge sitter" or "hedge rider"). As a "hedge or fence rider" (Old Icelandic *tun-rida,* Low German *walriderske*), she was a mediator between the worlds. Later, in Christian times, she was feared as a woman who is in league with the devil and has magical powers. We should remember that this

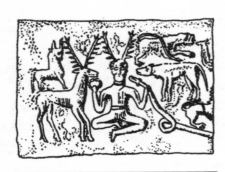

Cernunnos (from the
Gundestrupp Cauldron)

horned, goat-footed fellow (the devil) is actually an appearance of the Paleolithic master of the animals. In the European woodlands, he was present as the Stag God (the Celtic god Cernunnos). The worship of this horned forest god lives on unconsciously in the Christian legend of Saint Hubertus in which the Savior appears as a stag. The archetype resonates subconsciously with the image of the belling hart hanging in many living rooms over the sofa, or in the deer antlers on the gables of rural farms.

During the Middle Ages, it was believed that the deer knew all the medicinal plants and healing roots and used them to be healthy and stay young. In many parts of Europe, pharmacies are still named after the stag, in reference to its healing power. For the ancient Europeans, the stag was a symbol of the sun spirit visiting Earth and the forests; its antlers are golden, and it possesses the gold of wisdom. If it touches a spring with its antler, then the spring becomes a healing one. Those who have access to this divine being, such as the herbal woman does, will receive true healing inspiration. We will tell more about the wise woman, the companion of the Stag God, and their descendants later.

Feral Folk

In the realm of the hedge, on the edge of the settlement, the Neolithic border-walkers, "witches," shepherds, and hunters encountered not only deer and other timid forest animals, but they met also those intermediary beings—elves, nature spirits, or gnomes—who we otherwise meet in the dimension between sleeping and waking. Occasionally, the border-walkers and other dwellers of the Neolithic farmstead chanced upon the feral folk, or wild forest people. They live on today in legends and fairy tales, in folk tales and customs, as so-called "wild people," or *silvani* (Latin for "forest people"). Over time, the untamed nature people became ever more mythologized and pushed into the realm of giants, monsters, and hobgoblins.

Most likely these "savage people," the woods and moss people, the forest maidens and alpine spirits, were actually the indigenous people who had not taken the step into sedentary life. In legends, they are presented as follows: They have long, shaggy hair, carry cudgels, dress in animal pelts or even prefer to go naked, and rub their bodies down with fat to stay warm. They live "like gypsies" in caves or stone gaps. They don't like the sound of church bells ringing; they are shy and avoid people. But when happened upon, they are usually good-natured and friendly; only in the Alps they are often presented in a more threatening

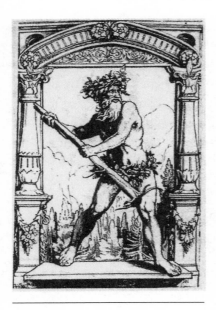

"Wild Man" (pen drawing by
Hans Holbein the Younger,
sixteenth century)

and wild manner. They protect the wild animals and sometimes are employed as dairymen and cow herders or shepherds. They eat herbs and roots but also will accept the farmer's butter, cheese, porridge, bread, fat, or barley for their services. They sometimes enter into marriages with sedentary people, as in the Wolfdietrich saga, in which a wild woman takes a knight as her husband. A Tyrolean legend tells of an alpine shepherdess who went with a shaggy-haired wild man and bore a strong, wild girl from him who always longed for the forest.

The wild people could predict the weather for the farmers; in fact, they possessed powerful weather magic. The dances of the wild men helped drive off the winter and bring fertility to the land. The memory of the indigenous people lives on in the alpine carnival customs, which include the dance of the wild men in the village of Obersdorf, Bavaria.

But above all, the wild people were knowledgeable herbalists. According to legend, they revealed a remedy for the plague to the frightened victims, namely angelica and pimpernel—indeed the roots of both *Umbelliferae* have an immune-boosting, diuretic, diaphoretic, and anti-inflammatory effect. The yarrow, one of the most important healing herbs, is also called "wild maiden herb." In the medieval tale of Gudrun, we learn that the old knight Wate was a good doctor and that he owed his knowledge of healing to a wild woman. And from the heroic story, *The Eckenlied* (around 1230 BCE), we hear of a *wilde vrouwelin* (wild maiden) who digs a root, grinds it in her hand, heals the wounds of Dietrich of Bern and his horse with it, and "swept away their pain and fatigue" (Hoefler

1911, 20). It seems that they existed for a long time; because still in the Middle Ages these people were persecuted by Church and State, and knights considered it a fun sport to hunt and kill them like wild animals.

Sedentary Lifestyle and New Diseases

The Neolithic farmers had a more diverse knowledge of medicinal plants than that of the Paleolithic hunters and gatherers. This has nothing to do with progress—rather the opposite. Farmers did not have as healthy a lifestyle as nomadic hunters and gatherers. The farmer's work is endless and exhausting; it is also more monotonous than hunting and gathering, which had determined peoples' lives for about three million years. The hard work in the field and stable resulted, for example, in the wear of their bones. Many Neolithic people in central Europe show degenerative changes of spine (spondylosis) and joint wear, and their teeth became bad. In some of these Neolithic cultures, two-thirds of the population suffered from food-related diseases—the one-sided carbohydrate diet and lack of vitamins and trace elements such as iron are responsible. Even malignant bone cancer was found several times in a southern German burial ground (Probst 1999, 229). Contrary to the Ice Age hunters who ate a lot of fish and fresh liver, rickets was frequently found among the farmers. People were a few centimeters smaller than their Paleolithic ancestors, and life expectancy, in particular among women, was lower (Porter 2003, 18).

The problems of a sedentary, farming lifestyle were not only the hard work, but also the accumulation of animal and human feces and other wastes. Excrement contamination in the water makes favorable conditions for infestation by intestinal parasites, amoebas, and worms. In addition, waste attracts flies, arthropods, and other vermin. The housefly (*Musca domestica*) did not exist in central Europe during the Paleolithic and Mesolithic eras; it was introduced with the pigs, sheep, and cattle of the first farmers from the Near East. Within permanent dwellings, fleas, lice, mites, and bed bugs nest easily in the sleeping area; stored cereals, dried meat, and other supplies attract mice, rats, beetles, borers, moths, and other unwelcome pests that may be vectors of contagious diseases.

The fly, for example, is involved in the transmission of cholera, typhoid, dysentery, anthrax, and other diseases, which were unknown to the Paleolithic hunters and gatherers.

Infectious diseases, such as influenza, smallpox, measles, leprosy, cholera, or tuberculosis, which were not known previously, were transmitted from the domesticated, suppressed, exploited, and castrated animals with which humans now shared a sedentary habitat. Viruses, protozoa, bacteria, and parasitic helminths need a high population density in order to spread, which did not exist among the wild hunters and gatherers. Only the population density in the longhouses and villages, and eventually even more so in the first cities, allowed the pathogens to jump the species barrier. Thus, we owe the flu to ducks and pigs, colds to horses, smallpox to cows, tuberculosis to cats and dogs, and bacteria such as salmonella to poultry, rats, and mice. The measles virus came from cattle, which causes rinderpest in cattle or is expressed as distemper in dogs (Porter 2003, 16; Diamond 1997, 207).[4]

Among the central European farmers, these infectious diseases were probably not as pronounced as in the overpopulated regions where people farmed with irrigation—Egypt, Sumeria, or China—and where periodic pandemics occurred. These are the "biblical plagues" with which the wrathful God of the Old Testament disciplined the Egyptian slave society.

Over the millennia, many of these diseases lost virulence and developed into childhood diseases, such as measles, mumps, rubella, chicken pox, or scarlet fever. Populations on remote Pacific islands or the natives of America, however, had developed no immunity against these European germs: for them, these "childhood diseases" proved deadly.

We can ask ourselves: What were, despite the obvious problems, the benefits of a sedentary agricultural lifestyle? Why did it spread over large parts of Earth? The answer is simple: agriculture makes it possible for up to a hundred times as many people per square area to survive, and larger population figures mean more power. By contrast, the small wild hunter-gatherer tribes could not assert themselves.

Compared to the farmers, who required as many helping hands as possible, the hunters and gatherers had a relatively low birth rate, and the children were breastfed for a long time. In addition, they had a high child mortality rate, so that a certain balance of the population with the natural resources was more or less guaranteed. As is the case with many hunter-gatherer cultures, the women of the Paleolithic hunters and gatherers certainly knew a number of fertility-regulating plants, such as mugwort, wild carrot seeds, savin juniper, polypody fern, and others. The reindeer hunters of Lascaux had huge quantities of mugwort, which in the correct dosage can trigger the monthly cycle (Beckmann 1997, 79), but we don't know whether these cave painters used it in this way, or as a ritual plant. Probably the Paleolithic peoples knew such a function, as today the Shoshone and other Native Americans do, in addition to estrogen-containing herbs, such as the gromwell, or stoneseed *(Lithospermum)* that prevent ovulation (Seyr 2009, 73).

Perhaps the women were also aware of other methods of regulating their fertility. It is typical for modern researchers to always look for material causes. The Cheyenne—descendants of Paleolithic big-game hunters—told me that they became aware in a dream, or in a visionary state, of the children in the spiritual dimension who want to incarnate. If the situation of the people is difficult, if hunger or war prevails, they tell the souls/spirits that they should wait. Souls appearing in pairs in the vision were not allowed to come in, because twins were too much of a burden for this nomadic hunting tribe.

Hunters and gatherers, like the traditional Cheyenne, saw themselves as part of nature, and animals and plants as their "relatives." As their brothers and sisters, they were approachable, and one had to ask for permission if one needed anything from them. Although the farmers also lived in nature, they saw themselves more as rulers over it, or as adminis-trators. For them, humans stood above nature. And the greater their number, the greater was their power, in the spirit of the Bible (Genesis 1:28):

> And God blessed them and said to them, "Be fruitful and multiply
> and fill the earth and subdue it, and have dominion over the fish
> of the sea and over the fowl of the air and over every living thing
> that moveth upon the earth."

Arable Weeds (Segetal Flora)

With the emergence of new diseases, healing lore naturally expanded, specifically the medicinal plant knowledge that went beyond that which had already been practiced by the hunters and gatherers. And just as new diseases emerged, new plants also showed up, which included the field weeds—so-called segetal flora (Latin *seges, segetis* = crops, arable field), the seeds that the Neolithic farmers brought to central Europe from the Fertile Crescent, Asia Minor, and the Mediterranean Basin.[5] These mostly annual or biennial herbs had perfectly adapted to the agricultural practices of plowing, hoeing, and harvesting and are actually the first field and pasture weeds. They include the blue-flowering cornflower, red-flowering corn cockle, scarlet as well as blue pimpernel, chamomile, mayweed, corn poppy, the pretty yellow-orange flowering toadflax, and others that once made the ripening grain fields and blue-flowering flax fields so bright and beautiful. Over the many centuries, these accompanying herbs have won a place in the hearts of Europeans. Until recently, they played a primary role in the seasonal customs as symbol bearers. They were present in harvest garlands and braided hair and banquet tables, and they decorated the images of gods (later, they decorated saints).

Belief in the grain spirit—folklorists speak of the "spirit of the vegetation"—is ancient. Until the early twentieth century, farmers knew the Grain Wolf, the Corn Mother or Harvest Queen (Celtic Cailleach, Slavic Baba), who embodied the fertility of the land. When the ripening field of grain swayed in the wind, people believed these spirits were passing through it. At the end of July or early August, the sweet, sunny, yellow-flowering tansy ragwort *(Senecio jacobaea)* begins to blossom. For the farmers, this was a sign to prepare for the harvest. In the times before machine harvesting conquered the fields, the men cut the sheaves of mature grain with their sickles and scythes while the women went behind them and bound the stalks together. The grain spirit fled in front of the reapers, and finally hid in the last sheaf. It was then ceremoniously decorated with colorful field flowers and carried triumphantly as a deity on the harvest wagon into the village where a harvest dance and feast were held.

Because of herbicides and intensive industrial agriculture, the community of old flowers that accompanied arable fields lost its habitat and ended up on various red lists of threatened species, such as the Red Data Book of the International Union for Conservation and Natural Resources (IUCN). The industrial field landscape has become a drab green (Storl 2006, 128–129). Of course, the rural population used these archaeophytes, these plants that had accompanied the expansion of early agriculture, as medicine. Although we do not know in detail how the Neolithic farmers used them, they are still part of the traditional medicine of the European forest peoples. Let's take a look at some of them.

Chamomile *(Matricaria recutita, M. chamomilla):* The sunny, light-loving flower from the daisy family is today the true queen of medicinal plants. Chamomile tea works wonderfully as an antispasmodic, anti-inflammatory, wound-healing, antifungal medicine. Tea made with the flowers is used for gastrointestinal complaints of all kinds, menstrual cramps, as a sitz bath for inflammation or candida infection in the anal or genital area, as steam inhalation for treatment of bronchitis, and more.

Common sow thistle *(Sonchus oleraceus):* In German, cabbage is Kohl, which also means "kale" or "cabbage." A plant that has "kohl" in its name in German is edible. Sow thistle (in German, Kohl-Gaensedistel) is not under threat of extinction and can be prepared as a vitamin- and mineral-rich vegetable in early growth stages but is less suitable as a medicine. In folk medicine, however, the milky sap is ingested for diverse ailments, such as liver problems, heartburn, or shortness of breath.

Corn cockle *(Agrostemma githago):* The grain-sized seeds of this rare herb companion in the cornfields are toxic and make the bread bitter. As a medicinal plant, it is used against worms, skin diseases, ulcers, and jaundice. Hildegard of Bingen made a gout ointment from the seeds with bear grease and olive oil (Riethe 2007, 466).

Cornflower *(Centaurea cyanus):* Today, the blue flowers are dried and mixed primarily for the beautification of herbal tea mixtures. The herb was once considered a healing plant for the eyes. Hildegard of Bingen put the crushed flowers over red eyes and other "fiery" ailments in order to cool them.

Corn poppy *(Papaver rhoeas):* This arable field plant has mainly symbolic value. In many places, the red symbolizes the blood of the fallen or the martyrs. The young leaves are edible in salads. The flowers are included in sedative teas or infusions for coughs—today, it is used to decorate herbal teas; the seeds are also edible.

Field cow-wheat *(Melampyrum arvense):* Whether or how this endangered arable plant was used as a healing plant is not known.

Field larkspur *(Consolida regalis):* This pretty, blue-blossoming field flower is described today as toxic and as having no curative effect. In the farmers' healing lore, there were many applications. Among other things, the tea was used to wash wounds, treat eyes, and as a diuretic and anthelmintic.

Field parsley-piert or colic-wort *(Aphanes arvensis):* This often overlooked tiny weed belonging to the same genus as lady's mantle is edible, and young leaves can be added to a salad; as a tea, it is used to treat bladder and kidney stones or enteritis.

Fumitory or earth smoke *(Fumaria officinalis):* These pretty flowers from the poppy family are toxic. However, that did not stop the knowledgeable herb women from brewing tea from just the right amount of the dry herb, which helps with spasms in the digestive tract, constipation, and scabies. The tea promotes the flow of bile.

Genuine toadflax or butter-and-eggs *(Linaria vulgaris):* This yellow- and orange-flowering weed of the figwort family was a particularly treasured herb. It was used as a tea to wash wounds and as a poultice for fistulas and poorly healing ulcers. It was a component of hemorrhoid salves and diuretic teas. Folk medicine also used the infusion to treat jaundice and dropsy.

Hedge mustard *(Sisymbrium officinale):* This yellow-flowering crucifer is still seen quite often. The young leaves are edible and taste like watercress; the seeds are used as a mustard-like spice. The plant is also known as singer's plant because the tea is used as a gargle to help with hoarseness, vocal cord infection, or laryngitis. As an ingredient in tea for a cough, the hedge mustard is an expectorant.

Pimpernel *(Anagallis arvensis):* The small, slightly toxic cowslip with brick-red, star-shaped flowers is now hardly used in phytotherapy. But when one sees how many conditions and diseases the country people used it for, then one knows that it was once an important healing herb. It was carried as an amulet against nosebleeds, "falling sickness" (epilepsy), and such diseases brought on by magic that tweak and pinch and are called "gout." The herb is said to clear the head of a foolish person, the "gowk" (northern English and Scottish dialect for a simpleton as well as for a cuckoo bird), thus its Dutch and German name, which translates as "healer of the gowk" (Gauchheil, Guichelheil, Ackergauchheil). It was hung up over courtyard entrances because it "wards off all sorts of gouts and ghosts" as is written in the old herbals of Leonhart Fuchs.[6] The bitter-tasting powder or tea was administered to treat melancholy and madness. Allegedly, pimpernel aids in stagnation in the abdomen, eye diseases, cirrhosis, dropsy, tuberculosis, and other illnesses. The decoction was also used to hasten the afterbirth.

Shepherd's purse *(Capsella bursa-pastoris):* The small cruciferous plant has always been considered a styptic. The tea has been used, for example, for abdominal bleeding.

Apophytes

In addition to arable weeds, which come from the Mediterranean and Asian regions, indigenous species of the late Pleistocene steppes also found niches to survive in field edges, in fallow fields, or along roadsides during the Neolithic era. Botanists call these "homeless species" apophytes, and among them are some of the best and most popular healing herbs and wild vegetables still used today. Incidentally, the elder bush that seeks the vicinity of human settlements, as well as the common juniper, are included among these apophytes. The following well-known species are described below (Hempel 2009, 132).

- **Black nightshade** *(Solanum nigrum):* The blackberries are edible when fully ripe.

- **Burdock** *(Arctium lappa, A. minus):* A liver and gall bladder tonic, lymph plant, and the young root is a wild vegetable.
- **Chicory** *(Cichorium intybus):* As a remedy for detoxing the liver and as a wild vegetable.
- **Dwarf mallow** *(Malva neglecta)* and **mallow** *(M. sylvestris):* The young leaves are likewise wild vegetables, and the plant is used as an emollient, mucilaginous, wound-healing remedy.
- **Goosefoot** *(Chenopodiaceae)* and **docks** *(Rumex; Polygonaceae):* Can be found in the spring and made into a vitamin-rich vegetable soup.
- **Mullein** *(Verbascum thapsus):* Emollient, expectorant, pulmonary medicine.
- **Nettle** *(Urtica dioica):* A wild vegetable (the young shoots) and a remedy with purifying, diuretic, and blood-building effects.
- **Silverweed** *(Potentilla anserina):* An antispasmodic gynecological medicine; also an astringent, wound-healing herb.
- **Soapwort** *(Saponaria officinalis):* The root acts as an expectorant, diuretic, cholagogue, and laxative.
- **Wild carrot** *(Daucus carota):* A wild vegetable; the seeds have a diuretic effect, help make milk for nursing mothers, and are carminative; the leaves are wound healing.

Tough Wayside Dwellers

In the village squares of Neolithic settlements, on the trails and the animal paths, the ground was trampled and compacted. Only the most tenacious species could survive there, such as plantain *(Plantago major),* common knotweed *(Polygonum aviculare),* and a few species of grass. The trample of hoofed animals, the rolling of crude cartwheels, and the constant comings and goings of people were of no consequence to these herbs. On the contrary, it gave them a survival advantage over delicate plants, for the kicking, trampling, and pounding nullified any potential competing vegetation. Also, these species produced seeds that became sticky with rain and moisture and stuck to the soles of the feet, hooves, and paws. In this way, they took advantage of their location to better multiply and propagate themselves. The Latin name of plantain, *plantago,* also goes back to *planta,* meaning "sole." Wherever European emigrants settled in temperate zones, in North America or New Zealand, the natives referred to the plant as "footsteps of the white man."

Pollen analysis shows that plants of trampling-resistant vegetation proliferated in the Neolithic era. In the Old Stone Age, they were rare. The tiny black seeds of plantain are tasty, and they are a vitamin- and protein-rich food. In the fall, when they are ripe, one can take the stems lightly between forefinger and thumb and strip the seeds off in large quantities. These small grains (Old High German for cereal grains, *gitregidi* = gathered together) were cooked with porridge or baked into bread throughout the Neolithic era. Plantain leaves, as well as the green shoots of the knotgrass, are suitable as a vegetable. "Vegetables" means something to cook with mush (in German, vegetables = *Gemuese,* the word for mush, or *Mus,* is still present).

Above all, these tread-resistant plants were valuable medicinal plants. In the pictorial world the ancient humans occupied, the herbs that could endure trampling and kicking certainly had special power. Both the broad-leafed plantain as well as knotgrass—"not harmed by footsteps" (*Unvertritt* as it is called in northern Germany)—are considered strong styptics. The Roman Pliny called knotgrass, as well as plantain, *herba sanguinaria*—referring to its use as a "blood stauncher." In folk medicine, knotgrass is now used to treat lung diseases and gout and, as a source of tannins, hemorrhoids as well as dysentery and diarrhea (Marzell 2002, 86).

Plantain, Burial Mounds, and Pathways of the Dead

Today, in the age of global trade dependencies, food is moved from one continent to another. By contrast, in the world of the Neolithic farmers, each village was self-sufficient and self-sustaining. What was traded—salt, amber, blades of flint, obsidian, or conch shells—could be easily carried along footpaths on the back or in boats along the rivers. Roads and fixed routes were unnecessary. Nonetheless, road-ways already existed during the period of megalithic structures and mounds. However, these cult roads led from the village of the living to the chambers in the grave barrows, or burial mounds where the departed ancestors lived. The megalithic tombs, popularly known as "barrows," were, at the same time, the access to the otherworld, where the Earth Goddess, the Neolithic Mother Goddess, lived.

In Ireland, these barrows are called *síd* (plural *sidhe,* from the old Irish *sid* = resident). According to the Irish legend, the Tuatha de Danann, the "people of the Goddess Ana," who once lived on Earth, have retreated to the otherworld. Dana, the Dea (goddess) Ana, is the ancestor, the primordial goddess, who later appears as Diana of the Romans, Goddess of the Wilderness, and as Anna Perenna, the nurturer; it is the Earth Goddess, Mother Holle, who guards the souls of the dead as well as the seeds of the plants in winter in their under-ground kingdom. In the vision of the ancient Scots, the Banshee, "the woman in the barrow," appears (Gaelic Síodach) as a washerwoman who washes the bloody clothes of those fated for death.

A straight road connected the grave mound with the Neolithic vil-lage. The deceased were placed on a cart with wooden wheels (tree trunk slices) or on a sled and carried in solemn processions into the realm of the dead. The carts were pulled by cows and sometimes even by a tame stag. For a long time, the British Celts believed that on special days, in the "interim periods," in the twilight before dawn, this hill opens and the otherworldly beings, the elves, fairies, and ghosts, move about. This occurs especially at the end of the year during the celebrations of the dead in November (Samhain), the May holidays (Beltaine), when the sun marries the flower-bedecked Vegetation God-dess, and in midsummer during the summer solstice.

Not only the elves and the deceased came out on special days, but also the goddess ascended to visit the village. The Roman ethnolo-gist Tacitus described how the Earth Goddess Nerthus (Hertha, Erda)

116

leaves her forest sanctuary in a chariot drawn by cows in order to pay a visit to the people. Harvest wagons full of the grain, the sheaves being the goddess's children who had fallen victim to the sickle of the harvesters, probably also traversed these sacred paths.[7]

Of course, these gods and ancestral pathways had to be kept meticulously clean. They were probably dutifully swept with birch-branch brooms—birch branches were even used in the Upper Paleolithic period to sweep away evil spirits. No herb was to grow on this sacred road. Nevertheless, the tough plantain and knotgrass spread out widely over the roads. Consequently, both are dedicated to the goddess who lived in the burial mound. Later, the Romans named both herbs *Herba Proserpinaca,* "Herb of Proserpina." Proserpina, the daughter of Demeter, is—like the Greek Persephone—the virginal flower girl who was raped by Hades (Pluto), the black god of the underworld, and forced to become the Lady of the Dead.

Thus, someone who is badly wounded and may bleed to death, or suffers from internal bleeding or hemorrhages—according to the view of the times—is on his way to the Goddess of the Dead, to Persephone or the Banshee. But along this path plantain grows, and its main therapeutic attribute is hemostatic.

Broad-leafed plantain *(Plantago major)* is the king of the road that leads into the subterranean realm of the Goddess of the Dead, Hel (she also appears as Mother Holle). Plantain has the power to avert the transition to the otherworld, the sinking into the Orcus. That's why it was highly revered, so much so that the ancient Germanic peoples called it *Laekeblad* (healing leaf) or *Læknisgras* (healing grass).[8] The Middle High German word lâchen means "to heal," and the *lâchen-aere* (old Germanic *lekjas, Anglo-Saxon *laece,* English *leech*) is the conjurer, magician, or healer.

So important was the plantain, or waybread, that the Anglo-Saxons (eleventh century) invoked it as the second of nine plants (mugwort was the first) of the Nine Herbs Charm, and it was addressed as follows (Pollington 2000, 215):

And you, waybread, mother of plants,
Open to the east, mighty within;
Carts ran over you, ladies rode over you,
Brides cried out over you, bulls snorted over you.
You withstood them all and you were crushed.
So may you withstand poison and infection,
And the evil who travels 'round the land.

The Anglo-Saxons made an ointment against "flying poison" (possible infectious diseases) from plantain, chamomile, sorrel, and other ingredients. Preserved in Latin from the eleventh century is a blood blessing spoken by a priest over a hemorrhaging woman *(Wiener akad. Sitzungsberichte,* no date, vol. 91, 528; cited in De Vries, 1989, 247). He placed plantain in her hand, saying "Herb of Proserpina! Daughter of Underworld King Hades! As you did to make the mule infertile, so close the wave of blood from the body of this woman!" Dioscorides, the Greek army field doctor during Emperor Nero's time who wrote the first herbal compendium in the Western world, devoted a whole chapter to plantain. He praised the astringent, drying qualities and recommended the plant for bleeding and ulcers of all kinds, and as a remedy for glandular swelling, fire wounds, dysentery, stomach disease, epilepsy, asthma, uterine disease, dog bites, malaria, and more. It was used throughout the Middle Ages. Hildegard of Bingen also recommended it to counter charmed love and protect against magic words (Mueller 2008, 198).

Plantain roots, seeds, and leaves also have broad medical and magical application in folk medicine in Russia, Mongolia, China, and the Himalayan regions. To describe them all would fill a thick book.

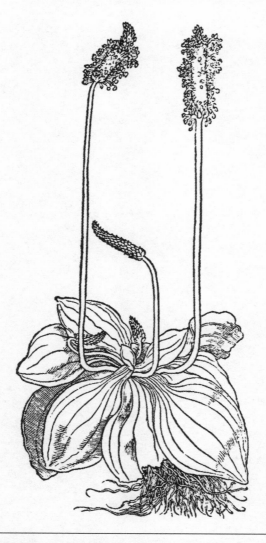

Plantain (Otto Brunfels, *Herbarium Vivae et Eicones,* Strasbourg, 1530, 116)

CHAPTER 5

Indo-European Roots

Take possession of this magic, which aims at immortality,
may your life last into old age, not be stopped by force!
I bring you new breath and new life:
Go not into the mist and into the darkness, go not sickly
there!
From the wind I have received your breath, from the sun
your eye;
I hold your soul close in you:
Be in your limbs, speak, by articulating with your tongue.
With the breath of two and four-footed
creatures I blow against you,
as Agni (the fire) does when it is born.

      –ATHARVA VEDA VIII, 2. PRAYER FOR EXEMPTION FROM THE
        DANGERS OF DEATH

As if from heaven
the herbs came down and said:
that when we meet the living
the man should remain unscathed.

      –THE SONG OF THE PHYSICIAN FROM THE RIGVEDA

The New Stone Age period was beginning to take shape. Megalithic
farming culture spread throughout northern Europe; their society was
probably organized along matriarchal lines such that the maternal line of

inheritance owned the land and the eldest woman of the clan possessed the most authority. Mother Earth, ever nourishing and eternally bearing, was probably the primary goddess. However, not all who lived in the large forested areas were farmers—hunters, gatherers, and fishermen still lived there too. Gradually, the farming villages and towns grew and people began burying their dead in megalithic tombs. The astronomically aligned megalith centers served as places of worship for the scattered settlements. Among other things yet, they served as calendars to correctly determine the agricultural year and the times for sowing and harvesting.

The Appearance of the Nomads of the Steppes

Around 2000 BCE, bronze gradually came into use in central Europe, ushering in the Bronze Age and the end of the New Stone Age. The warm period, the so-called Holocene Climactic Maximum (the Atlantic period) that had favored the first farmers, was long over. Toward the end of the Bronze Age, the climate became cooler and less stable. Crop yields were low, there were more military conflicts, more palisade castles were built, and sacrificial cults increased.

The climactic deterioration affected the grass and forest steppes of western Asia (southern Russia and Ukraine) so that the endless wide pastures, on which large livestock depended, became ever drier with ever less yield. The nomadic pastoral tribes were thus prompted to leave the steppes to look for newer, greener pastures, so to speak. With their four-wheeled covered wagons (pulled by oxen or horses), steeds, cattle, and sheep, they moved off in all directions, far beyond the borders of the steppes, as far as Iran and northern India, to Mesopotamia and east to China's borders. In the periodic climate fluctuations, these so-called Kurgan people also migrated in several waves into green, forested Europe.[1] The Bronze Age farmers who lived there could put up little effective resistance to the shepherd tribes who were mounted on horseback and had better weapons. Sometime during this history, the Indo-European–speaking inhabitants of the steppes had tamed wild horses and put on bridles and tack to ride them, or harnessed them to two-wheeled chariots.

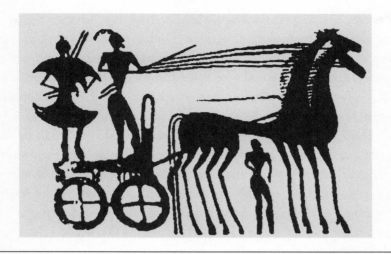

Indo-European war chariot (Mycenaean, second millennium BCE)

Other peoples knew horses only as wild game. The horse gave the steppe peoples immense superiority. And several centuries later, they were the also the first ones to possess iron weapons.

The diet of these livestock farmers, which consisted of plenty of animal protein, suited their warlike lifestyle. The meat diet made these men strong, energetic, and combative, similar to the cowboys who captured the Wild West on horseback with the motto, "Shoot first, ask questions later." In India, it is still the case that eating meat and drinking alcohol is the privilege of the Kshatriya, whose members are descendants of the warrior caste of Indo-European steppe horsemen.

Pastoral tribes who need to move their flocks to new pastures are warlike and tough by nature. They must drive the herds in wind and weather and protect them from theft and predators. They are forced to mercilessly disperse other nomads who want to dispute the use of the grasslands. All this is traditionally men's business. The survival in the steppes requires tough warriors who are blood related—fathers, sons, brothers, uncles, nephews, cousins—and who can rely on each other unconditionally. Equally important for these herding tribes is the charismatic tribal leader, the *Reg*, who must be able to make intelligent, quick decisions. The *Reg* (Latin *Rex,* Gallic *Rix,* Irish *Rig,* Sanskrit *Raj*) is the governing one, the king, and one who is rich in cattle, who *reg*ulates and corrects, who is in harmony with the cosmic law (Sanskrit *ritam*) and the *reg*ion (Latin *regnum*), and who defends his tribe. However, the power of this *reg*ent was not absolute; it was moderated by the Indo-European council of tribal elders (the Senate, from *senex* = old).

The society of the steppe nomads was shaped by patriarchy. The wealth and the herds were owned by the male lineage. The man was the lord, and the women were subservient; their work consisted of milking the cattle and sheep, making cheese and churning, cooking and sewing, and caring for the children and the sick. With other nomadic peoples who kept livestock, such as the ancient Hebrews, Arabs, Berbers, Mongols, and Turkic peoples, the pattern was similar.

Two worlds clashed as these riders from the steppes arrived in the western corner of the Eurasian landmass. Although the Kurgan livestock herders also grew them, crops played a very minor role. The self-confident, proud Kurgan warriors had nothing but contempt for the matriarchal farmers who "rooted around in the ground like pigs." In the tripartite Indo-European society, the farmers found themselves on the lowest rung, even below merchants and craftsmen, while the warrior nobility, the cattle owners, as well as the priests who controlled the relationship to the gods, occupied the highest level. Men on horseback made an impression and demanded respect; the knight, the Spanish caballero, the French chevalier, or the Italian cavaliere are still considered superior people—all these names refer to the horse (Latin *caballus*).

The most important divine powers were no longer the Earth Mother and her dying and resurrecting son and lover, but heavenly powers and forces of nature, such as God the Father, the *Dyeu Peter, or later, Jupiter, (Greek Zeus Pater; Sanskrit *diaus pita;* Latin Deus; Baltic Dievs), and fire *(agni, ignis),* which played a central role in the sacrificial rituals, as did the Thunder God with his lightning bolt and likewise the divine horses.

Over the course of time, the Kurgan people intermixed with the original inhabitants. The immigrants from the grasslands of the east, where the sky reached from horizon to horizon, had to adapt to the woodland

and its *genii loci,* that is, the spirits and deities that occupied the area—or, as we would probably say today, they had to adjust to the given morphogenetic field. Whether tolerated or taboo (such as was also the case in India), there were nevertheless marriages between the immigrants and local men and women. In this way, customs and cultures blended, as did forms of societies, worlds of the gods, and particular healing traditions.

Finally, the synthesis came about that characterizes European culture in modern times. The Celts represent the most successful amalgam of these two traditions. The goddess cult continued to survive in the worship of Demeter, Hestia, Freya, Šiva, Saule, and countless other indigenous goddesses, who then were also often married to Indo-European gods.[2, 3] Even Mary, who was pregnant by Deus, the sky father, in order to give birth to the Savior, is one of these archetypes. But the Stag God, the Bear God, and other forest gods also remained. The ancient Europeans took the Indo-European language of the proud intruders like the African and American colonial peoples assumed the language of their conquerors. However, many words, rhythms of speech, and expressions were maintained in the newly created languages. Nearly thirty percent of the vocabulary of Germanic languages is not Indo-European, but comes from the older base layer of the indigenous people.

It is not possible to speak of an exclusively pure Indo-European healing lore. The nomadic, Indo-European tribes of the steppes emerged from the shamanic late Stone Age hunter-gatherer culture of the post-glacial period. At the same time, the medicinal techniques of the Indo-European herdsmen have mixed so much with the indigenous peoples, whom they overran, that they are difficult to tell apart. The Arya (the "noble" and "free"), the Indo-Europeans on the Indus and the Ganges rivers, tried to keep their language (Sanskrit), rituals, and medicine (Ayurveda) pure from alien contamination. Nevertheless, over the centuries, many elements of the indigenous Dravidian population of the Indian subcontinent have trickled into Vedic Aryan culture. In Europe, the two cultural currents—the ancient Europeans and the nomads of the steppes—mixed so that they are hard to disentangle. The therapeutic procedures of both cultural traditions are the roots of modern European indigenous folk medicine.

Here we will try to emphasize the similarities between the various Indo-European peoples, especially the Vedic Indians, in order to understand how they influenced the medicine of the forest peoples.

Illness Is a Bad Spell

Today's physicians see diseases as defensive reactions of the organism to bacteria, viruses, toxins, and other external injurious influences or as a disorder—a rather mechanistic view—of normal somatic or mental functions. The Indo-European healers—regardless if they were Celtic, Germanic, or Baltic people or Vedic Indians—saw it differently. For them, disease was mainly the effect of an evil spell, a hex or enchantment. It is based on a false, disconnected consciousness.

The Proto-Germanic word *spellam* is the key to understanding this. It means "to create images with words" and is related to the terms *split* as well as *spiel* (Old English *spelian*), which means "to play," or "to tell, to say aloud, recite, to produce ideas with words, to tell a story." The playing is not a reality of its own, but an "as if." A master musician is capable of playing the lute, using songs to captivate the entire court, and making the audience laugh or cry. The obviously related word *spell* itself illustrates the concept best: death magic is a death spell; someone who is bound by a spell is spellbound; weather-magic becomes a spell of weather. Witches and warlocks "weave" a spell with a magical song and words, or they brew one up by stirring herbs while muttering magic words into their witch's cauldron. A good, positive bit of magic is a "good-spell"—hence the word *gospel;* in other words, Christian missionaries referred to their message as "good magic" or the "gospel." The verb "to spell" goes back to the Germanic practice of making runic magic by casting staves cut from beeches carved with runes and colored with sacrificial blood or ocher.

Thus, if sickness and infirmity are due to enchantment or bewitchment, then the healing spells must be stronger than the disease-bringing magic. The healer must have spiritual power, the power of truth, because this is always stronger than that of lies and deceit. A healer must be able to see through the illusion and master the rituals and chants, which could transform the illness into health.[4] Healers are given this magical power through their connection with the gods and the cosmos. This spiritual strength is necessary, for the healing ritual is a magical battle with hostile beings.

For example, when bewitchment or enchantment was present, the Latvians turned to an *atbureis* (magician or shaman) who could undo bad magic *(atburt)* or conjure it back; or they sought an *atkodejs,* who was capable of avenging harmful magic *(adkost* = make harmless by a counter-bite), or the intercessor *(aisluhdseijs)* and similar people in possession of spiritual strength (Kurtz 1937, 22).

Agents and Causes of Disease

Diseases can only afflict humans when suitable means exist. These means are provided by immoral behavior, for instance, selfishness, greed, injustice, disrespect, dishonesty, and other weaknesses. Then, the disease demons appear like flies, attracted by filth. They come as the *erinyes* or furies of Greek and Roman mythology. In the hair of these goddesses of vengeance hang venomous snakes; their eyes drip with blood, and their breath is as hot as fire. These imaginations purport the idea of karma: just as one calls into the forest, so it echoes back.

The ailments of pets, dogs, cows, or horses were believed to be caused by a curse or jinx for reasons of envy or revenge, or that they suffered from the loveless indifference or carelessness of their owners, within the meaning of the proverb "the pastor's children and the miller's animals rarely thrive, if ever" (meaning they are both too busy in the church and in the mill to take good care of their own families and animals—similar to the adage, "the cobbler's children have no shoes").

The healer must have a clear mind in order to recognize which spirits, gods, or demons or which negative magic is causing the disease. This requires an accurate empirical observation of symptoms and external circumstances combined with inner vision. The "mirror of the soul" that perceives the interior side of the phenomena must be smooth and clean. The soul is like the sea: When it is quiet, then even the most distant star is

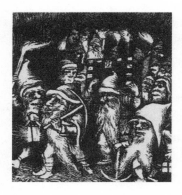

Gnomes underground
(G. MacDonald,
nineteenth century)

reflected in it. When the soul, however, is agitated by, for example, passion and greed, it neither reflects nor perceives anything.

One should emphasize that, for these people, the presence of the disease agents was not a matter of faith—or in modern terms, it was not a "cultural construction"—but they "saw" the contaminator in prophetic, visionary states, in lucid dreams, as well as in trance. In some ethnic groups, entheogen plant substances were used to perceive the otherworld. Since they are not part of the objective world "out there," they belong to the "intermediate world"—to the twilight zone, as we say. These mental images, these imaginings, are shaped by cultural tradition as well as the surrounding nature. This is why the angels in the Christian tradition have white wings, similar to a dove, to represent their flying abilities. Other cultures represent these divine messengers in different ways, such as floating or with dragonfly wings. Thus, the dwarves and gnomes in central Europe wear pointed caps that once belonged to the costume of the Celtic miners who chiseled and mined underground ores and rock salt in the Hallstatt period.

These images are not at all subjective psychological projections in which an empty, soulless nature is clothed, but culturally influenced perceptions of metaphysical (Greek *metá physikós* = beyond the physical) realities. Similar or related cultures share similar images and mythologies, just as they speak similar languages. Thus, the Indo-European peoples share pictures of those metaphysical entities, which have to do with illness and disease. Here are the transcendental causes of disease as understood in the Indo-European cultural tradition.

Demons (Sanskrit Yakshmas, Rakshas)

For the Vedic Indians, there were many categories of disease-bringing demons, spirits of the dead, ghosts, and vampires that bring fever, pain, and decay. In particular, the yakshmas sneak into the body and cause tuberculosis and severe internal diseases. They are attracted by sin and the breaking of taboos (Zysk 1996, 15–16).

These Vedic demons, elves, and spirits of the dead are also no strangers to the cousins of the Indo-Europeans in the West. A nightmare can make people sick with slashes, stabs, blows, or shots. A nightmare (from Old English mare = a mythological demon who torments people with frightening dreams; Polish mora; Wendish murawa; Russian *kikimora;* Irish *Morigain*) can ride a person at night like riding a horse, as an oppressive night ghost, so that one wakes up exhausted and drenched in sweat, or send a person terrible dreams (French *cauchemar*) or weigh on one's chest until one can hardly breathe. Gnomes and elves can hunt down and strike humans with sickening and even deadly magic arrows ("elf shots"; Anglo-Saxon *ylfa gescot,* Norwegian *alfskud*); they can make a person faint from their breath (Norwegian *alf-gust, elfblæst*) or cause a heart attack with one malicious blow, such as in the Danish legend of the fairy king *(Ellerkonge).*[5]

Worms (Sanskrit: Krími)

The disease-bringing demons often take the shape of worms, leeches, crabs, weevils, beetles, little dragons, or snakes.[6] In the Vedas, we read that some krímís can be seen, others are invisible; they can be black, brown, red, or white in color. There are dark brown ones with ears, black ones with white limbs, spotted, whitish ones with three heads and horns, and ones similar to vultures or wolves; there are also male and female worms (Zysk 1996, 64ff.). The European forest peoples knew these "small worms, skinless and without body and substance," as defined by the famous medieval doctor, Paracelsus. A large number of these nightmarish worms were known to them: the nagging, biting worms; the piercing, boring, tapping, sucking worms; the hair worm; the tooth worm that lives in rotting teeth; the brain worm; the heart worm that has deer-like antlers on its head; the mawworm (stomach worm); the tape worm; the nettle worm (chronic gout); the voracious appetite worm; the hand worm (scabies); the skin worm (scurf); the bone worm; the marrow worm; the rump

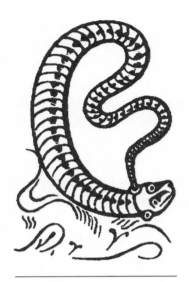

Old Germanic
representation of a worm

worm that rots cows' tails; and many, many others. The Norwegian peasantry knows the *hvidorm* (white worm), whose evil eye can make a person crazy, and the *blaswurm* (blow worm) that can blow its poison even through seven church walls. Most of these evil spirits in the Vedic imagination are black, brown, red, or white in color (Storl 2005, 115–125).

According to Celtic and Germanic mythology, the first human couple was created out of trees. Elvish worms can therefore infest both humans and trees. They often nestle under the bark of forest trees, flying out from there and then nestling as diseases in humans. That is why the shamanic healer could reverse the process and put the diseases back into the trees again (Mannhardt 1875, 12).

Magical Intrusions, Magic Arrows, Elf Shots

These are visible or invisible foreign bodies sent by spirits or sorcerers—such as bone splinters, sharp stones, thorns, straws, nails, and so on.

Poisoned Drink and Food

These include, for instance, the poisoned apple that the envious, wicked queen gave to Snow White.

Curses and False Words

For the ancient people, words were not empty sounds arbitrarily created by people.[7] Words were considered beings that have the power to make things happen. That is why spells, healing chants, mantras, and curses were considered effective. Among the ancient Indians, the curse of an ascetic, holy hermit, or wandering monk, one in which spiritual power was concentrated, aroused great fear. During conversation, words are expected to be true; they should correspond with reality. Pointless babble is harmful because it creates an ethereal dress for the disease-bringing spirits of falsehood. It is said that a person is as good as his or her word—until recently, that was also the belief in our culture.

Wrath of the Gods and Ancestors

Not only demons can be dangerous, but also the ancestors, if they are not honored. If they are not remembered and food and drink is not sacrificed to them, then the deceased find it difficult to send their offspring blessings and protection. Especially the fallen warriors, who sacrificed their young lives for the community and therefore were not able to produce sons and have those sons carry out the funeral rites for them, deserve to be remembered. For this reason, in India, the daily *puja* (ritual) for the ancestors and other dead is performed by pouring water toward the west—the direction of the setting sun. Even in European culture, there were periodic occasions for feeding the dead: the Samhain festival in October/November, the "hallowed night" (Halloween = hallowed evening) celebrated the dead among the Celts; the dead were invited in late autumn to a feast, often in the bathhouse, among the Baltic people; and they were fed with millet and hemp seeds at the winter solstice among the Germans and Slavs. As we have already seen, during the still time of the winter solstice, shamans sometimes also used sacred mushrooms to deepen their connection with the ancestors.

The gods are powerful, full of magic and—just like the change of the seasons, like day and night, like the tides—they are relentless. They are not to be trifled with. Although they guide and protect people, they can also punish or harm them. The hyperborean Sun God Apollo, who otherwise appears as a healer, can shoot arrows of disease and death with his bow. Even the Vedic Storm God Rudra, otherwise a master of medicinal herbs and donor of curative urine, can shoot his arrows and slay people, including virtuous Aryan priests, like fleeting deer. It can be dangerous for strong-willed ascetics who acquire too much spiritual power through their abstinent life, penance, and self-sacrifice, which disturbs Indra, the

131

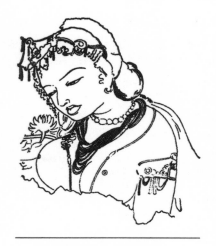

Apsarasa, seductive
heavenly dancer

Vedic Thunder God, because they could challenge him and take his throne. To prevent such a coup, the jealous god may punish them with disease or madness. Or he sends the penitents a charming divine nymph (apsarasa) to entangle them in sensual passion and thus cheat them of being rewarded for their asceticism. The Germanic central and northern Europeans knew about the elf shot *(ylfa gescot)* and the witch's shot *(haegtessan gescot),* as well as the plague-bringing "gods' shots" *(asa gescot).*

Natural Causes

Not all suffering had supernatural causes. Space was granted for other causes, such as accidents, wounds, snake bites, scorpion stings, and the like. The shaman, *bhishàj,* the Anglo-Saxon "leech" (Old English *laece*), the Latvian *burwis,* or by whatever name the clairvoyant healer was called, would be able find the cause.

Healing Gods

It is not easy to bring the various healers and medical practices of the different Indo-European peoples under a common denominator. Still, there are enough similarities. For the appointed healer, knowing the magic chants and rituals was not enough as we have seen that healers also must have the spiritual power to banish the disease and rectify again what is not right. Second, in addition to locating the disease demon that had taken root in the body and shied away from the light of day, the healer must also know its name and how to call it out. Because the name is, as already described, always a part of the essence. Just like in the fairy tale Rumpelstiltskin—"Little does my lady dream. Rumpelstiltskin is my name!"—the evil worm tries to keep his name secret! The name gives the healer a handle so that the monster loses its magical power. Thus, we read in a Swiss house blessing (tenth century):

> Well wight, you should know that I know that you are called wight, so that you do not understand, nor know how to say: Chnospinci.

In the Atharva Veda, a collection of magical rituals (1500–1000 BCE), the healer uses the smoke of the aromatic kúshta plant.[8] The demon Takman, who in particular plagues people with fever and jaundice in the sweltering heat of the monsoon season, is first courted and flattered because he is a powerful being. Then, he is addressed by his secret name Hrúdu: "Be thou flame or hot glow . . . you, O God of the Yellow, are named Hrúdu! O Takman you all knower, pass harmlessly over us and move on without doing any harm" (Atharva Veda, 1.25). He should rather jump into the cold-blooded amphibians or fly away with the yellow-feathered birds. Hrúdu probably had the shape of a worm; the name is definitely reminiscent of the Latin word *hirudo* (leeches)—maybe there exists an etymological connection.

Finally, the healer also had to know how to call the good spirits and healing gods to help. Here are the most important of the Vedic Aryan gods of healing whose equivalents can be found among other Indo-European peoples.

Agni

Agni is the Vedic Aryan god of fire. His name is related to the Latin word for fire, ignis. The Slavs knew him as Ogoni or Agoni. He is pure and purifies everything he consumes. He is present in the hearth fire where herbal infusions and decoctions can be prepared; he is active in the hot therapeutic bath and in the dugouts heated with burning dried cow dung patties where patients sit to sweat out their illnesses. People offer him butter and cereals into the blazing flames. He himself is the sacrificial fire into whose ravenous jaws the offerings are given and sent to the sky gods.

And he is the funeral pyre on which man, when he dies, also sacrifices his own body.

Vayu

Vayu is the Vedic god of the wind who races through the air in a chariot pulled by stags. In all breathing and living beings, he is the breath of life. The healer uses the power of Vayu to blow away the disease of the patient during the healing ritual. When the healing priest kindles the fire and blows on it, he uses the wind that flows from his lungs "so that Agni can be born."

Surya

Surya, or golden-handed Savitri, is the Sun God worshiped by the Indo-Europeans and is drawn in a golden chariot by seven horses, which moves across the sky and overcomes the darkness.

Ashvins

The two Vedic gods called Ashvins (Sanskrit for horseman, *ashva* = horse) are handsome young men, twins, whose father was the sun and whose mother was a mare. They are the dispensers of medicinal plant remedies and the restorers of youth. The divine young physician pair appears every morning in a golden chariot drawn by horses and birds just before the sun rises. It is in this sacred twilight, when the birds begin their morning concert and herbalists gather their healing plants and roots, that these two doctors of the gods send down their blessings. They were worshiped throughout the entire Indo-European region and appeared to the Greeks as the two Dioscuri (Greek *dio* = god, *cyrus* = sons, youths), masters of equestrians and charioteers, who were regarded as helpers of people and who were set into the night sky and shone down to Earth as Castor and Pollux in the sign of Gemini. In Baltic mythology, they appear as the Ašvieniai (Lithuanian *ašva* = horse); they are the charioteers of the Sun Goddess Saule, and are represented as two crossed horse heads (similar to the Anglo-Saxon Hengist and Horsa), which can be found on the gables of Baltic farmhouses and also often seen on farmsteads in northern Germany, Denmark, and Holland. They can still be seen in Germany as the logo of the Raiffeisen banks (rural credit cooperatives).[9]

In their Christian metamorphosis, these healing gods live on as Saint Cosmas and Damian, who are revered as patron saints of physicians, nurses, and pharmacists. These two saints are also invoked for treating equine diseases. In hagiography, it is said they healed the sick free of charge in order to convert them to Christianity.

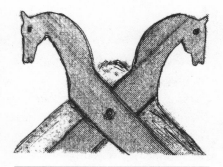

Crossed horse heads on a gable

Arundhati

Arundhati is associated with the Morning Star and mentioned in the Vedas as the kindly, mild "queen of healing herbs." She reveals herself in various medicinal plants and also in *laksha* or *lac,* that red juice or remedy of red resin used by healers to treat and seal wounds and fractures in people and animals (Zysk 1996, 74–75). Arundhati is probably a goddess of the Dravidians, the pre-Aryan inhabitants of northern India. The local, mostly subtropi-

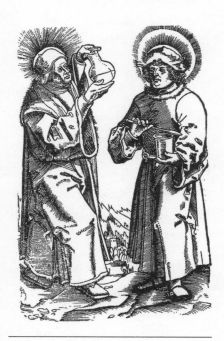

Cosmas and Damian (woodcut, H. v. Gersdorff, Feldtbuch der Wundarztney, Strasbourg, 1526)

cal plants were not yet known to these Indo-European conquerors, and they had to learn about them from the local population before they could incorporate them into their healing rituals.

Soma

Soma, the Moon God, is treasured in the Vedas as the lord of the water of life, the plant juices, and the psychedelic substance of the same name, the beverage that makes the gods immortal and inspires singers and princes. Soma is also Oshadhi-Pati, the guardian or lord of the healing herbs. The Moon God, who has twenty-seven wives (days of lunation), is always ready to mate and give fertility; the hare—you can see his picture in the full moon—is his animal.

Dhatr

The "bonesetter," the "builder" or "binder," was invoked for bone fractures. He is the Vedic lord of the animals who also heals horses' hooves.

Healing Arts

Because descriptions of the many healers and healing methods of the various Indo-European peoples or the traditions of the indigenous peoples among whom they settled could fill a book on their own, we will limit our inquiry to the medicine of ancient India, the *bhishàjs,* and the Anglo-Saxon leech doctors. In this way, we can span the wide arc of the Indo-European peoples, which ranges from Iceland in the far west to Bengal in the east.

The Healing Rituals of the Bhishàjs

The *bhishàj* was often a *vipra,* a shaker (from Sanskrit *vip* = shake, rotate; related to "vibrate"); that is, he was also a dancing, singing shaman, who—similar to the American Shakers—attained an altered state of consciousness through sustained strong shaking of the entire body. Often these healers were wandering ascetics—similar to today's sadhus (wandering monks)—who knew the medicinal herbs and effective, powerful incantations. They healed, as the leech doctor did, with words (charms, incantations) and herbs (medicinal plants) as well as with water and fire. Thereby, they called the demons by name and lured them out—because spirits cannot be killed—and transferred them to animals (birds, frogs) or enemies. Here are some essential elements of the *bhishàj* healing séance:

- Before the séance, the sick person was incensed with aromatic plants, in other words, cleansed. The medicinal plants themselves were invoked, sung to, and blessed. Since plants are powerful beings and manifestations of the Great Goddess, her presence alone already helps.

- The healer waved a bundle of herbs over the sick or brushed them over the body—similar to the methods of the Mexican limpia. He brushed the herbs over the body from top to bottom so that the disease would disappear into the ground.

- While doing this, magical chants (mantras) were sung over the patient.

- The healer sprinkled water (or cow urine, which is considered sacred) on the wounds and diseased areas.

- The patient was touched on the head, ears, eyes, chin, nostrils, or aching areas with ritually prepared clarified butter (ghee) to which herbs had been added. Butter, the noblest thing the sacred cow of man bestows, played an important role in healing for all Indo-Europeans. The patient was also swabbed with red powder, with *laksha*, or ochre. Traditional peoples considered ochre to be "the blood of the earth," as blood is the essential fluid of life; with ochre, or *laksha*, life force is transferred to the patient. The association is ancient; Neanderthals smeared their bodies, including those of the dead, with red ferruginous earth.

- With bundles of *darbha* grass, or *kusha* grass (big cordgrass, *Desmostachya bipinnata*), healing water was sprinkled onto the ailing person. Grass is of course a particularly powerful plant for herding peoples because it is the fodder for very important horses and cattle. Seats of the gods were decorated with sacred *kusha* grass in Vedic sacrificial rituals; and as Gautama Siddhartha sat under the sacred fig tree *(Ficus religiosa)* to attain enlightenment, he is supposed to have sat on a mat of *darbha* grass. The Indian legend tells that snakes have forked tongues because they have been licking the sharp edges of the blades of such grass.

- The spirit of the disease was forced to leave the sufferer. It was driven out through the orifices by vomiting, sneezing, or flatulence (Zysk 1996, 97).

- The healer gave the sick person milk with butter and put a salve made from a decoction of ghee and *laksha* on the wound. During recovery, healing herbs might be administered in the form of powder, infusion, decoction, or ointment. They were often worn as an amulet, as a poultice, or just placed on the body. During the application of these remedies, the *bhishàj* spoke mantras to boost the herb's potency. At the beginning of the healing ritual, the surrounding area was cleaned and the floor swept with sacred grass brooms or twig brooms. The best time for the ritual is the dawn, when the stars are waning, or at dusk. The position of the planets and constellations in the sky are also taken into consideration (Zysk 1996, 9).

The healing was achieved with what we now refer to as a "magical ritual" due to our lack of understanding, but objective methods were also just as important. For instance, a catheter made from a fine reed was used for urine blockage, boils were lanced, wounds were cauterized with astringent resins, and blood was stopped—the healing plants applied had an empirical effect even when judged by the criteria of today's analytical chemistry.

The Healing Rituals of the Leech Doctors

The healers of the forest peoples used similar means and methods to address the issues. They also sang, burned incense, lured out the disease-worm, disposed of it, and used medicinal plants, their allies, for healing.

Among the Germanic peoples, the healer, the leech doctor, was called *lachsner* or *lachsnerin,* in Middle English, *leche,* and in Old English, *læche.*[10, 11] As already mentioned in the discussion of the hemostatic plantain, the name *laekeblad,* or leech's leaf, has to do with the color red, the lifeblood. The original Indo-European word **lak* means on one hand "to sprinkle, spot, mark" and on the other, "red." The salmon (*Lachs* in German; Yiddish *lox;* Scandinavian *lax*), the fish with red flesh, the magic fish, symbolizes wisdom for the Celts; the Indian goddess Lakshmi is the red goddess and is the female counterpart of the supreme god Vishnu. And the Grail Knight Lancelot du Lac does not refer to Lancelot of the Lake, but Lancelot of the Pool of Blood—the one who bathed in the red blood of the dragon, which he had slain (Gardner 2000, 51).

Rudolf Schmitz, founder of the Institute for the History of the Pharmacy in Marburg, Germany, writes: "Originally, lach meant a red color, as well as common ochre *(taufra),* that was used for magic. The blood-red color was used by the medicine man as he sang chants and marked the places where the disease demons had invaded" (Schmitz 1998, 85). Here are a few elements of the healing ritual, as mentioned in the Anglo-Saxon *Lacnunga.*[12]

- The healer calls to the cardinal directions.
- He finds the painful area where the "worm" is sitting or has penetrated, touches it with the leech finger, marks it with ochre or sacrificial blood, and breathes or blows on it.
- He then sings over the sick person, as well as the "worm," with magical songs or *galdor,* which in Old English means "spell, enchantment, or an incantation".
- He sings close to the body and the body orifices of the patient. He sings near the face, near the mouth, into the right and left ear, and over the wound.
- The worm or serpent is lured out with magical song or power words.
- He blows the disease back in the direction from which it came.
- The disease spirit, the worm, can also be grafted onto trees, bound to the elder tree, or shot to the otherworld on an arrowhead.

- The evil spell can also be washed away with boiled "invoking or magical" herbs.
- Subsequently, an herbal ointment, usually macerated in butter, is applied. Amulets are made, and a cure with medicinal plants is prescribed for the continuing, final healing and recovery.

Destroying "Worms"

The disease spirits reveal themselves in many forms in the visionary experience. They often appear as careworn, unhappy, cranky, suffering beings—as dry, pale, bent figures, crippled or hunchbacked, ugly old people. One can tell they lack something—the fullness of life and love; they are not whole and hunger and thirst for what they lack. Sometimes, however, they might make an appearance as seductive, beautiful young men and maidens, but those who fall for them and let themselves be kissed will be invaded by disease and pain. Mostly, however, these demonic beings come in the form of worms, snakes, crustaceans, or dragon-like, cold-blooded animals. The manifestation of diseases as wormlike creatures is almost universal; thus, in almost all traditional cultures, so-called sucking shamans specialize in sucking out these beings with their mouth and then disposing of them.

One can well understand how the image of disease-bringing worms is a common theoretical model since countless teeming maggots can occupy festering wounds or corpses, roundworms and flukes can suddenly appear in the stool, woodworms gnaw under the bark of trees, blood-sucking leeches lurk in standing water, and sneaky snakes with poisonous bites slither through the grass. For the soul, they are appropriate images of pathogenic entities, which bustle on the non-physical level, in the otherworld or astral realm. As such, empirically, diseases do not have the appearance of snakes or worms—unless it is on a microscopic spirochete level. But this imaginary form corresponds most to the insidious, sneaking, invisible, hostile nature of disease. As William Blake (1977, 123) puts it:

O Rose, thou art sick.
The invisible worm
That flies in the night
In the howling storm
Has found out thy bed . . .

Even today, this idea is reflected in the language. We still say "something has wormed its way into me," or "the worm at the core." In German, people might say that you "have a worm in your head" if you have stupid thoughts, and so on. One still speaks of the worm of hatred or envy that infects the soul and causes disease. In France, it is said of someone who is constantly sick that they "have the worm" *(Malade toujours, il a le ver!)* or "everyone has his pet worm" *(chacun a son ver coquin)*.

The Indo-Europeans overwhelmed the demonic worms with magical power. They sang over the worms with magical chants and charms and drew them out of their animal or human victims. The higher powers, the devas (Indo-European **div* = radiant, celestial being; Latin *divus* = deity), were called upon for help, and especially the lightning- and thunderbolt-carrying Sky God. The gods of light are all enemies of worms and vipers, which creep around in damp, dark places. Indra's lightning bolt *(vajra)* destroys the serpentine *vrita,* which blocks the water of life, just as it destroys the disease-bringing demons; Thor stands with his lightning hammer in the fight against the Midgard serpent and other worms; the stag, which the ancient Europeans revered as the "sun in its in animal form," as well as the celestial eagle, were considered enemies of the disease-making, relentless, creeping things. And in the Anglo-Saxon herbal blessing from the eleventh century, the so-called Nine Herbs Charm, we learn of how Woden (Odin), the shamanic, magical god, triumphed over the disease-bringing snake with three-times-three powerful medicinal plants:

A worm came crawling, to destroy a man;
Then Woden took up nine wondrous staves [herbs],
struck the adder so that it flew apart into nine parts.

In the Vedic Aryan healing chants of ancient India, the worms are ritually ground, pounded, and buried under heavy stones or burned. It is reported that the wise Rishi (seer) Agastya, the father of Siddha (magical) medicine, drove away the worms at dawn with magical chants. Such a song is described, for example, in the collection of magical texts, the Atharva Veda (2.31, translated by R. Griffith in *Hymns of the Atharva Veda*, 1895):

A Charm against All Sorts of Worms

With Indra's mighty millstone, that which crushes worms of
    every sort,
I bray and bruise the worms to bits like vetches on the
    grinding stone.
The Seen and the Invisible, and the Kurñru have I crushed:
Alāndus, and all Chalunas, we bruise to pieces with our spell.
I kill Alāndus with a mighty weapon: burnt or not burnt
    they now have lost their vigour.
Left or not left, I with the spell subdue them: let not a single
    worm remain uninjured.
The worm that lives within the ribs, within the bowels, in
    the head.
Avaskava and Borer, these we bruise to pieces with the spell.
Worms that are found on mountains, in the forests, that live
    in plants, in cattle, in the waters,
Those that have made their way within our bodies—these I
    destroy, the worms' whole generation.

Another typical example (Atharva Veda 5.23, translated by R. Griffith in *Hymns of the Atharva Veda*, 1895):

A Charm against Parasitic Worms

I have called Heaven and Earth to aid, have called divine
    Sarasvati,[13]
Indra and Agni have I called: Let these destroy the worm, I
    prayed,

O Indra, Lord of Treasures, kill the worms that prey upon
this boy.
All the malignant spirits have been smitten by my potent
spell.
We utterly destroy the worm, the worm that creeps around
the eyes.
The worm that crawls about the nose, the worm that gets
between the teeth.
Two of like color, two unlike, two colored black, two
colored red.
The tawny and the tawny-eared, Vulture and Wolf, all these
are killed.
Worms that are white about the sides, those that are black
with black-hued arms,
All that show various tints and hues, these worms we utterly
destroy.
Eastward the Sun is mounting, seen of all, destroying thing
unseen,
Crushing and killing all the worms invisible and visible.

The forest peoples worked in the same manner against venomous
worms. A ninth-century verse charm in Old High German is a good
example, the so-called Tegernsee Charm:

Get out, worm, with nine little worms,
go out of the marrow into the veins,
go out of the flesh into the skin,
go out of the skin into this arrow.
And [pray] three Our Fathers.

In this manner, the healer sings the worm gradually out from the bone
marrow, the innermost core, up through the skin and into an arrowhead.
This arrow is shot far away into the world of the afterlife, into the astral
world. This practice of shooting away the disease is encountered among

the forest peoples over and over. The native people of North America are also familiar with this practice (Storl 2010b, 172).

An instruction and a charm *(galdor)*, "Against a Worm," recorded in northern England shortly after the conversion to Christianity, shows how the old pagan tradition continued on.

> If a person or animal swallowed a worm:
>
>> If it is a male, sing this song into the right ear,
>> if it is a female, sing into the left ear:
>> I wound the beast [worm], I smite the animal, I slay the animal . . .
>> Sing this nine times into the ear and say the Lord's Prayer once.
>> This same charm can be sung against any invading worm. Sing it often into the wound and rub the wound with your saliva; take grene curmellan [possibly the centaury plant], pound it, place it on the wound, and cover it with warm cow dung (*Lacnunga*, "Remedies," Harley 585, British Museum).

Another typical banning of worms from the Middle Ages is as follows:

> Jesus and Peter plowed in a field,
> plowed three furrows
> plowed three worms:
> One is white,
> the other black,
> the third red.
> Since all the worms are dead. In the name of . . .

Instead of Jesus and Saint Peter, it would have certainly been Odin and Freyr, or the goddess Freya, or other healing deities that roam Earth in the older pagan banning charms. These are the gods who repeatedly reveal themselves to humans—when they are tired or in a state of rapture. The

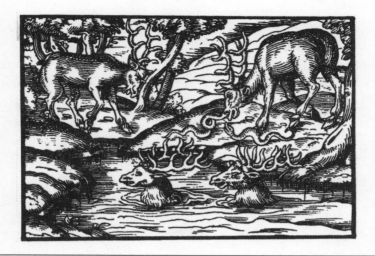

Stags with healing abilities destroying "worms" (anonymous woodcut, 1582)

word "field"—like also the Sanskrit word *kshetra* (field)—is a metaphor for the human body from which the disease is plowed out.

The color of the worms, white, red, and black, are, as we shall see later, also the colors of the Earth Goddess, because these creeping creatures are also her children. They nest in the maternal ground of the earth, in the trees and the people.

Similarly, an old Swabian saying from the southeast corner of Germany refers to the "worm field."

> The Lord God went to the field;
> he plowed the whole acre; he plowed three worms,
> one white and the other black, the third red,
> here lie all worms dead.

In the French-speaking world, if an evil worm infested a human child, one implored Saint Médard: "Saint Médard, you who possess all the power, take the worms from this child. They are cohabitants who are constantly out to strangle the child. They come out of the nothingness; you can send them back there again" (Loux 1978, 222).

Vermifuges in Folk Medicine

Folk medicine includes many different methods of deworming with local, antiparasitic herbs (anthelmintics). Some of them, such as tansy and male fern, although effective, are rather toxic. An extract from the male fern *(Dryopteris filix-mas)*, in earlier times called wormfarn, is ineffective against roundworms but can paralyze tapeworms that can then be excreted with the administration of a laxative. The dosage is, however, difficult to judge. At high doses, it can affect the liver and cause severe jaundice, or the optic nerve can also be damaged. Tansy *(Tanacetum vulgare)* expels pinworms and roundworms, but it also acts abortively; in high doses, because of thujone, it can even cause fatal poisoning. Wormwood, called "wormdeath" in a Germanic dialect, also contains thujone and does not kill the intestinal worms but paralyzes them so that they can be excreted. Milder acting are chamomile, elecampane, wild garlic, garlic, brewed walnut leaves, maiden hair fern, and mint. Even in my childhood, mothers still grated carrots and gave them to the children when they suffered from roundworms.

In addition to these more or less effective anthelmintics, folk medicine has an arsenal of worm-killing, worm-expelling herbs. However, they do not stand up to scientific and pharmaceutical analysis. Most of these anthelmintics turn out to be completely ineffective. Well—let the scientists smile knowingly—at that time, in the Dark Ages, people had indeed neither the analytical munitions, nor knew the physiology of parasitic helminths. But folk medicine initially had nothing to do with that, for it had not only the visible intestinal inhabitants in its sights but also the invisible demonic "small worms, without legs or skin"; the "worm herbs" were to get rid of these. Thus, for example, garlic was also used—especially in Slavic countries: it keeps blood-sucking vampires and other "vermin" away from the body.

Incidentally, one should know that an occasional infestation of intestinal worms is not a disease. The visible worms, the roundworms and pinworms, have inhabited our intestines for over a hundred million years. We live in co-evolutionary cohabitation with them. The same applies to the worms in the feces of cattle, horses, and dogs. Studies have shown that

146

these unwelcome guests have trained and stimulated the immune systems of mammals. Those who were occasionally afflicted by intestinal worms as a child later suffer less from allergies and other autoimmune disorders, and have a lower risk of inflammatory bowel disease (Crohn's disease, ulcerative colitis) or colorectal cancer (Zuk 2008, 37–38). It is also known that the maggots of blowflies clean the gangrenous rotting tissue of flesh wounds in humans and animals better than even the best surgeon, and that they also excrete the active ingredient allantoin in their feces, which helps heal wounds. Allantoin is, indeed, the potent wound- and bone-healing ingredient in comfrey.

Chants for Dispelling Diseases

The Brahmins of the Vedic Aryans, as well as the Celtic Druids, made every effort to orally pass down from master to student their long magical incantations and sacred songs with careful precision. The secret knowledge—including the sacred songs—had to be learned by heart, and it had to come directly from the heart. It was only in later times, when they had concerns that changes could creep into the recitations, that they were written down in India as Vedas (Vedas = wisdom teachings). The magical power of song is based on the fact that they are recited verbatim.

The magic and healing chants of Germanic people, the *Galsterlieder* (Old High German galen = sing—the *gale* in nightin*gale* is related—or bewitch; Old Norse *galdr;* Anglo-Saxon *gealdor*) also demanded accurate recitation. They were sung in magical tones and with alliterative rhyme. Odin, the Shaman God, was considered the master of these songs, as *Galders Fadir,* "father of the magical songs." The second Merseburg Incantations from the ninth century testifies to this.

Phol and Wodan rode to the woods[14]
there Balder's foal wrenched its foot
Sinthgunt charmed it, Sunna's sister,[15]
Frija charmed it, Volla's sister,
Woden charmed it as he well could,
as bone wrench, so blood wrench, so limb wrench,

bone to bone, blood to blood,
limb to limb, so they are joined.

By the Middle Ages, it was no longer Phol and Wodan, but Christ and Saint Stephen who healed horses with charms: "Christ and St. Stephen came to the castle of Salonae. Then St. Stephen's horse was caught. As Christ healed St. Stephen's horse from entrapment, so I heal this horse with the help of Christ" (Stroem and Bieszais 1975, 91).

A more or less congruent healing formula as in the Merseburg Charm is found in a charm to heal bones in the Atharva Veda (4.12).

> Thou art the healer, making whole, the healer of the broken
>   bone:
> Make thou this whole, Arundhatī!
> Whatever bone of thine within thy body hath been
>   wrenched or cracked,
> May Dhātar set it properly and join together limb by limb.
> With marrow be the marrow joined, thy limb united with
>   the limb.
> Let what hath fallen of thy flesh, and the bone also grow
>   again.
> Let marrow close with marrow, let skin grow united with
>   the skin.
> Let blood and bone grow strong in thee, flesh grow together
>   with the flesh.
> Join thou together hair with hair, join thou together skin
>   with skin.
> Let blood and bone grow strong in thee. Unite the broken
>   part,
> O Plant (Griffith 1895).

The elvish worms, snakes, and arthropods that are sung out by shamans—by the Germanic *galsterer*, the Vedic *bhishàj*, the Baltic *burwis* (magician) or *wahrdotjs* (blessing speaker), and other healers—cannot be killed; they are spiritual entities that have no physical body. They must be, as Paracelsus said, transferred to a suitable medium.

In Vedic medicine, diseases are conjured upon enemies—such as the swarthy dasas, natives who disrespect the Aryan sacrificial rituals. Jaundice is summoned to sit on yellow birds and fly away or go into the yellow sun. Hot fever is transferred to the cool, damp frogs. Other diseases are magically transferred into running water, so they float away. The following is a charm against jaundice (Atharva Veda, 1.22).

> As the Sun rises, let thy sore disease and yellowness depart.
> We compass and surround thee with the color of a ruddy ox.
> With ruddy hues we compass thee that thou mayst live a
>   lengthened life:
> So that this man be free from harm, and cast his yellow tint
>   away.
> Devatyās that are red of hue, yea, and the ruddy-colored
>   kine,
> Each several form, each several force—with these we com
>   pass thee about.
> To parrots and to starlings we transfer thy sickly yellowness:
> Now in the yellow-colored birds we lay this yellowness of
>   thine.

Takmán, the demon who shoots lightning arrows during the rainy season, which brings body aches and fever, is sent under the ground by the healer back to where it comes from. The earth detours its magical potency and discharges it. The Cheyenne medicine men work in a similar way: In breaks between the treatment of the sick, they incense their hands and touch the ground to dispose of the negative energy. Even into relatively modern times, a battle victor would touch the earth with the flags and banners of the defeated enemy army to "unload" them of their power. According to general Native American belief, the trees also take suffering and disease away from humans. This applies not only to the lofty giant trees of the forest, but also especially to those trees that grow near the house and share an energy field with the people.

In Indian or Nepalese villages, one can occasionally encounter trees decorated with flower garlands. The reason is usually the following: If the astrologer discovers, when comparing the horoscopes of an engaged couple, that the bride could bring, for some sort of dark karmic reason, her husband or her in-laws misfortune, she is first married in an elaborate wedding ceremony to a tree that is decorated like a typical groom. The tree husband then takes everything bad from the woman. Later, she will be married to her human husband. In this way, happiness and domestic peace are secured (Mehta 1998, 190).

Transferring Sickness onto Trees

Pests can be handed over to trees, which was common practice among the western European forest peoples in rural areas and even into modern times. A hole is drilled in the trunk and the disease is put therein. Fever is tied with a knot on a willow branch, and the following is spoken: "Dear Willow, I beseech thee, seven and seventy fevers are plaguing me." Because the evil spirits come along as unwanted guests, one takes bread and salt so that the tree becomes their host. At the same time, people say the following to the tree, and the evil spirits are then confused and are sent away with the birds (Mannhardt 1875, 21):

> Tree, tree, I shake you,
> the fever I bring to you.
> The first bird that flies over,
> shall take away the fever.

Sick people were also pulled through trees—young oak, ash, or fruit trees—whose trunks had been split down the middle, or they were pulled through the arc of a root so they could wipe off the disease.

It is not so very long ago that in England children with fractures or rickets were healed by splitting a young ash tree and pulling the sick, naked child through it three times, with the head in the direction of the rising sun. The tree was bound back together with mud and rope, and, if it grew back together, the child would heal. But if the tree did not grow together and heal again, then the child would remain sick (Chamberlain 2006, 149). The ash was, like the oak, sacred to the pagan Anglo-Saxons. It was consecrated to the Shaman God and healer Woden (Odin). For a long time in England, a piece of ash wood was laid in the birthing chamber and the newborn was given a drop of ash juice on the tongue. Other than that, the bitter-tasting, diuretic, laxative decoction of the bark and leaves is administered in cases of fever and rheumatism in folk medicine. Another typical magical cure for chills is to transmit them to a shrew then drill a hole in an ash, put the poor animal in it, and cork the hole. "When the shrew is dead, the chills are gone" (Chamberlain 2006, 146).

Until the early twentieth century, farmers in central Europe transferred their sufferings onto trees with a charm—especially onto a spruce or the house elder. For instance, in Frankenwald, Germany, white stockings from a person with a lame leg were hung from a hawthorn bush. If you were attacked by a fever, you could go out at night during the waning moon and tie the disease to an old elder. In Brandenburg, you said this at the same time:

> Good morning, elder,
> I'll bring my fever,
> I bind it to you,
> Now I'm departing in God's name.

In Mecklenburg, to treat gout, three days in a row before sunrise one walked to the elder bush and spoke (Marzell 2002, 249):

> Elder, I have the gout,
> You do not have it.
> Take it from me,
> so I don't have it.

For toothache, one went to the elder bush before sunrise, cut a splinter of wood from under the bark, picked the gums until they were bloody, and said:

> My teeth hurt me,
> A black, a red, a white worm.
> I want them bleeding to death,
> In the name of the Father . . .

The ethnobotanist Miriam Wiegele told me that there are still farmers in the mountains of Austria who are wart-healers *(Warzenwender)* and speak a charm while etching papillae on an elderberry branch and then throw the branch into water or bury it in the ground. For conventional medicine, it is a mystery that this activity leads to success.

In the Alemannic region, there are still so-called *Besenkapellen* (broom chapels) to which the sick make pilgrimages in order to transfer their diseases to the healer Jesus Christ. These pilgrims offer a broom made of birch twigs (bound for them by a neighbor), which symbolizes cleaning and a new beginning. Interestingly enough, often an old elder grows beside these chapels. Originally, the diseases were hung on the elder, so it is as if that has remained unconscious in the memories of the local population. If the Savior does not want it, then the old Mother Holle will surely dispose of the disease.

The Baltic people were also convinced that diseases could be transferred to other living beings—humans, animals, and plants. In 1825, for example, a pastor in Latvia reported enthusiastically in his notes about a healer, a "blower" *(puhschlotajs)* who breathed on the patient's wounds, blew salt, water, or beer on them, and then spoke this healing charm:

> All unclean spirits are to stand up and depart from off of this sick person (or animal) and go to the dense trees, wide fields, and great hills, to the storms, seas and hurricanes, 3 times 9 men should come with the same force, and, speaking the same words, cut them down; 3 times 9 storms will come and smash all unclean spirits,

so that they become detached from this man and go onto dense trees, rowans, aspen and roots, to be stretched, to shed their skin, and to remove themselves from this sick person (or animal), so that he may be healed. (Kurtz 1937, 33)

The ritual was then completed with The Lord's Prayer said three times.

There is another Latvian healing charm that should be said three times: "Fall into the stump! There it does not swell, there it does not hurt. Fall into the stone! There it does not swell, there it does not hurt! Fall into the holy Mahra Church![16] In the name of . . ." Or: "Go away to the sea, nibble white stones in the sea, don't nibble my body! May all evil disappear like mist, like fog, like frost in the morning sun, like the old moon! My health shall shine, like the sun in the sky! A white snake swims through the sea, gnawing pebbles. The fire swells, the water flows through, the damage no longer swells. In the name of . . ." (Kurtz 1937, 48).

The Magic of the Elder

The herbalist Hieronymus Bock wrote in his *Kreutterbuch (Herb Book,* Strasbourg, 1539), "In Teutscher [German] nation indeed the elder is known to all / wherefore not many words / how / where or when are necessary / forasmuch as everyone knows the elder." Everyone knows it and yet does not know that the black elder is sacred to the archaic grandmother under the earth, the Earth Goddess. Its German name, *Holunder,* connects it with the Mother Holle or Mother Elder of fairy tales and the hidden folk, the dwarves who wear magic hats that make them invisible.

The house elder is the gateway to underworld realms; it is a threshold tree. René Strassmann, a Swiss chemist and mediumistic person who has traveled far and wide in ethereal worlds says the elder protects the beings living on the earth from attacks by creatures of the netherworld. The elder draws the boundary between the underworld and the middle world (Strassmann 1994, 153). He says elderberry—wood, bark, root, flowers—are suitable as incense to establish conscious contact with the shadow world. In fact, it is so that when one meditates under the elder, one has the feeling of being pulled downward. In the meditation under the birch, one experiences precisely the opposite—it is as if one is lifted up into the light.

If one is so daring as to sleep under the elder, then one can feel the constant coming and going of gnomes, goblins, and dwarves. The little people, whose queen is Mother Holle, may be in a good mood and ready for games, but they can also be ornery. Under the elder, one can also encounter *Hoelderlin*, the *Hollabiru*—which is a name of the "devil," the Paleolithic, horned Nature God, who is the companion of the elder mother (Danish *Hyldemoer* or *Hillefro*). Hillefro is pictured in Danish folklore as a crone dressed in black with a white shawl.

In the Middle Ages, the once revered old Earth Goddess mutated into the "devil's grandmother," who still stirs her boiling cauldron under the roots of this tree. This connection can be interpreted as an indication of former pagan worship of the tree. Until the twentieth century, rural women still sacrificed under the elder next to the house. In East Friesland, for example, when children or even adults were sick, bread and wool were placed under the branches of the house elder. Elsewhere, beer and bread were laid under the elder bush for the wee folk or spirits.

Just as it seems to pull the soul down during meditation, the elder soaks up all negativity and illness and passes them down into the earth, into the cauldron of the ancient goddess. According to rural beliefs, the house elder, thus, gets rid of the negativity of the entire house, barn, and stall. That is why one hung purulent dressing cloths, fallen out teeth, and the like in the elder. The shirt of a child made sick through magic could be buried under the tree because it would "consume the evil." This custom is also one of the reasons one could not trim or cut the elder, because the disease could jump back out, a yearlong toothache could plague the patient (a belief from the Transylvanian region), the horses could go lame (from the Altmark region), or you even may soon die.[17]

154

But if cutting or trimming it cannot be avoided, when the elder bush threatens the entrance way for instance, then one goes at full moon to the tree, sacrifices some beer, flour, and milk, and says, "Mother Holle, give me of your wood and I give you mine, when it grows in the forest." The wood in this charm, however, was nothing other than one's own dead bones; it is clear from the English version of the charm: "Old Gal, give me of thy wood, and I will give my bones when I am dead." (In fact, here and there, such as among the ancient Friesians, it was the custom to bury the deceased under the house elder.)

The legend that Judas hung himself out of shame and regret on an elder tree after he had betrayed the Savior for thirty shabby silver coins, illustrates that the elder tree attracts evil. As proof, one points to the beige-brown, slimy, ear-shaped elder sponge *(Auricularia auricula-judae)*, the parasite on old elder trees that is similar to the ear of a corpse. This "judas ear" remained hanging in the branches as the traitor went down to hell.

If you want to get rid of a fever, you can go to the elder and say:

Oh elderberry tree, beloved,
a fever plagues me,
Because Judas hanged himself from you,
the fever is given to you.

Elder is medicinal, but also has a toxic side; its blossoms are creamy white, but its berries are black and purple. Like Mother Holle, it has two sides; it is not only the goddess of life but also of death. So it was in many places the custom that the coffin maker used an elder shoot as a yardstick or that the coachman of the hearse carrying the coffin drove the horses with a switch made of an elder branch.

Elder also played a role in the natural annual calendar. In Westphalia, the women danced outdoors on Candelmas—once dedicated to the goddess of spring, Brigit—and held elder whips in their hands with which they playfully whipped the men who approached the dance (Aigremont 1910, 42). In Thuringia, Germany, an elder branch is placed in the windows of unchaste women during Pentecost. In central Germany, it was the summer solstice:

> To midsummer! The elder is flowering!
> Now lovemaking will be yet greater!

A maiden in Carinthia, Austria, might shake the elder bush on Saint John's Night and then speak the verse:

> Elder bush, I shake thee,
> Saint John, I beg thee,
> Let it in my dream appear,
> Which man will be mine here.

The elder bush, as the goddess of recurring life, stimulates desire and sends the souls of children into existence. In "Ringel-Ringel-Reihe," the German version of the well-known charm, "ring-around-the-rosie," the little souls dance around under an elder bush:

> Ring around the elder tree
> we are children three,
> dancing under the elder bush,
> we all go hush, hush, hush.

At midsummer, when the elder flowers blossom in many regions, umbels are still deep-fat fried in batter and eaten for the solstice festival. In peasant culture, it was once said that anyone who eats many elder fritters will be able to jump over the midsummer fire, and then the flax and the crops will grow tall. Syrup and wine are also made from elder flowers.

When the elderberries in autumn turned dark purple, it was a sign that it was time for the winter crops to be sown. A sweet, purple soup from the berries was a ritual food that protected people against winter colds and was eaten in preparation for the dark season.

In Lower Germany, the elder is also called *Elder* or *Ellhorn,* and the elder woman is known there as *Ellermutter,* which can be translated as grandmother. In England, the elder tree is known as the Elder Mother, and in Lincolnshire as Old Gal or Old Lady. It was believed that the elder supports women in labor by lending them a helping hand in their hour of need.

Ladybugs and Beetles

Not only could diseases be moved to trees or transmitted to animals by the right charm or sickly children be pulled through split tree trunks to strip off the disease, but in northern Europe, the illnesses also could be attached to a beetle, in particular to the ladybug or rose chafer. These pretty insects crawl up the healer's index finger while the healer recites a charm; at the top of the finger, they usually then fly away and the curse or the sufferings are carried off into the otherworld. As with so many rhymes and sayings, they lived on in children's culture. In English-speaking countries, it may go:

> Ladybug, ladybug, fly away home
> your house is on fire,
> your children are gone.
> All except one,
> And that's little Ann,
> For she crept under
> The frying pan.

One of the most well-known sayings in German goes:

> Maybug [usually meant ladybug] fly,
> father is at war,
> mother is in Pommerland [or Engelland],
> Pommerland has burned,
> Ladybug, fly.

"Pommerland" in this charm does not refer to Pomerania on the Baltic Sea, and "Engelland" is not England but the otherworld, the land of the angels (German = *Engel*) and the elves. A charm in Low German is as follows:

> Heavenly child, fly up,
> Fly up to the highest heaven.

And in France one says to the beetle:

> *Vole au ciel, ton père te demande.* (Fly to the sky, your father
> is calling you.)

The cute ladybug, with its seven black dots on the red wings and white cap (pronotum), was particularly sacred because, as the swan or the stork, it had the three colors of the primordial goddess Holle. It is to her womb, her cauldron, that the spirits of disease, the incarnated spirits in general, return when they leave the world. It is also she who sends the children into the world. The stork brings the souls of children from the otherworld and drops their spirit down the chimney into the house where the expectant mother receives them. And just like the stork, ladybugs—also called beetles of Mary, ladybirds, sun child, Mary's chafer, and so on—can also bring the children's souls into the world. An old Swiss nursery rhyme says it:

> Ladybug, fly up,
> fly up into heaven,
> bring down a golden basket,
> with a golden swaddled baby in it.

Other species of beetles were also used. If someone suffered from colic (*wambe-wœrce*), the pain could be transferred to the black dung beetle (*tordwifel*), as we learn in the Anglo-Saxon *Bald's Leechbook*.[18] For this purpose, the dung beetle had to be picked up with both hands together with the earth in which it burrows, shaken, and spoken the following charm to three times: *Remedium facio ad ventris dolerem* (I am the remedy for stomachache). Then one had to throw the beetle over the shoulder without looking back at it and hold the abdomen with both hands. It is interesting that the spell was not written down in the native Anglo-Saxon but in ecclesiastic Latin. For the common peo-

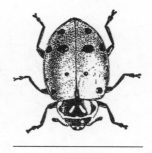

Ladybug

ple, the unintelligible language of the priest and later the robed physicians had an aura of mystery and magic.

The Essence of Healing Herbs

According to current views, plants are soulless, mindless organisms characterized by chloroplasts and are able to build organic matter from inorganic substances (Schubert and Wagner 2000, 417). There is nothing mystical about these growth and reproduction processes; they can be understood as complicated chemical-mechanical processes and reactions.

Neither the ancient Indo-Europeans nor the archaic forest peoples would come to terms with such a definition. Plants appeared to their visionary awareness, especially healing herbs, as lofty, powerful entities. The healer was able to communicate with them and ask them for help. The Rigveda, the oldest evidence of Indo-European literary culture, and the Atharva Veda outline the importance of the healing herbs.[19]

- Herbs are the elders; they were born three ages before the gods.

- They are called Mother, and they have immense amounts of knowledge, especially where it concerns the health of humans and animals. Yajur Veda sings to the plants calling them goddesses.

- Sacrifices are made to the medicinal plants. The Vedic healer promises to sacrifice a cow to the medicinal plants when they heal a sick person (Rigveda 10:97, 5). Similarly, when the Celtic

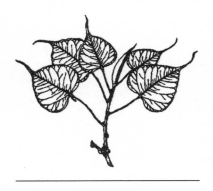

Pipal leaves

people harvested a branch of golden mistletoe, they sacrificed two white bulls. The Celtic mistletoe harvest ritual was no ordinary gathering of herbs, but part of the elaborate enthronement ceremony of a new king; the mistletoe's white, slimy berries were considered drops of the cosmic bull's semen and granted the new regent potency. The king, then, was no longer a simple man but became the husband of the goddess of the land and responsible for the fertility of the fields and herds (Storl 2009, 247).[20] In today's traditional medicine, offerings such as milk, cereal, beer, blood, bread, a copper coin, or similar things are often still brought to healing plants when asking for their help. All Native Americans sacrifice tobacco to the healing herbs.

- The powerful herbs meet for council, as would a king and his knights, and advise the competent physician.

- The herbs stream out, like cows out of the gate, in order to cure the sick person. They have the power of horses; they are filled with soma and increase the vitality of the patient. Like thieves who climb over the fence, they overcome all obstacles.

- Simply holding the medicine plant in one's hand has a healing effect. Brushing a tuft of herbs over the patient retrieves the patient's life spirit as the herbs penetrate, limb by limb, joint by joint.

- Medicinal plants are heavenly beings. Although they descend from heaven, they are at the same time referred to as children of Mother Earth in the Atharva Veda (12: 1.17) because the earth gives the plant devas their physical body.

- Soma, the moon, the giver of the water of life, is the "master of herbs" *(Oshadhi Pati),* and wise Brihaspati, the planet Jupiter, is their teacher. Brihaspati is considered guru of the gods *(Deva Guru)* and conveys all the insights that lie beyond the mind. He is, like Odin, master of the magical word; he conveys the power of the word, with which the herbs are invoked and their strength is called forth.

- The plants, these powerful beings, are to be approached with considerable caution: "Let the root digger who uprooted the plant to heal a person, not come to harm" (Rigveda 10: 97.19). Thus, one apologizes and explains, as the Cheyenne do, that they come with humility and good will, or as the Chinese do when they dig wild ginseng, that they approach the medicinal roots with a refined and pure soul. Or one tries to move the responsibility of digging up a root to someone else: "The gandharvas [angels, divine musicians] have uprooted you." Or, as it says in the Atharva Veda (5: 14.1): "An eagle found you, a wild boar dug you up with his muzzle." Elsewhere, even Jupiter or the moon is responsible:[21] "Brihaspati dug you up!" or "Oh herb, Soma, the wise king has liberated you from the demon [Yákshma]!"

In modern phytotherapy, one is accustomed to using healing plants for specific health problems based on the combination of molecular active ingredients present in the plant. But that is a very narrow understanding. The plants, as communicative beings, can do much more when they are asked. In the Vedas, one hears that they not only heal wounds, fevers, and faintness, but that they also work against poison and increase longevity; they can remove curses and allow victory in conflicts; with the help of certain herbs, a woman can eliminate her rival, secure the love of a man, and attain fertility; with plants, one can detect witches and secret enemies; men can increase their masculinity; and bad ghosts can be kept away from the body with their help. Written down over three thousand years ago, these applications are shared by other cultural traditions as well as the forest people.

The great vision—in which the plants appear as goddesses and fever and pestilence were demonic powers against which the appointed healer could proceed with herbs, power words, songs, and rituals—began to fade in the middle of the first millennium BCE when a paradigm shift took hold of all Indo-European cultures, at least as far as the Great Tradition is concerned. In the urban civilization, a new zeitgeist made its appearance: scholar doctors, such as Charaka (cofounder of the Ayurvedic teachings) and Sushruta (founder of surgery) in India and Hippocrates in ancient Greece, tried to provide an empirically rational basis for medicine. The great cosmic vision faded, and the material dimension moved into the foreground. Although the gods were still acknowledged, the attempt was made to determine which environmental factors were effective and what role objective things such as lifestyle and diet played in sickness and health. Not ghosts and demons, angry gods or ancestors, but an imbalance in the body fluids, the *dathus* and *humors,* was now blamed for illness. In the rural areas, though, among the illiterate farmers and herders, the magical worldview of the Little Tradition was maintained for a long time.

Signatures and Signs

In the Indo-European tradition, as almost everywhere among people who live close to nature, all plants harbor healing qualities within themselves (Findly 2008, 21). Each plant actively heals, and usually its healing quality can be perceived in its outer appearance, its peculiarities, or the location of its growth. Physical features provide information about the plant's effects. Hairy plants are used to combat hair loss; wormlike roots against "worms"; bitter herbs for stomach and bile complaints; milky plants for increasing lactation; those with yellow juice for jaundice; plants with distinctive red parts for hemostasis; herbs with thorns, like the thistle, against side stitches; and so on. The plants thus carry signs or signatures. This way of "reading" the plant's appearance was referred to as the "doctrine of signatures" during the Renaissance. Its principle is homeopathic: like heals like.

Of course, this interpretation of the signatures also played a role among the Celtic people, but it took visionary skills to recognize them.

Diancecht was the name of the Irish-Celtic god of healing. He had a cauldron called the "Sea of Herbs," in which the water contained all medicinal herbs. The cauldron could even bring the dead back to life, except if they had been decapitated. The cauldron was put to the test when Nuada, king of the goddess Ana's people, the Tuatha de Danann, lost his arm in a battle (as a cripple, he would never be allowed to be king among the Celts). The wise Diancecht made him an artful arm prosthesis of silver. Nevertheless, Nuada's right to rule was put into question.[22]

Diancecht had a son named Miach who could also heal, and indeed even better than his father. They say he healed with plants and charms. He performed the incantation "bone to bone, muscle to muscle, tendon to tendon" and in three times three days created a new arm of flesh and blood for the maimed king. But old Diancecht was jealous. In his anger, he hit the son and wounded his scalp. But Miach healed himself. Then Diancecht beat him again and wounded his skull. Again Miach healed the wound. Then the father hit his son so hard that he injured his brain. Against this, the son with healing wisdom could do nothing. His sister Airmed mourned the dead body of her brother with many tears, whereupon 365 medicinal herbs sprung up out of his corpse. Airmed gathered these herbs, arranged them according to their effects, and hid them under her cloak. But Diancecht nevertheless caught her and tore the herbs from her, scattering them. Although each plant has its signature, since that time, they could not be interpreted easily. No one can read them unless the information is revealed to them by the Holy Spirit—or the goddess Airmed, the elves, these beings of heavenly light, or the ancestors.

Even in the sixteenth century, Paracelsus wrote of his aversion to school knowledge and did not shun learning from herbal women, traveling people, and modest peasants:[23] "Nature designs a plant so that it emanates what it is good for" *(De Natura Rerum)* and "Nothing exists that was not marked by nature, and by understanding the signs, one can recognize what is concealed in it" *(Philosophia Sagax).*

But "it is not only with the external senses and the mind that one recognizes the signs and signatures, but they should be recognized the way animals do it, in an intuitive way . . ." According to Paracelsus, everyone can see the signatures—but few have the gift to understand them. The illiterate peasant sees the script in an old book, just as the scholars do, but cannot read it. It is love, the loving look that transforms figures into significant and understandable symbols (Braun 1993, 69–70).

The signature of the plants plays a role in Rudolf Steiner's anthroposophic medicine as well, in which the nature of the sick human has its counterpart in the medicinal plant. Both are expressions of the same processes. What is excessive in the plant is sickness for humans.[24]

The belief that the plant's appearance, its signature, says something about its healing powers is universal—apart from the point of view of today's natural sciences. I found this to be true with Native Americans, Indians, and Nepalis as well as among Africans. Amazingly, the validity of the medical application of the plants based on the signatures has often been demonstrated to be true by scientific research. Cultural anthropologists argue that the reason for this is that the healers in illiterate societies use mnemonic devices to remember the therapeutic potential of the various plants. But it could also be interpreted as follows: The plant devas reveal themselves to the finer senses; they say: "Mark these signs so that you do not forget my strength."

The Signatures of Indigenous European Healing Plants

With its appearance, its color and shape, and the nature of its location, a plant attracts the attention of the healer and indicates its potential healing power. For shamans and medicine people, this is an invitation to approach the plant meditatively and to get to know its innermost being. That was the case with the forest people. Later in the Middle Ages, the doctrine of signatures corresponded to the characteristics of the saints and martyrs, then in the Renaissance to one of the seven visible planets or "planetary gods" (the moon, Mercury, Venus, the sun, Mars, Jupiter, and Saturn).

Autumn crocus *(Colchicum autumnale):* Also known as meadow saffron and naked lady, this dangerous, deadly poisonous crocus in the lily family shoots up its ghostly, pale pink-purple–colored flowers out of the ground in the autumn. The bulbs have been said to resemble toes with gout. In the Middle Ages, they were used externally as an effective painkiller for gout.

Bistort *(Polygonum bistorta):* This knotweed that grows in damp meadows with its sinuous, serpentine, ringed roots, having the thickness of a finger and with pinkish flesh inside, has the signature of the colon. A decoction is used for diarrhea, dysentery, bloody stools, and rectal varicose veins—rightfully so, because bistort, also called snakeweed, is one of the best tannin-containing drugs.

Burdock *(Arctium lappa):* Burdock is powerful; its fruits have claws like a bear and the bear is similar to the human being, only hairy from head to toe. A bear plant of this kind, as in burdock oil, can promote hair growth. Its common names include lappa, fox's clote, thorny burr, beggar's buttons, cockle buttons, love leaves, philanthropium, and cockleburs.

Celandine *(Chelidonium maius):* This plant from the poppy family, with rich yellow juice that tastes sharp and bitter like bile, has a signature that indicates it is a remedy for liver problems and is used to treat jaundice. In fact, it has a favorable effect on liver and biliary diseases. It contains active ingredients that are antispasmodic and act on the biliary pathways and stimulate the bile flow. (It is a powerful plant that should be used under the guidance of a knowledgeable herbal practitioner.)

Comfrey *(Symphytum officinale):* Another common name for comfrey is knitbone or boneset, which points to its ability to heal broken bones. The interwoven veins serve as a signature because the pattern is similar to the tissue of old bones when they are found decomposed after they have been in the earth for a long time.

Dandelion and bitter herbs: All non-poisonous herbs that taste bitter have, therefore, the signature of bile and can help in liver and biliary complaints, which indeed applies.

Eyebright *(Euphrasia officinalis):* The small flowering figwort is said to resemble bleary eyes. An eye bath with the tea helps, indeed, with conjunctivitis, styes, and the tired, red eyes of people who have been at the computer for too long.

Figwort, woodland figwort *(Scrophularia nodosa):* This plant that smells of wild game is, as the Latin name suggests, full of nodes. The rhizome is knotty, and the flowers resemble nodes. Therefore, they have been used successfully as an ointment for scruffy skin, lymph node infections, boils, skin tuberculosis, and similar "knotty" diseases.

Goldenrod *(Solidago virgaurea):* The bright yellow flowers all along the stem are a signature of a healthy urinal flow. In fact, this diuretic herb is one of the best remedies for inflammation and stones in the urinary tract.

Herb Robert, herb Rupert *(Geranium robertianum):* The many common names of this species of cranesbill attest to its popularity—storksbill, wild geranium, red robin, death-come-quickly, dove's foot, crowfoot, Robert geranium, old maid's nightcap, and so on—as well as its wide range of therapeutic uses. It was also used to fulfill a couple's wish for children due to the signature of its seedpod, which is reminiscent of the beak of the stork, who delivers the babies.

Horsetail, shavegrass *(Equisetum arvense):* The regular, rhythmically articulated, siliceous stalks are reminiscent of the human skeleton, particularly the segmented structure of the spine. In fact, a decoction of horsetail strengthens and heals bones, strengthens the connective tissue, and promotes the synovial fluid that nourishes the cartilage.

Lesser celandine *(Ranunculus ficaria):* This yellow flower in the buttercup family is one of the earliest among spring blossoms. It is also called fig buttercup because the root nodules resemble warts (papillae) and figs (piles); the root tubers are still sometimes processed to treat hemorrhoids. Another signature of the acidic plant juice was that it causes redness and "burning" on the skin. Therefore, it was also used to treat wounds and "hot fire" (festering ulcers).

Linden: Both the large-leaved linden, basswood, or lime tree *(Tilia platyphyllos),* and the small-leaved linden *(T. cordata)* have heart-shaped leaves, so they are good for the "heart." Of course, the heart, at that time, did not refer to a muscle with a pumping function as we see it now, but the seat of cheerfulness and courage, as well as the center of our being in which the divine resides. Heart disease was considered a state of being disheartened, despondent, merciless. The mere presence of the linden could help and cheer the mind (Storl 2010c 161).

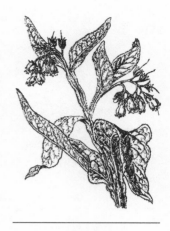

Comfrey

Lungwort *(Pulmonaria officinalis):* The leaves of this white-flecked, bristly plant in the borage family are said to resemble spots on sick lungs. Why should the lung-wort—as it was named by Hildegard of Bingen—help in diseases of the respira-

tory system? In part, because of its high content of silica and some mucilaginous ingredients.

Meadowsweet *(Filipendula ulmaria):* Meadowsweet prefers moist, cold locations. Like the washerwomen, the herb constantly has its "hands" in cold water but gets no rheumatism. That is why they brewed a tea from the white-flowering meadowsweet (*Herba et Flores Spirea ulmariae*) to counter rheumatism and joint pain. Today, we know that this indication is true. Both willow and meadowsweet contain salicylaldehyde, which is synthesized in the body to acetyl-salicylic acid—a natural, pain-relieving aspirin. Other common names include lady of the meadow, bridewort, and queen of the meadow.

Milk thistle *(Silybum marianum):* Also called holy thistle or Marian thistle, the milk thistle, as well as other spiky thistles, was considered a remedy for "side-stitches." If "stitches" (on the right side) meant disorders of the liver, then that would be true. The seeds of the milk thistle (*Fructus Cardui Mariae*) are indeed one of the best liver remedies.

Mugwort *(Artemisia vulgaris):* The stems of the mugwort plant turn red when they grow in the full sun, a sure sign that mugwort can stimulate menstruation.

Saint-John's-wort *(Hypericum perforatum):* When the flower bud is squeezed, a spot of red "blood" comes out, and the leaf looks as

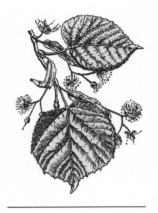

The heart-shaped linden leaf

if it has been poked with needles when held up to the light. Paracelsus determined the signature indicated it was a medicinal herb for stab wounds. The herb may, in addition to many other uses, be effectively used in wound healing.

Saxifrage *(Saxifraga spp.):* The saxifrage, which means "rock-breaking herb," as the name suggests, grows on stony and rocky soils; therefore, it is said to have the ability to "break up" bladder and kidney stones. Current science denies this effect, although meadow saxifrage *(Saxifraga granulata)* is given in homeopathy and in folk medicine for kidney stones.

Teasel *(Dipsacus sylvestris):* The opposite, exstipulate leaves are joined together at the stems, forming a basin, commonly referred to as "Venus's bath" in which water accumulates. The water in this Venus's bath is considered cleansing and rejuvenating. Like other herbs from the teasel family *(Dipsacaceae),* it is used as a tea with a "cleansing" and purifying effect on the lymph system. Teasel has been used as a remedy for Lyme disease since its emergence. Again, one could speak of a signature, because a symptom of spirochetes is the wandering redness *(erythema migrans),* which, after the tick bite, spreads on the skin like a ring. When teasel begins to bloom, a reddish "ring" appears that begins in the middle and "wanders" up and down the egg-shaped, cylindrical flower head.

Shamans and wise women work in a state of lucid consciousness and receive direct messages from the plant spirits. In the course of historical development with increasing civilization, this kind of dialogue became increasingly rare, but the healers still recognized the outward signs, the signatures of the plants. Even if the plant spirits do not disclose it directly, they offer in form, color, smell, location, season of blossoming, and so on,

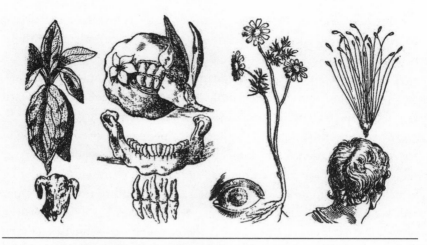

Pseudo-scientific signature theory of the Renaissance
(copper engraving, seventeenth century)

the opportunity to recognize their attributes in an intuitive manner. In the sixteenth and early seventeenth centuries, scientists tried to empirically and rationally substantiate this symbolism. The scholar Oswald Croll (1550–1609) devoted seventy pages of his work to the doctrine of signatures. Giambattista della Porta (1538–1615), the inventor of the camera obscura and explorer of witch's flying ointment, tried to scientifically systematize the signatures as well. For these researchers, the world was a book in which the scholar could read.

The walnut, for example, is likened to the human brain: The hard shell indicates the skull bone, so an extract obtained from the shells is good for skull injuries. The skin surrounding the core, similar to the membrane that encases the brain, and the core itself are the best brain medicine. The arum *(Arum maculatum)*, also called lords-and-ladies or cockoo-pint, is a good medicine for the genitals, for the bulbous flower heads are like a penis in the vagina. Fenugreek pods resemble the stinger of scorpions, and were thus considered a good remedy for scorpion stings. Seeds of rose hips and hawthorn fruit are hard as rocks—a sure sign that they dissolve kidney stones. Writhing earthworms help against gout, as they are twisted like gout fingers. The attempt to capture the signatures systematically and scientifically remains superficial, however, and has lost the direct access to the underlying spiritual essence—so, though not completely without insight, it ultimately turned out to be a dead end.

Nonetheless, the doctrine of signatures is still not completely obsolete. The principle is found, for example, in the flower essences of Edward Bach. The fast-growing Indian jewelweed *(Impatiens glandulifera)*, whose seed heads suddenly explode after ripening, are used as a remedy for states of impatience. The loose, puffy, feathery seed stocks of clematis, which in winter can be seen high up in the trees, represent the floating white clouds common to the floating state of mind of the daydreamer and are used as the flower remedy to treat it. Another example is the now-fashionable chaga mushroom *(Inonotus obliquus)*, which attacks the white trunks of birch trees like a black canker and is traditionally used in Siberia for cancer cures.

Roots and Wortcunners

If the Vedic Indians needed a medicinal plant, they used the whole plant: root, leaf, and flower, part of the respectful manner of dealing with plants—nothing should be wasted (Zysk 1996, 247). The Cheyenne and many other indigenous peoples do it in the same way. Even if the entire plant is used, generally the root is considered the most powerful healing part. In many cultures, herbalists are called root diggers—*rhizotom* (root diggers) by the ancient Greeks; *oertkaennare* in Sweden and wortcunners in English; and, even today in the Alps, as rooters *(Wurzer* and *Wurznerin)*, root men *(Wurzelsepp)*, and root maids (Wurzelweib). It was understood that the plant's root, which penetrates easily into the dark depths of the earth, penetrates easily into the dark interior of the body and with its strength can drive out the "worms" and render them harmless.

Plants are, as stated in the Rigveda, beings of light (devas) from heaven. The worm beings are averse to light; they cannot bear the light of heaven that the plants possess. That is why they must yield and disappear. The healers support the plants with the power of the word. Both "worm" and "root"—and also "word"—can be traced back to the Indo-European word *uert,* which means "wind, turn, screw."[25] The healing word is similar to the root: It winds out of the depths of the soul of the speaker and penetrates the soul and the body of the patient. Together, the root (Anglo *wyrt,* Old English *wort,* Old Norse *urt*), or the herb and the word, the healing chant, or incantation, bring healing (Storl 2012, 15–16). For this reason, the strongest plants are called *wort*—adderwort, banewort (belladonna, *bane* = deadly poison; Old High German *ban*), mugwort, lungwort, figwort, liverwort, elderwort, bloodwort, motherwort, Saint-John's-wort, feltwort (mullein), nipplewort (the flower buds have the signature of nipples and were thus used as a tea to wash inflamed nipples), tetterwort (celandine, used against the tetter worm, meaning various skin problems, such as eczema, etc.), and so on. Thus, one can see how much cultural history already lies in the name of the plants.

CHAPTER 6

The Transitional Period and the Christian Middle Ages

Destroy the web of the nettles' roots,
destroy the burrows of moles, adverse to light
and heave the earthworms into the light of day.
> WALAFRID STRABO, DE CULTURA HORTULUS,
> EARLY NINTH CENTURY

I invoke with Christ's words and
with a corpse's hand I stroke away all diseases and pain.
Your faith can help you
and may the Lord Jesus Christ bless you
and strengthen and rejuvenate
in the name of . . .
Amen!
> CHRISTEL LEHMANN-ENDERS, WAS DIE SCHWARZE KUH SCHEISST
> DAS NIMM ...: VOM ABERGLAUBEN, HEILEN UND BESPRECHEN IM
> SPREEWALD, 2000

The Latvian healing charm at the beginning of this chapter is spoken three times, while the patient is stroked with the hand of a recently deceased person.

In 391 CE, Emperor Theodosius I declared Christianity the state religion in the Roman Empire. Polytheism was banned and the pagan temples were destroyed. Although there seems to have been a few Christian monastic communities in Gaul, and some of the Germanic mercenaries who had served in the Roman legion had included Christ as one of their gods, on the whole, the conversion of the barbarians would drag on for several centuries; Christianity was initially confined, for the most part, to the former Roman Empire. The Irish Celts voluntarily accepted the new doctrine in the seventh century in order to use it as an ideological weapon against the heathen Angles and Saxons, who had settled in Britain after the departure of the Romans. Gregory the Great, pope in Rome from 590 CE to 604 CE, sent the first missionaries to Britain to convert the Saxons who worshiped the "devil Wodan." When the Romans finally succeeded, the converted Saxons themselves sent missionaries back to the continent in order to bring the gospel to their tribal relatives who still lived there ("the good magic of the gospels"). The best known of these missionaries was Winfrid, who was canonized as Saint Boniface and was under the protection of the Frankish-Merovingian rulers. The Baltic and Slavic missions occurred later, and it wasn't until 1200 CE that paganism was extinguished in Scandinavia.

In the former Roman Empire, Galenic medicine (humoral pathology), the classification of medicine into "hot" and "cold," "dry" and "wet" qualities, persisted. Benedictine monks practiced this sort of Galenic medicine less to liberate the sinner from their just punishment than demonstrate Christian charity. However, the majority of the clergy had no tolerance for medicine that thwarted the plan of God. God alone will heal if He wills it. Had he not spoken, "I am the Lord who heals you!" (2 Moses 15:26)? Who should presume to interfere?[1] Pope Gregory the Great took the view that the suffering of the body leads to the purification of the soul. Man should be educated to endure suffering. The health of the soul is more important than the health of the body (Stille 2004, 25). Disease is, then, the natural consequence of sin, so it is virtually sinful to do something about it, save for the recitation of the apostolic prayer and the sprinkling of holy water, which shoos away the devil. Pilgrimages to chapels and churches, in which the relics of martyrs are kept, were also legitimate responses to illness. As recently as 1229 CE, the English bishop William Blois said that it would be enough if patients took communion once a week and received the Anointing of the Sick once a year (Chamberlain 2006, 37).

The use of healing herbs and healing chants was considered a sure sign of paganism. It was also assumed that, among the non-believing barbarians, the Celts and especially the Germanic people, the healers, usually women, could only be evil. Had not the church father Tertullian said that women were the gateway to the gates of the devil? Did not sin and death enter the world through a woman? Tertullian wrote that the daughters of men had been courted by fallen angels and had received the knowledge of the secret power of the plants, so to speak, in payment for their prostitution (Tertullian, *De cultu feminarum*, Chapter II). In general, the Church did not think much of the abilities of women. Had not Hippocrates recognized that women are governed by their uterus (Greek *hysteria*)? Obviously, they are naturally hysterical and incapable of logic and rationality. The chatter of healing chants with which they addressed herbs and the sick is an expression of their weak brains and could only be based on the inspiration of the devil (Chamberlain 2006, 48).

Herbalism and healing spells were thus considered not only stupid, but also unchristian. Healers have sinned against God's order. Many Church synods and councils forbade healing with such "occult" means, including the Synod of Ancyra (Ankara, 314 CE), the Council of Laodicea (364 CE), the Council of Agde (507 CE), and several others. The Holy Synod convened by Boniface Liftinae (743 CE) in Hennegau prohibited collecting so-called Freya's bedstraw (aromatic, sweet-smelling herbs placed in or near the bed of mothers and their newly born child; Latin = *petenstro;* see page 182 for more details). The penitential books, such as that of Bishop Burchard of Worms, give insight as to what and how the old customs were forbidden. The bishop asks in his penitential (Poenitentiale, 9.3): "Did you collect herbs while speaking prayers other than the singing of the Creed and the Lord's Prayer? If so, you have to do penance with ten days on bread and water."

Bishop Gregory von Tours (539–594 CE) demanded the abolishment of all medicine in general, allowing only Christian miracle cures. Miracle cures would incidentally also be more impressive to the barbaric infidels than the rational Galenic medicine. It would amaze the stubborn, recalcitrant pagan nations. For example, near Lake Constance, Saint Gall healed the daughter of an Alemannic chief and stood henceforth under his protection. Thus, the monastery of the Abbey of Saint Gall became the nucleus for the conversion of the entire southern German region and all the way to Vienna. Saint Martin allegedly brought two dead people back to life again. And the Anglo-Saxon missionary Walburga, the niece of Boniface, calmed a rabid dog when she was abbess of the convent in Heidenheim (Germany), saved a child dying of starvation with three stalks of grain, and calmed storms. Every year a drop of precious healing oil drips out of her reliquary shrine. If that didn't impress the heathens!

Cloister Gardens

Despite the threat of hell and the lure of heaven, despite pressure and ban, the common people continued to go to the wise old women knowledge-able in healing when illness plagued them, and still used the traditional herbal remedies in connection with the healing incantations and sayings. That must have driven the religious brothers almost to despair. In order to not lose the new converts, concessions had to be made. Even the Holy See, Pope Gregory the Great, wrote to the missionaries in England (*Registrum epistolarum* 11, 37) that they should not destroy the sanctuaries of the pagans but should purify them with holy water; only the idolatry should be eliminated.[2] "And since they are wont to kill many oxen in sacrifice to demons, a festival should be designed for them, so that on the day of the dedication or on the anniversaries of the holy martyrs whose relics are deposited there . . . they may make for themselves tents with the branches of trees around these temples that have been changed into churches, and celebrate religious feasts" (Mone 1823, 105).

These were clever tactics. Furthermore, the idols that could not be Christianized were to be made into fiends, and the interest that the converts still had for these degenerate gods would be neutralized by the Church by providing remedies to protect against these powers or, on the other hand, portraying the idols as in need of redemption and offer possibilities for their salvation (Baechtold-Staeubli and Hoffmann-Krayer 1987, Vol. 3, 1635).

The Church began to make other compromises. As we have seen (page 53), the four-armed cross became ever more dominant in Christian symbolism, and the monotheistic divinity evolved into the Trinity. The Christian festivals were fitted to the annual rhythms, adapted to the natural calendar, so, for example, the birth of the Savior Jesus now fell on the winter solstice, although no one knows when the Rabbi Yeshua was truly born. The annual pagan herbal blessing became Christian and was placed on Assumption Day (August 15th); the blessing formula had been established since the ninth century. The saints took the place of the old

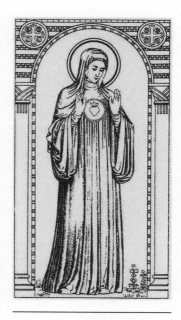

Saint Gertrude

deities, such as the bringer of gifts, Saint Nicolas, who replaced Old Man Winter, Father Christmas, or Little Father Frost;[3] and John the Baptist, who took the place of the Sun God or the Sun Goddess at the summer solstice festival. In Germany, Saint Gertraud (English Gertrude), daughter of the Frankish ruler Pepin of Landen, took the place of Ostara, the ancient goddess of spring. Her name day (March 17th) marks the beginning of the agricultural year. It is in the farmers' almanac even today:

> Gertrude
> leads the cow to the grass,
> the horse to the plough
> the bee to its maiden flight.

Every day became consecrated to a Christian saint, and some of them still showed quite a few characteristics of the pagan deities that they had replaced. It all went far beyond the contents of the Greek-Hebrew

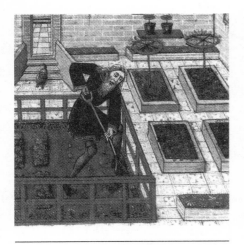

A monk gardening

Bible. Simple clergymen from the lower classes also brought many pagan ideas into the theology. For them, weather, magic, the presence of giants, dwarves, and elves was not strange. So in terms of cultural anthropology, one can speak not only about the Christianization of the forest cultures, but also of a "Celtic-ization" and "Germanization" of Christianity. The village wise women knowledgeable in healing could now confidently, under the guise of Christianity, continue with their healing.

As part of this development, the monks now planted herb gardens in their cloisters. Of course, they did not grow the wild herbs and roots that the old herbal women and leech doctors used, but such plants that grew in the Holy Land and that are mentioned in the scriptures. The herbs that grow around the Mediterranean Sea, in Asia Minor, and that are at home in Greece and Italy, where the sacred feet of the apostles had touched the ground, were suitable as medicinal plants. Benedictine monks coming from sunny Italy brought seeds and roots with them in their bags and backpacks to the north. Some of the plants that originated from southern countries and were common to cloister gardens include dwarf elder (*Sambucus ebulus*), pyrethrum (*Chrysanthemum* sp.), hibiscus, lovage (*Levisticum offinale*), parsley (*Petroselinum crispum*), rue (*Ruta graveolens*), and sage (*Salvia* sp.) (Marzell 2002, 18).

Unfortunately, the plants were quite foreign to the moist, harsh biotope north of the Alps. Time and time again, in the winter, like the breath of the devil, icy winds swept over the land and killed the poor plants. Was that not similar to the newly converted and baptized? The "neophytes"—Church Latin for the "freshly baptized" or "fresh converts"—were like the herbs in the small, square beds, vulnerable and in need of protection. Only too easily could the delicate flame of faith be blown out again. Both needed special care. High walls were needed to protect the Mediterranean, heat-loving herbs— fenugreek, rosemary, sage, pennyroyal, southernwood, wormwood, clary sage, and so on—to keep the cold at bay and radiate warmth.[4] The plants grew in neatly separated, tidy, and well-kept

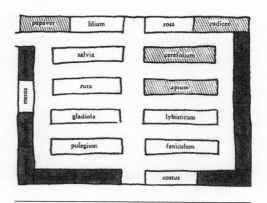

The *Herbalius (Herb Garden)* in the St. Gallen Cloister plans

flower beds from which the weeds—the symbols of sin—had to be carefully exorcised. The battle raged especially against nettles, as we learn from the diligent gardener Walafrid Strabo, the squinting monk.

The model for the emerging monastic gardens was the enclosed herb garden (herbularius) shown in the Abbey of St. Gall plans.[5] There, one can see, similar to the converts on church benches, the plantlets alien to the biotope in sixteen square beds. However, in most monastery gardens, such as in the *Hortulus* of the cloister of Abbey of Reichenau, such herbs eked out an existence in twenty-four beds. These monastery gardens were later models for farmers, and many of the cloister plants, including boxwood hedges, can be found in traditional farm gardens.

The herbs found in the monastery gardens and later also in the farmstead gardens, are the same ones that Charlemagne ordered cultivated in his country estates. This emperor's decree *(Capitulare de villis vel curtis imperialibus)* was given in 812 CE. These plants and trees were native to the natural vegetation of the Roman Empire but were not originally indigenous to northern Europe.

Fortunately for the monastery gardens and the emperor's venturous plans, the climate warmed during this time. The cold spell that had set the Migration Period in motion and forced the barbarians to the south was over; Greenland became ice-free, and the Vikings who had settled there were able to farm and even grow crops. The cultivation area for wine stretched northward from southern Scandinavia to Scotland. It was not until the fourteenth and fifteenth centuries that it become colder again (Behringer 2009, 106–107).

The Pharmacopoeia of Lorch, Germany

During the reign of Charlemagne, who was crowned by the pope as emperor (Caesar) of the newly arisen "Roman Empire" (as he believed it to be), the industrious Benedictine monks in the Lorsch Abbey (at Worms) wrote an herbal book, the *Macer Floridus*. In this work, some five hundred recipes and eighty-five plants (partly local) are listed. This book announces the new acceptance of medicinal plants, which were previously reserved for the heathens. The monks defended themselves successfully against critics of the book, who had long claimed that medicine is an intrusion into God's plan. The *Macer Floridus*, which is based on the medical teachings of antiquity, on Dioscorides, Hippocrates, and Galen, became the most influential work of monastic medicine for centuries and had even more impact than the writings of Hildegard of Bingen.

Religious Legends

The country people did not permit their medicine to be taken away, and they held on to their herbal traditions. For them, the native flora, the herbs near the doorstep, still played a major role in their lives. For the clergy, it became more difficult to demonize the commonly used herbs. By means of pious legends, the ancient common plants growing freely on the edges of the forests and fields were therefore incorporated into the Christian cosmos. Here are some examples.

Elder

Not only is the tree addressed in English with the respectful name of elder—and in German its name *Holunder* still evokes Holle, the ancient Earth Goddess—but under its branches also live the spirits that inhabited the farmstead, who still receive sacrifices. In addition, the elder proves highly effective as medicine. And sometimes, as in Scotland, the deceased would call on Sundays and sit down under the house elder when they wanted to visit with their descendants and relatives. They wore pointed hats made of birch bark to make it clear that they weren't evil spirits. Under these circumstances, it came to no good when the priests condemned the elder as a "witch's tree." So a pious monk thought up the legend that as the holy family was fleeing to Egypt, Mary hung the diapers of the Christ child to dry on the branches of an elder sapling. And how could a tree that bore the swaddling clothes of Jesus be a witch's tree?

Today, fever, gout, and toothache may still be discarded under an elder bush. Thus, another legend was needed to justify this practice, namely as already mentioned that Judas hung himself from one of its branches. Or it was told that the Savior banished seventy-seven "gouts" into the elder—all the conjured diseases that tweak and twitch here and there. A Swabian peasant is said to have seen it with his own eyes. As Odin and Freyr in ancient heathen times, it was now Christ and Peter who were walking in the countryside when suddenly the terrible gouts came shooting out from behind the bushes. Christ asked them, "You gouts, where are you going?" They hissed and giggled with their unpleasant falsetto: "To destroy the people, to bend crooked their limbs, to sew cracks on their skin, to poison their lives!" The Savior said, "You gouts, give yourselves up to the elder," and then they raced off to be captured by the elder and pulled by its suction into the depths of the earth. If not before, at least since then, we know that the elder can capture and destroy disease.

Ground Ivy

This tangy plant, which was already sacred to the heathens, flavored the daily ale and was consecrated to the Thunder God, protected the milk and the udders of cows, healed purulent ulcers, was worn at the midsummer festival as a wreath in the hair, and found its way into the Christian cultural cosmos. When the aromatic herb was collected before sunrise, one now said:

> Ground Ivy sprouts,
> I break you in in honor of our dear Lady

And in honor of our beloved Lord Jesus Christ. In the name
of . . .

The spicy herb continued to be used for dairy magic. If the cow, the
most important domestic animal of farmers, was not producing milk, a
bouquet of ground ivy was picked before sunrise and thrown into the
air with the following words:

I throw you into the clouds,
that our dear Lord Jesus Christ
will give me back my cheese and my whey. In the name
of . . .

Then some salt was sprinkled on it, and it was put into the cow's
fodder. A pious legend tells the following about the creeping, aromatic
plant: John met Jesus. Jesus asked, "John, why are you so sad?" "Why
should I not be sad," he replied, "my mouth is rotting!" The herb-wise
Savior advised him, "Get thee creeping jenny vines [one of the many
other names for ground ivy] and let them float about in thy mouth, and
thy mouth shall be healed" (Marzell 2002, 196).

Lady's Bedstraw

In English, the term "lady's bedstraw" refers to a yellow herbaceous
perennial plant *(Galium verum)* growing in meadows. However, lady's
bedstraw, Mary's bedstraw, or Virgin's bedstraw refer also to various aromatic herbs that were gathered for use in the childbed. When the time of
labor approached, the midwife prepared a bed of fragrant herbs—lady's
bedstraw, oregano, wormwood, Saint-John's-wort, wild thyme, ground
ivy, woodruff, betony, enchanter's-nightshade *(Circaea lutetiana)*, chamomile, sweetgrass, and others that were originally dedicated to the goddess Freya (Hoefler 1911, 116). These herbs for women in childbed were
expressly prohibited by Saint Boniface at the 742 CE Synod of Liftinae;
they contain aromatic oils and coumarins that have a calming effect on

mother and child, as well as an antibacterial effect. For the women of that time, the fragrance indicated the presence of the goddess. Also impossible to prohibit, Freya's bedstraw hence became Our Lady's bedstraw. The pious legend tells these were the same herbs in the manger in the stable in Bethlehem, which the ox and ass had not eaten, and upon which Mary laid the baby Jesus down to rest.

Linden Tree

The leaves of linden are delicate, light green, and full of light. They are heart-shaped, and, when the tree flowers in midsummer, swarms of bees are attracted to the sweet scent that emanates from the flowers. The buzzing of the bees sounds as if the lovely goddess herself were singing and humming. Linden tea sweetened with honey conjures up summer bliss again during the winter and warms the soul and the body so that colds vanish. It is no wonder that the forest peoples believed that the linden tree embodied the goddess. For the Germanic people, the tree reveals beautiful Freya herself; for the Baltic people, Laima, the goddess of fortune and destiny; for the Scythians, the oracle-speaking goddess of love; and the Slavs worshiped the linden tree as Libuse (Old Slavic *l'ub* = dear, lovely).

Christian missionaries cut down these "witch's trees" that often stood in the middle of villages and built chapels to Mary in their place. Statues of the Virgin Mary were carved from the soft, light wood, and soon the tree itself returned with the name Mary's linden. Not long after that, people started telling the legend that the holy family had rested under a linden tree during their flight, and that is why linden trees are a safe haven during lightning storms.

Mullein

Already during Celtic times, the tall flower stalks of mullein were immersed in pitch and then used as torches for religious ceremonies, especially at the summer solstice. The plant has been used as medicine since Druidic times. As they pulverized the herb, the Celtic healers sang this charm (Hoefler 1911, 266):

Sky above,
Earth below,
in the middle the healing plant.

The plant should actually be referred to as "queen's candle" (in German, it is called *Koenigskerze* = king's candle) because it was once dedicated to the Great Goddess. For herbal ordination on Mary's Ascension (August 15th), mullein is put in the middle of the herb bundle. In Lower Bavaria, healers sprinkled holy water on the flowering *Fackelkerze* (torch candle) or dipped it in spring water and then touched the sick while reciting the charm:

Our Lady moves about the land,
she carries the torch candle [mullein] in her hand.

It is reported that spontaneous healings took place thereby.

Ragwort, St. James Wort

This daisy family plant with its radiant, sunny yellow blossoms begins to bloom in the second half of July. Among the Celtic peasants, it was part of the natural rhythm of the seasonal calendar, well adapted to local climate. The opening of the flower petals was a sign that the grain harvest was imminent. Now was the time to sharpen the sickles, whet the scythes, and sweep the threshing floor. The flower is connected to the Celtic *Lughnasadh* festival—the harvest festival—and was consecrated to the Harvest God Lugh and the Grain Goddess Cerridwen. In other words, it was an important plant. Even medicinally, it was probably used by well-versed herbalists as a gargle for sore throat and tonsillitis and a tea to treat diarrhea as it was later still used in folk medicine (a practice that is not recommended without exact knowledge because ragwort contains toxic pyrrolizidines). As an amulet, the flower protected against enchantment. Christians dedicated it to the apostle James the Elder, whose name day falls on July 25th;[6] thus, one of the English common names is St. James wort. He is, among other things, the patron saint of grain.

Grazing animals avoid ragwort and will not eat the fresh, green plant, but if it gets into the hay or especially the silage, the pyrrolizidine alkaloids contained therein, and which the animals can no longer smell, can damage the liver. Therefore, it is now no longer a sacred plant but is strongly combated with herbicides. However, the use of heavy agricultural machines and overgrazing favor the germination, resulting in the increase of this weed in the fields.

Stinging Nettle

The stinging nettle practically embodies paganism and, in early Christian symbolism, was believed to contain the "heat of sinful passion" and likened by the afflicted convent gardener Walafrid to darts "tainted with a coat of corrosive poison." It was reinterpreted as one of the best means to expel ghosts and witches (Birkhan 2012, 114).

Saint-John's-Wort

When the yellow flowers that blossom proficiently at midsummer are crushed between the fingers, red "blood" swells out. For the Germanic heathens, it was the blood of Baldur, the mortally wounded Sun God; for the Celts, it was the blood of Belenos (Bel). Christians dedicated it to John the Baptist, whose blood was transferred into the plant when he was beheaded during the time of the solstice. So it happened that the devil cannot stand the herb but is forced to flee. *Fuga daemonum,* "demon flee," is one of its names. Even Paracelsus writes that Saint-John's-wort has the power to drive away imagined illnesses *(phantasmata)* and "worms." The Dominicans shared this belief; they ordered it burned as incense while questioning witches during the Inquisition so that Satan could not whisper any answers to them as they were being interrogated and tortured.

The small oil glands in the leaves make it seem as if they have many tiny holes, which were believed to have come about when the frustrated devil, in his rage, maltreated the leaves with a needle. Its signature, therefore, pointed toward the healing of stab wounds.

Herbs Consecrated to Mary

At Assumption, on August 15th, it is still a custom in many places in Europe for the women to gather a large bouquet of the strongest healing herbs and bring them to the church to be blessed. On this Day of Assumption, it is said, that the Mother of God goes to heaven, leaving back a blessing in the form of healing plants.

Before the pills and preparations of the pharmaceutical industry and the medical doctors gained the upper hand, a bundle of these healing plants was always in the household medicine cabinet with which the housewife kept the family members and the barn animals healthy. Not only did they bring relief for physical suffering, but they were also used for magical purposes. Some were placed under the roof to keep lightning from striking and hail from doing damage; others were hung in the barn to thwart the evil doings of the milk-witches; and still others were placed under the bed so that the joys of marriage remained. The calving cow was given an infusion of the healing herbs to drink. It was burned as incense during the Christmas holidays, and certain herbs from the bundle were even put in the coffin to protect the deceased.

What appears as a typical Catholic tradition here is much older than the Church and Christianity. The Hindus also celebrate the Festival of Nine Herbs (navapatrika) in the fall, when the goddess Durga visits the human world and then departs. Again, the women collect the healing and magical herbs that they need for the year; here it is said that the goddess returns to the heavens to Shiva, but her blessing remains in the herbs.

The choice of mid-August for the herb consecration is not arbitrary. It is the heat of the hottest month of the year that stimulates the plants to produce particularly large amounts of essential oils and synthesize active ingredients. The forest peoples believed that, at that time of year, the Fire God, the fulfiller of all things, radiates healing powers into the herbs and then makes them available to the goddess. There is no better time to collect healing herbs. The composition of the herb bundle varies somewhat from region to region (Baechtold-Staeubli and Hoffmann-Krayer 1987, Vol. 5, 442).

The Palm of Palm Sunday

In many places in all of Europe, it is an old custom in the spring to walk around the fields "with the sun," or clockwise, with all of the members of the farmstead, including servants (in earlier times) and the cattle. A wheel cross (sun wheel) decorated with flowers and evergreen foliage is carried along. Folklorists who have compared these processions of various peasant cultures are convinced that the custom can be traced back to the European megalithic period. Originally, participants were naked, drumming, dancing, and singing, between midnight and sunrise, to stimulate the growth of the fields in this way. This custom for the blessing of the fields was continued as a procession on Palm Sunday or Ascension under the auspices of the Church.

The Palm Sunday processions in southern Germany and in parts of Switzerland contain archaic elements. The "Palm," which is supposed to represent the palm leaves with which the people cheered Jesus when he rode on a donkey into Jerusalem, consists of a wheel cross, embellished with seven plants: evergreens like yew, juniper, white fir, spruce, and common box, as well as the fresh green shoots of willow and beech. The green twigs are braided into a wreath and fastened to a cross made from elder wood—this elder has to be peeled, however, so that no "witch" can hide between the wood and the bark. The green wheel cross is attached to a long hazel rod; for the ancient pagans, hazel was always an intermediary between the mundane and the otherworld, between the humans and the spirits. Here, we see yet another ancient pagan custom that continued in Christian garb.

Blackthorn (Sloe)

This thorny shrub with black bark, suddenly erupts at the spring equinox in white efflorescense, even before any of its green leaves appear. It was once consecrated to the gloomy Winter Goddess (Celtic Morrígan), who turns into the White Goddess of spring at this time of year. The ancient Britons considered blackthorn a witch's shrub. The witches made death spells by muttering curses while thrusting the sharpened thorns into wax dolls that represented their victims; and a blackthorn winter is a phrase for a relapse of winter, which can freeze the spring flowers.

Although it was considered a witch's tree, the blue sloe fruits are edible (only after a frost) and have been a popular wild fruit since the Stone Age. Although sloe berries were used as an ingredient in beer brewing, it was considered a tree of misfortune. The black, thorny branches were used as a crown of thorns for crucified Jesus in Christian iconography. The legend, however, says that the blackthorn protested its role in Christ's passion, so God took pity and showered it overnight with thousands of white flowers.

Chicory (Blue Weed)

With chicory, we are dealing with a plant that probably already had a sacred status and was revered in megalithic times when the sun was imagined as a cosmic stag with golden antlers. The blue flowers open at dawn and, like sunflowers, orient themselves to the sun. Like a hind, they follow the cosmic Sun Stag through the year as he jumps across the heavenly mountain—germinating and sprouting at the spring equinox when he takes the first leap. The higher the sun rises in the first half of the summer, the higher grows chicory and then flowers in response. In the fall, chicory follows the sun back into the depths, wilts entirely, and withdraws. Chicory, which opens its bright, sky-blue flowers in the sun and then closes them again around noon, embodies like no other plant the Vegetation Goddess, mistress of the Sun Stag. The chicory's blue eyes gaze only at the sun. When it rains and the sky is overcast, the flowers remain closed. Old names of chicory are *Hindlauf* (hind's run), *Sonnenwirbel* (sun whirl), or *Solsequium* (*sol* = sun, *sequi* = follow). In the Middle Ages, the root was dug as a medicinal plant or for magical purposes with a deer antler or a gold-plated tool (gold is the metal of the sun).

In the Middle Ages, one no longer saw the chicory as the daughter of the goddess of vegetation and the beloved of the Sun Stag. Instead one told the story of a girl who was standing by the roadside and always looking with her blue eyes to the east for her dearest, a young knight, who had ridden in that direction in the crusade to liberate the Holy Land from the Saracens. The others in the village teased her and said she should rather take another. But she remained faithful and declared, weeping, "I would rather become a flower on the wayside than stop crying." God heard her and turned the maiden into beautiful chicory flowers, also called "blue sailors."

Another legend, told by priests for pedagogical reasons, tells of Jesus as he was traveling with his disciples on a hot, dusty day and came across a maiden by a well. "Please give us some water; we are thirsty," he said. "Am I your servant?" she answered cold-heartedly. "Fetch the water yourself!" At that, Jesus cursed the maiden to become a wayside flower until judgment day.

Cowslip

The cowslip has many common names including key flower, key of heaven, and Our Lady's keys because it resembles the bundle of keys, which was the prerogative of the housewife, the *hûsfreyja,* to carry. Freya—the name means "free woman" or "lady"—unlocked the heavenly gate with this beautiful yellow-blossoming flower so that the warm spring rush came in and brought gladness to all hearts.[7]

Other common names include herb Peter and Key of Heaven because the missionaries of the new faith took this key away from Freya and gave it to Saint Peter, who had replaced Thor, the god of weather. However, the saint did not open the door for seasonal change but to the pearly gates of heaven so the blessed could enter when their time on Earth was over.

The legend tells that the devil one day climbed the ladder into heaven to see what the competition was up to. When good old Peter saw the sneaky, ugly, horned, furry devil, he was so startled that he dropped his key ring. When the ring fell to the ground, the keys turned into cowslip flowers. Since Saint Peter had once held it in his holy hand, it is said that the plant still has the power to expel demons— (and it also is said to help acrobats and roofers from getting dizzy at great heights). So, when the cattle became ill and the reason was not known, one picked cowslips early in the morning before sunrise on Saint Walpurgis Day (April 30th), made a powder from the plants, and put it in the cattle's fodder (Marzell 2002, 176).

Herb Robert, Storkbill, Robert Geranium

Since Herb Robert has seedpods reminiscent of stork beaks, it is dedicated to the crane or the stork that brings little bundles of joy (children). The stork's colors, black and white plumage and red beak and legs, are the colors of the goddess and show it to be a bird of Mother Goose. The stork fetches the children from the world of the returning ancestors, from the Holle pond.

In addition to its use for erysipelas and as a hemostatic, an astringent wound-healing agent, the herb was also worn as an amulet or placed under the bed as a signal to the spirits that one is ready to receive a child. The herb became known as Herb Robert after the conversion; its namesake, Saint Rupert or Robert, was a Franciscan evangelist from Salzburg, Austria, who died in 715 CE. He is regarded as the apostle of Bavaria and protector of salt. He is invoked for erysipelas and pediatric seizures.

Fireweed, or Willow Herb

In folk medicine, this circumpolar plant of the evening primrose family is used as an emollient and a dispersing and slightly astringent remedy. As part of the psychedelic fly agaric ritual, the Siberian shamans, and possibly even the Germanic and Slavic peoples, drank a tea from fireweed leaves. Whatever other uses it may have had are unknown. Since the lovely red-flowering plant appears after a forest fire and densely covers the area, Americans named it fireweed. Because sufferers appealed to Saint Anthony for help when they were afflicted with St. Anthony's fire (erysipelas, also called *ignis sacre,* or holy fire and ergot poisoning), the plant was also called St. Anthony's herb (French *ossier de Saint-Antoine* = St. Anthony's willow). Ergot poisoning leads to vasoconstriction, the dying off of fingers and toes, and, because of an LSD-component, hellish hallucinations. Since Saint Anthony, the holy hermit, had himself withstood an onslaught of hordes of terrible demons, the afflicted prayed to him for help.[8]

Greater Celandine, Swallowwort

This plant is called "goldwort" or "golden plant" in many Slavic and Germanic languages for its orange golden juice and is used widely in folk medicine for healing everything from hepatitis to cancer. It is not to be recommended, however, as the sap is toxic. In ancient times, it was called swallowwort because it was believed that swallow mothers carry it in their beak back to their nests and then brush the eyes of the newly hatched swallow chicks so that they could see well. The juice, diluted with milk or morning dew and rubbed around the eyes, is said to heal eye diseases of all kinds.[9] In the folk medicine of Maria Treben and Maurice Mességué, it is still used in this way but only by a knowledgeable healer. Since Christ made the blind see, greater celandine was dedicated to the Savior himself.

Juniper

As we have seen, juniper has been used since the Paleolithic era as medicine, as wood for the funeral pyre of the dead, and as sacred incense. After being initially demonized, this evergreen also found its place in the Christian cultural cosmos. For Estonians, it is said that Christ went to heaven from a juniper bush. In the Baltic regions, it is also said that Christ's cross was made of juniper wood; therefore, a stick from the wood also has the power to chase the devil into flight. And in an Italian legend, Mary took protection in the tree during her flight to Egypt (Marzell 2002, 49). A Norwegian blessing formula says:

> I eat juniper berries blue,
> and show the cross of Jesus.

Yarrow, Milfoil

Yarrow was one of the most powerful pagan healing plants. It is one of the best wound healers and gynecological herbs. Some of its common names are staunchweed, sanguinary, and nose bleed. In German, the most common name is *Schafgarbe*. The word *garbe* (Germanic *Garw*) as well as its English cognate "yarrow" (Old English *gearwe*) can be interpreted as "fast and complete healing." As a gynecological herb and love oracle plant, it was dedicated to the goddess Freya. This herb also found its way into the league of "Christian" plants with a sentimental legend: when Joseph hurt himself during carpentry work, the child Jesus ran to the meadow and fetched him the hemostatic herb.

Even the love oracle of young women who want to know who their paramour will be took on Christian traits. When picking the plant, they said:

> Yarrow, sweet yarrow, the first I have found,
> In the name of Jesus Christ I pluck it from the ground,
> As Jesus loved sweet Mary and took her for his dear,
> So in a dream this night,
> I hope my true love will appear.

The Saints and Their Plants

The heathen people saw aspects of the gods and nature spirits or their effects in the vegetation. The Great Goddess was present in most plants. Freya, as a Vanir goddess, was not only the goddess of love and the joy of life, but also the lady of the plants. Her necklace, *brisingamen,* is said to have consisted of sparkling gems; a rather far-reaching interpretation of this fine jewelry is the glowing green band of vegetation that is laid around her neck in early spring. The legend tells how, in autumn, Loki, the Harvest God, steals this necklace. In the spring, she gets it back. Freya, the lady of life-giving greens—the *Viriditas* as Hildegard of Bingen called it—was honored by the Germanic women who tended "leek gardens" with fresh green herbs, just as the gynecological herbs and yarrow, lady's mantle, chamomile, or the "goose herbs" (for example, the anticonvulsant, contractive silverweed cinquefoil and daisy) were consecrated to her as well.

Thor (Anglo-Saxon Thunar, German Donar), the thunder god in his appearance as the hairy Bear God Osburn (German *Goetterbaer,* Norse *Asbjoern*), was responsible for hairy herbs or those that encourage hair to grow, such as burdock or nettle. Since Thor is as powerful and strong as he is honest, the strongest and most powerful healing herbs were consecrated to him: bear plants such as bear root *(Ligusticum meum),* meadow hogweed *(Heracleum),* wild garlic, clubmoss *(Lycopodium),* or bearberry *(Arctostaphylos).* Since he bears a lightning hammer, plants that protect against lightening, such as thunder beard or houseleek *(Semper pervivum),* were dedicated to him. Plants with red flowers or fruits, such as the mountain ash (Scandinavian *Þorbjoerg* = Thor rescue), were also under his protection as well as herbs that are suitable for brewing beer, such as ground ivy, yarrow, sweet gale *(Myrica gale),* and wild rosemary *(Ledum palustre).* Just as his counterparts are—Zeus, Jupiter, Perkunas, or the Vedic Indra, who also possess lightning and thunderbolts—he is the lord of intoxication. The thunderer was the most popular god of the common people; he was like a great farmer, and in his hall the best beer was brewed. The oak, the tree most often struck by lightning, also belonged to all of these thunder gods.

Charms and shaman herbs, and hallucinogenic plants were, on the other hand, dedicated to shifty, unpredictable Odin, insofar as they were not associated with Tyr or Tiwas (Old High German Zius), the guardian of the true word.[10] Tyr was lord of all toxic or corrosive "wolf plants," such as daphne, wolf berry *(Belladonna),* spurge, and wolfsbane (monkshood, *Aconitum).* A German name for Arnica is "mountain wolf" *(Bergwolf),* because a wolf had bitten off Tyr's arm. Why? This is revealed by the story of the Fenris Wolf: The gods (Aesir) found a cute little wolf cub and took it with them to their castle. The little pup was incredibly voracious and grew from day to day. Gradually, the gods feared that he might become too strong and dangerous for them. They decided to put him on a chain, but he bared his teeth and would not allow it. So they invented a ruse: the dwarves were to forge a chain, finer than spider's thread; then, they would tell the wolf it was just a game to put this chain around his neck. But the mighty wolf distrusted the gods. He would only allow it if one of the gods would be willing to put his arm between his jaws. If they captured him, he would bite off the arm. Courageous Tyr volunteered. The filigree bondage held, and the god of the true word lost his arm.

All useless or smelly plants are classified as "dog plants." In German, they still call the scentless chamomile that has no healing power "dog-chamomile." The "dog rose" is the common rose and not a superior cultivated one; the tansy is a "dog fern," and berry bushes whose fruits are unwholesome are referred to as "dog cherry."

Horse plants are coarse, massive plants, like the "half a hack" (worn-out old horse) referring to the broad-leaved dock that is the bane of some farmers' fields, the horse fennel (meadow hogweed), or the horse chestnut, which cannot be eaten.

Besides these, there are toad plants, which have to do mostly with the uterus and birth—it should not be forgotten that the toad was a sacred animal for the heathens, which was not to be killed. Fox herbs, calf herbs, sheep herbs, snake herbs, and several others took the name of animals related to how their properties were classified.

These classifications are not rigid, however; they are fluent and have a poetic streak. Most plants have multiple names, and many of them refer to nature spirits, ancestral spirits, elves, or dwarves, which the wortcunner recognized in them. There were no academic botanists back then and there was no scientific, scholarly writing fixing a system of classification. Plants were their own beings. From what I have learned from modern indigenous or preliterate people, the various healers also had their own personal access to nature and plant spirits and often even had their own names for the herbs and roots with which they healed.

In the course of proselytizing, the missionaries replaced the many local deities, nature spirits, or, as they were called in the Baltic region, the many "little mothers" that populated nature with Christian saints and martyrs. Not only was there a saint for each institution and for each disease, but also the most important healing plants were assigned to them. The Church tried to give each herb a Christian name. The daffodils were changed to Joseph flowers, boneset to Saint Kunigunde's herb, bugleweed to Saint Catherine's herb or Saint Laurentius's herb, chamomile to Saint

Magdalene's herb, Freya's mantle to Mary's mantle, saxifrage to Jehovah flower, violets to Jesus floret, alpine leek to Saint Barbara's root or Saint John's root, anemone to Saint Gertrude's roses, calendula to Mary's gold (later marigold), geranium to Saint Robert's herb, and wild breastwort became the angelica consecrated to archangel Raphael. White wort was changed to Solomon's seal, forget-me-not became Mary's eyes, and so on. The aromatic forest herbs, which the monks later very gladly worked into their herbal brandies, fell under the protection of Saint Hubertus and the sacred stag, the solar animal that became associated with Christ, the bringer of light. Some of these names remain to this day, but most do not.

The saints and patron saints were responsible for healing those diseases and ailments that they had themselves suffered during their life or martyrdom. The Church tried to associate all healing plants with a matching patron. Today, we ask ourselves which molecular compounds—essential oils, tannins, alkaloids, flavonoids, glycosides, bitter substances, and so on—or active ingredients are contained in a medicinal plant. In the Middle Ages, they asked which saint was connected to the plant, which also told about its effects—if one knew the name of the saint of a particular plant, then one also knew what healing effect was to be expected. If the herb had the name of Saint Benedict, then one knew it would benefit the liver; were it the name of Saint Gerard, then it was known that it would expel gout; were it dedicated to Bernhard, it helped with a sore throat. Here are some examples that will help us understand the medieval vision of the medicinal plants.

Saint Apollonia

Already during her lifetime, Apollonia was known to possess miraculous gifts. She had blown her breath onto the idols of the heathens, who then fell to dust. As punishment, the "elderly Christian virgin" had all of her teeth broken out with sharp stones. Later legends say that, since she refused to deny the true Christian God, her teeth were individually torn out with red-hot tongs or her cheeks were maltreated by the hangman's servant for so long with a stick that her jaw broke and her teeth were shattered. In this way, she became the patroness against dental

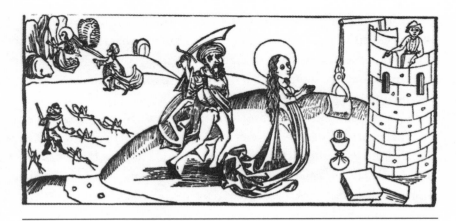

The saints stood by to help with whatever suffering they themselves had endured

complaints—with whatever suffering the saints had to endure themselves, they stood by to help.

Thus, Apollonia ruled over plants that help for toothache. Among them, the main one is the poisonous henbane *(Hyoscyamus niger)*, also called Apolloniawort and toothachewort. The seed pod of henbane carries the signature of molars. To kill the evil tooth worm, seeds were placed on hot coals or in hot pans. The suffering person sucked the smoke into the mouth via a funnel (Storl 2004b, 111ff.). (The smoke, being very poisonous, was not inhaled into the lungs.) In Bavaria, the "small, hairy tooth worms" were also driven out with the vapors of the "Apolloniawort"—which could refer to either henbane or monkshood *(Aconitum napellus)*—collected at midsummer. Using these plants was very dangerous business. No other root is as poisonous as monkshood (Baechtold-Staeubli and Hoffmann-Krayer 1987, Vol. 1, 552). In Upper Bavaria, the seeds of peony are called Apollonia grains and were strung on a string for teething children to bite on.

Saint Barbara

The three "holy Virgins," Saint Barbara, Saint Catherine (see below), and Saint Margaret, are really the Christianized versions of the three Celtic Matrons, the Beden of Gallo-Roman culture, the three Fates. In

196

German-speaking countries, they also appear as the three Beths (Anbeth, Warbeth, and Wilbeth or Ambeth, Wilbeth, and Barbeth), who once embodied the three women, as well as the three classes of Indo-European society:[11] Catherine, the Pure, the teaching class (priest Brahmins, druids, and scholars); Barbara, the military class (warriors); and Margaret, the class of common folk, the farmers and craftsmen. The colors of the three virgins are black (Barbara), white (Catherine), and red (Margaret)—these are the colors of the primordial goddess. Black Barbara, whose name day is celebrated around the beginning of winter (December 4th), is a warrior. She is symbolized by a tough crucifer plant that defies the icy winter like a warrior, the herb Barbara or winter rocket *(Barbara vulgaris);* no matter how cold and how much snow, the fat, shiny, mustard oil–containing leaves remain green. They are rich in vitamins and prevent the old winter disease, scurvy. In the late spring, as in a victory celebration over old man winter, this cress blossoms in sulfur-yellow flowers.

Yarrow *(Achillea millefolium),* one of the best wound-healing plants, which was once dedicated to the warrior Achilles, was also called a Saint Barbara herb in the Middle Ages. Saint Barbara also had "Barbara branches"—cherry twigs or hawthorn branches. On her name day, women cut and place some branches in water in the house. If they bloom for Christmas, then that is a good omen for the year: cattle and fields will be fertile, or the young woman will find a good man. According to an old Germanic and Slavic custom, the branch symbolizes the rod of life, life carrying on during the dark, "dead" time of winter. The flowering hawthorn branches of Glastonbury, the most sacred place of worship in England, which are delivered at Christmas to the British royal family each year, belong to this ancient pagan custom.

Saint Benedict

Saint Benedict is a heavyweight, which can already be seen by his name day, March 21st, the day of the spring equinox. In 529 CE, he founded the first monastery in Europe (Monte Cassino). The motto of his black-clad monks was "pray and work" *(ora et labora).* He was stern and drove the monks mercilessly. Several times, often having been put in the monastery

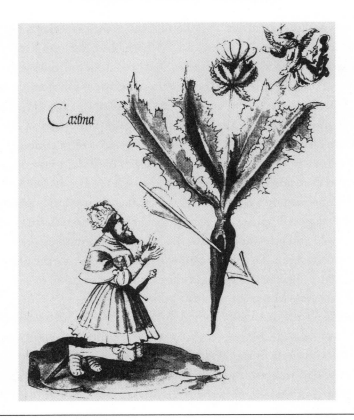

Charlemagne with carline thistle

involuntarily as a child, they tried to kill their strict disciplining abbot but to no avail. Then they developed a ruse: They laced the sacramental wine with the deadliest poisons, arsenic and monkshood; thus, when he would take a sip from the "blood" of the Lord at the celebration of mass, he would fall over dead. But when he then lifted the communion chalice, so the story goes, the poison balled up—thanks to his sacred aura—and crawled in the form of a poisonous viper over the edge of the cup. The cup, from which a snake is escaping, is still one of Saint Benedict's symbols.

Medicinal plants that are consecrated to him act exactly in this manner. They concentrate the poison in the body or in the liver and flush it out.

To these belong, in the first place, wood avens (herb Bennet, *Geum urbanum*), which is also called Saint Benedict's herb and the blessed thistle or Saint Benedict's thistle *(Cnicus benedictus)*. The roots of these herbs should be collected on March 21st, this saint's name day. The time around the spring equinox is indeed a good time to dig the root because the herb has not yet sent out a shoot and the active ingredients are concentrated in the root. The liver detoxifier, the silver thistle *(Carlina acaulis)*, is also assigned to this saint. The latter is also called carline-thistle because, during a plague, an angel appeared to the Emperor Charlemagne and instructed him to shoot an arrow into the air. The root of the plant where the arrow would hit the ground was the right remedy; Charlemagne's arrow landed near a silver thistle.

Saint Fiacre

Saint Fiacre (Fiacrius, Fèvre, Ficker) was an Irish monk who settled in the forest near Paris. There, he stuck his walking stick into the ground, and it became a beautiful garden. He became the patron saint of market gardeners. Since he did not like women, he gave them no access to his garden; whether the holy man therefore suffered rectal pain and rectal varicose veins cannot be said. In any case, all herbal remedies for hemorrhoids are dedicated to him, which include lesser celandine *(Ranunculus ficaria)* and knotted figwort *(Scrophularia nodosa)*, also known as greater figwort. As we have already seen, "fig" meant either piles or warts. Another figwort was tormentil *(Potentilla erecta)*, which has an astringent, styptic, and drying effect.

Incidentally, in Vienna, the horse carriages are named *Fiaker* after Saint Fiacre, and the stalls where Parisian coachmen once parked their teams is today's Rue de Saint-Fiacre, the very place where the saint had his garden.

Saint Gerard

Saint Gerard (Gerhard) was a Lombard, who proselytized in Hungary. It is said that he was martyred there by being placed into a barrel studded with nails and rolled into the Danube where he drowned. But even before his martyrdom, he suffered from violent pain—namely from gout (podagra). That's why all gout herbs, primarily the goutweed *(Aegopodium podagraria)*, are also called "St. Gerard's-herb," and are consecrated to Saint Gerard.

Saint Catherine

The name of the martyr Catherine (Katharina) means "the pure" (Greek *katharos* = pure, clean). She is said to have been a highly learned, beautiful king's daughter to whom the Christ child appeared in a dream and on whose finger he put an engagement ring. She received an invitation from the Roman emperor to a sacrificial feast, but, when she came to meet him, she proved to him with learned words that his gods are idols. The emperor then called fifty philosophers to debate her, but she defeated them all and converted them to the "one and only true religion." The angry emperor had her tortured on a wheel with pointed knives and nails, and finally beheaded. Her symbol is characterized by a piece of the wheel, a sword, and a palm frond (Keller 1979, 309). The sword symbolizes her mental sharpness, among other things. Of course, all cleansing herbs are consecrated to her, such as the toadflax *(Linaria vulgaris)*, which was once called "Catherine-herb" because it cleans "within and without" (Marzell 1979, Vol. 2, 1324). She was tortured and beheaded, so her herbs also work against migraines and are wound-healing plants, such as the marsh yarrow *(Achillea ptarmica)*, the Roman chamomile *(Anthemis nobilis)*, or the creeping bugle *(Ajuga reptans)*. She is the patron of barbers and surgeons.

Saint Lawrence

Saint Lawrence, or Laurentius, has his name day in the middle of the very hot "dog days" of summer, on August 10th. But not only that: The Roman emperor who wanted to force him to do pagan sacrifices had him beaten with lead blocks and set him between red-hot plates. Then, he was put on a grate over a constantly maintained fire and slowly roasted to death. It's no surprise that he is connected to the herbs that relieve burns. These include common bugle (Lorenz herb, *Ajuga reptans*), sanicle *(Sanicula europaea)*, or the more toxic white swallowwort (St. Lawrence herb, *Vincetoxicum hirundinaria*), which was considered a diaphoretic means.

Saint Lucian

Saint Lucian, or Lucius, attempted to convert the wild mountain people in the Graubuenden region of Switzerland.[12] But not all seemed to have been in agreement with the message of the gospel because they threw him into a well and threw stones in behind him. Apparently, because some converts saved him, he did not die. However, he suffered from severe bruises; therefore, medicinal plants that assist in such contusions are dedicated to him, such as arnica *(Arnica montana)*, which is also called Lucian's herb (Dutch *Sint Luciaans kruid*, French *herbe de Saint-Lucien*).

Saint Mary

The Virgin Mary appeared, as we have seen, to replace the Vegetation Goddess, the flowered bride of the Sun God. For the Germanic people, she took the place of Freya (Frigg, Erda). In medieval art, the Mother of God is shown in flowering meadows, in rose bushes, in grain fields, or with healing plants, especially with mullein, red or purple dead nettle, lily of the valley, daisy, speedwell, columbine, lady's slipper, and silverweed. The white spots on the leaves of milk thistle were said to have come from a few drops of milk from her chaste breast. The spots on the early purple orchid *(Orchis maculata)* are the traces of the Mother's tears as she wept for her crucified Son. Many hemostatic plants are dedicated to her, such as burnet-bloodroot or pimpernel *(Sanguisorba officinalis);* the dark crimson color of the flower head came—it is said in the Allgaeu region of southeastern Germany—from one drop of her menstrual blood when it fell to the ground as she was on her way to Elizabeth to tell her of her immaculate conception and pregnancy.

Saint Roch

Saint Roch (Rochus, Rocco), who gave away his inheritance and became a simple monk, was one day infected with the plague. He became an outcast and retired to a modest hut deep in the forest. A dog came, brought him bread, and licked the sores on his leg. Even an angel—it could have been a raven—descended from heaven to help him. With his wide-brimmed pilgrim's hat, broad cape, long walking stick, and a dog at his side, he has

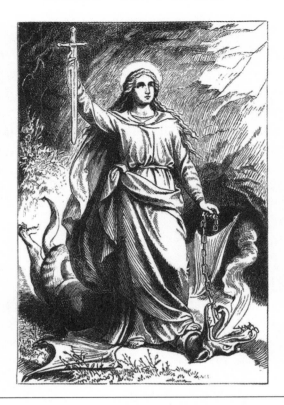

Saint Margaret

a similar appearance to Odin, the wanderer. Of course, he was destined to become the patron saint of the plague, and also for pain in the knees; butterbur *(Petasites hybridus)*, which, as herbalist Leonhart Fuchs wrote, "forces the poison of the pestilence out through sweat," is dedicated to him. Other plague plants, like the poisonous herb-paris *(Paris quadri-folia)*, were also dedicated to this plague saint. The poisonous blueberry of herb-paris, which has the signature of a plague boil, was sometimes placed in the house altar under the image of the saint.

Saint Margaret

Saint Margaret is said to have been the daughter of a pagan priest in Antioch. In prison, where she was tortured with iron combs and torches, a huge dragon appeared that swallowed her. In his belly, she crossed herself, whereupon the dragon burst and she came out again unscathed. This miracle made her the patron saint of women in labor. Her cult spread in northern Europe from the sixth century. She was one of three holy virgins, the successor to the triple goddess (see also above, Saint Barbara). At the same time, she became the patroness of the common people and the peasants; illegitimate girls were also under her protection. It was a common practice to name such girls Gretel, Greta, or Margaret in German and in English, Margaret (or Margret), Peggy, or Maggie. Not only did she protect women's fertility, but she also protected the fertility of the fields and meadows. And since the peasant people, compared to the knights and clerics, are so numerous, the oxeye daisy *(Chrysanthemum leucanthemum)* and the common daisy *(Bellis perennis)* are dedicated to her for there are many of them as well. Other aster family flowers with yellow centers and white ray petals such as feverfew *(Chrysanthemum parthenium)* or chamomile also belong to her. The latter two played an important role in birth.

Saint Veronica

Saint Veronica is known for the veil with which she, full of mercy, dried the sweat off the face of the Savior, when he, in his bitter Passion, had to carry the heavy cross through the streets of Jerusalem. He had such a powerful radiance that his face is preserved as in a photographic plate on the cloth.[13] To Saint Veronica are assigned diaphoretic, detoxifying herbs such as veronica or speedwell *(Veronica officinalis)*.

The Comeback and Metamorphosis of Heathen Customs

The Church thus conformed to fit in with the folk ethos. It Christianized and incorporated what had always been part of common culture. In this way, the midwives, wise old women, and leech doctors who had the basic knowledge could continue to carry out their vocations. Healing continued to be done with incantations and herbs. For the simple village priest, that was not a problem as long as the people were baptized, came to church on Sundays, and participated in the sacraments. The ancestral healing spells, the evocation of healing plants, the spells, and the incantations now became prayers and benedictions and were carried out in the name of the Father, the Son, and the Holy Spirit. And the few who did not participate, the renegades, retreated further into the wilderness and heath.

The transition period was long. For a few centuries, the old gods and spirits rumbled on in the rural areas. In modified form, they played into the customs and into the so-called superstitions. Let us take for an example a current superstition about horseshoes. Horseshoes are nailed on goalposts, houses, barn doors, and ceiling beams with three nails to keep away bad luck, lightning, evil spells, and the devil—"Let the devil get stuck there by his claws!" Probably, it goes back to the widespread custom of the Indo-European horse sacrifice after which, as we have heard, the horse's skull was nailed to the gable boards of the house. It is said that the ground that Odin's horse touches will be fruitful. The hoof print was believed to bring blessings, although in medieval superstitions it became a sign of the devil.

One saying recorded in 1850 in Lincolnshire, England, still bears distinctly pagan elements of the transitional period. When nailing a horseshoe to the bedpost to keep away chills, nightmares, and the fiends that ride people in their sleep, one recites (Chamberlain 2006, 144):

> Father, Son, and Holy Ghost
> Nail the devil to this post.
> Thrice I mite with Holy Crok,
> With this meil I thrice do knock,
> One for God,
> And one for Wod (Woden)
> And one for Lok (Loki).

There are many examples of this kind, in which pagan elements in folk medicine mingle with Christian Mediterranean tradition. A further typical example, recorded in the eighteenth century in England, has to do with the collection of clubmoss for the purpose of curing eye diseases; Pliny (23–79 CE) had already written that the Celts used it to treat such conditions. The common clubmoss (*Lycopodium clavatum*) was probably not intended but rather the northern firmoss or fir clubmoss (*Huperzia selago*). The ointment was applied to the eyelids. English wortcunners took the northern firmoss on the third day after the new moon, when the crescent moon is just visible again. Just in the period in which the crescent moon goes down beneath the horizon, wortcunners would make a cut in their hand with a knife, show the bleeding wound to the moon, and say,

> As Christ healed the issue of blood,
> do thou cut what thou cuttest for good.

They then took some northern firmoss and wrapped it in a white cloth. From the nearest spring, they drew the water they would use to cook the herb. To make a salve, it could be cooked with butter from the milk of a cow milked for the first time (Chamberlain 2006, 149).

Lacnunga and the Anglo-Saxon Lay of Herbs

A collection of various texts, called *Lacnunga* (Anglo-Saxon for "therapeutic products"), gives an insight into the healing of West Germanic Anglo-Saxons. The charm *wid færstice* (against a sudden stitch) mentioned therein is actually a shaman charm, which philologists did not detect because, for a long time, they knew nothing or little about shamanism.[14]

The charm is about the wild female demons who come rushing over the hills with loud cries. The leech doctor (*læce*), the shamanic healer, deflects the hail of their magical, disease-bearing arrows by taking up a shield of linden wood.[15] Whatever works for warding off real arrows and javelin projectiles, works for warding off magical arrows.

> Shield yourself now so that you may escape this attack.
> Out little spear if it be in here.
> [I] stood under the linden tree, under a light shield,

when the mighty women (mihtigan wif) declared their might
and yelling sent their spears (gyllende garas)
(*Lacnunga* 135, Charm against a sudden stitch; Pollington 2000,
229).

Shamans deflect the spirit spears and send them back to where they came from. Then, they turn to the stricken patient and sing out the spirit arrows. They threaten them with the power of the blacksmith, who makes iron structures with lightning (hammer blows) and fire and was indeed always considered a magical personality among the ancient peoples. Perhaps the archetypal magician Wayland is meant or Odin the Shaman God himself, who strikes the nine-herbs disease worm just as the blacksmith strikes the iron on the anvil. The shaman sings the charm three times in the mouth of the patient, in the right and in the left ear, and on the spot penetrated by the magic arrow:

> Out, little spear, if it be in here.
> A smith sat, hammered a knife,
> a small weapon iron, a serious wound!
> Out, little spear, if it be in here.
> Six smiths sat, wrought slaughter spears.
> Out, spear, be not in, spear,
> if there be in here a piece of iron
> the work of a witches, (hægtesse) it must melt away.

The leech doctor turns to the patient:

> If you were shot in the skin, or you were shot in the flesh,
> or were shot in the blood, or were shot in the bone
> or were shot in the limb,
> may your life never be threatened,
> If it were the gods' shot (Æsir gescot)
> or it were the elves' shot (Ylfa gescot)

or it were the witches' shot (Hægtessan gescot), I will
help you.
This is a cure to you for the gods' shot,
this is a cure to you for the elves' shot,
this is a cure to you for the witches' shot.
I will now help you.
There it [the disease] fled to the mountain; no rest did
it have.
Whole be you now, may the Lord help you!
Then take your knife and put it into the liquid (Pollington
2000, 229).

The herbal ointment is then applied, consisting of feverfew *(fefer-fuige),* red dead nettle *(reade netele),* and broad-leafed plantain *(weg-brade)* cooked in butter.

Another example from the transitional period, in which the heathen (Germanic-Celtic) and Christian-Mediterranean (Greco-Roman) elements were mixed in healing charms, is the Nine Herbs Charm *(Nine Worts Galdor)* from the eleventh century, in which Odin kills the "worm" with nine herbs. Let's look at the nine herbs—some have already been mentioned (see page 117)—in detail.

Mugwort *(Mugwyrt):* The herb consecrated to Mother Holle, known as an incense and a shaman's and midwife's herb since the Paleolithic age, is mentioned with good reason as the first in the Anglo-Saxon herbal charm.

> Remember, Mugwort, what you made known,
> What you arranged at the Great proclamation. You were
> called Una, the oldest of herbs,
> you have power against three and against thirty,
> you have power against poison and against infection,
> you have power against the loathsome foe roving through
> the land.

Plantain, waybread *(Wegbrade):* This plant, open to the forces of the East, which are light and healing, this tenacious, hemostatic, and wound-healing leech doctor's herb (Læce-wyrt), is mentioned in second place.

Stune: About this mysterious plant, the charm says:

> This plant is called stune, it grew on a stone;
> it stands against poison, it attacks against pain,
> Stiðe it is called, it attacks against poison,
> it drives off harmful things, casts out poison (Pollington 2000, 229).

Linguists have puzzled in vain about which plant stune could be. Candidates are the following:

- hairy bittercress *(Cardamine hirsuta),* a small cruciferous, edible in the spring;[16]
- the nasturtium *(Nasturtium officinale)* that grows near fresh spring water and was once important as a sacred healing plant for the Celts;17 and
- field pennycress *(Thlapsi arvense)* (Raetsch 2005a).

Atterlothe: The charm says the following about this plant:

> Now, Atterlothe, the lesser shall drive out the greater,
> The greater the lesser until the cure for both be with him (Pollington 2000, 213).

As with stune, it is not certain which plant atterlothe is. The Anglo-Saxon word attor (Germanic *aithro*) means "pus" or "poison." *Atter* could also possibly have to do with a poisonous adder. And *lathe* means "to loathe" (from the Germanic *laithoz*, which is related to the German *leid* = misery, and French *laid* = ugly). What plant could this one be?

- Barnyard grass *(Echinochloa crus-galli)* is a commonly encountered wild grass in root crop fields.[18]

- Betony *(Stachys officinalis)* is an herb that has been used magically elsewhere in *Lacnunga* "against night spooks, wicked elves, and nightmares."[19] Since ancient times, it has been basically used as a panacea and could be found in every monastery garden.

- Blueweed, viper's bugloss *(Echium vulgare),* due to its signature[20]—the cleaved scar looks like a snake's tongue—was used as a healing medium for snakebite.

- Christian Raetsch (2005a) suggested male fern or tansy.

- My personal candidate would be bistort *(Polygonnum bistorta)* whose astringent and antitoxin tannic effects have been treasured, and its roots also have the signature of a rolled snake, or the colon.

Chamomile: Chamomile, or mayweed, is the most popular medicinal herb in central Europe. It is used for wound healing and as an antifungal and antispasmodic; it helps with gastrointestinal discomfort, colic, internal and external inflammations, and is a gynecological healing plant. In Rhineland, Germany, it is said: "A good cup of chamomile tea helps more than three doctors do." The Anglo-Saxons called the plant *maythen* and *mægthe,* "maiden herb." In the charm, it says:

> Be mindful now, chamomile (maythe), of what you made known,
> of what you finished at Alorford, so that he should never give up his life for disease, once chamomile was prepared for his food (Pollington 2000, 213).

It is interesting that the healing plant is called upon to remember its characteristics, which is also the case with mugwort: "Remember, Mugwort, what you have proclaimed . . ." This rousing, this call to the plant, to remember is found in other traditional herbal medicine, such as that of the Native Americans. The plant spirits or devas are far away in the otherworld—they are not as present as animals are, for instance; they have to be awakened and reminded of their power.

The place mentioned in the charm, Alorford, is not necessarily a certain geographic name. In modern English, it would be Alderford, "Alder Ford." In ancient Europe peat bogs and alder fens were considered places haunting by the dead; in the Germanic-Celtic sagas alders were associated with the world of the dead or the otherworld, and a ford is a crossing point over a river, in this case, the river that separates the dead from the living world. Chamomile is, therefore, a lifesaver.

Chamomile as well as the similar-looking daisies and oxeye daisies were sacred to the forest peoples and were dedicated to the sun gods, such as the Celtic Bel (Belenos) or the Nordic Baldur, who embodied the spring sunshine. In Scandinavia, flowers with yellow centers and white ray florets are still called "Baldur's eyelashes." According to folk customs, one must collect chamomile flowers before midsummer because, after that, "flying crabs" would destroy them.

Ethnobotanists are not sure whether *maythen* meant the annual German chamomile *(Matricaria chamomilla)* or the perennial Roman chamomile *(Anthemis nobilis)*. Maybe there was no great difference made between them. The Roman chamomile is originally from North Africa; the plant does not like wet, moist soil and does not grow in a cold climate. Their healing effect is similar but not quite the same.

Maude Grieve (1858–1941), the luminary of the new British herbalism, was sure that it is exclusively the Roman chamomile referred to in the Nine Herbs Charm and not the German chamomile. During World War I, when drugs formerly imported from Germany and Austria were in short supply, Grieve collected and published information on useful medicinal herbs as a substitute for pharmaceutical products. If you read her work (Grieve 1931), you would get the impression that the great herbalist was in synch with the zeitgeist and had little sympathy for German things, and that included the "German" chamomile. The result of this attitude still resonates in that, nowadays, *Anthemis nobilis* is used in particular in the English-speaking countries where Grieve's book remains one of the most important references regarding healing plants, while the true German chamomile hardly gets any notice.

Stinging nettle *(Urtica dioica):* Nettle appears in the Nine Herbs Charm under the name *wergulu.* It was long speculated what the plant could be. Some believed it was the crab apple *(Malus sylvestris).*[21] Others wondered if it could be chicory (Raetsch 2005a). In the meantime, it has been established beyond doubt that it is the nettle, namely with respect to the *Werg* (Old High German *werc*), obtained during the processing of the fibers. Nettle was also, besides flax and hemp, an important fiber crop.

> This is the herb that is Wergulu,
> A seal brought it back over the sea,
> as an aid against the wickedness of the other poisons.
> It stands against pain, it dashes against poison.
> It has power against three and against thirty,
> against the hand of a fiend, against clever scheming, against
>   the magic word [spell] of evil creatures.

The seal that bore the nettles over the sea remained a mystery to philologists for a long time. Maude Grieve suggested it means that, in 43 BCE, the Romans had introduced and sown nettle because they rubbed the stinging herb on their arms and legs to combat the harsh, cold climate of Britain, which caused numbness and stiffness (Grieve 1931, 575). However, this argument is far-fetched because nettle is one of the island's native plants. It already grew there even before rising sea levels separated the islands from the European mainland community 5,500 years ago.

Not only were nets and clothing made from nettle fibers back then (the resulting durable cloth is similar to hemp and linen) and the young leaves were used as vegetables, but nettles also had important psychoactive functions. Lunatics and epileptics were brushed with fresh nettle branches "to bring them back to their senses," so as to bring their mind back to the present. Ancient tales also tell of nettles, such as in *The Six Swans,* the story of the six king's sons whom a sorceress had bewitched into swans. The swan, a bird more at home on the water or in the air and less on the solid earth was for forest peoples a creature of the otherworld.

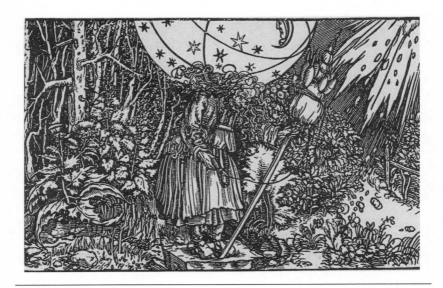

Witch with weeds, including nettles (from Petrarch Master, *Von der artzney bayder glueck des guten und des widerwaertigen,* from the Bayer pharmacy for happiness of the good and destitute, Augsburg, 1532)

In Slavic tales, the souls of the dead fly as swans along the Milky Way; swan maidens are clairvoyant and connected with the spirit world; and swan knights in the Celtic legends hail from a mystical dimension. The king's children in the fairy tale of The Six Swans are not in the here and now; only after their sister makes them shirts of nettle fabric can they return to a normal state.

The Nordic god that was always in a state of waking consciousness in the here and now is Heimdall, the guardian of the Rainbow Bridge, which leads to the high heavens. He is described as watching the bridge so that no demons go over the rainbow, and that is why he is always awake.

He sleeps neither day nor night. His senses are so sharp that he can see hundreds of miles, and hear the grass growing in the pasture and the wool growing on the sheep. This glistening god with gold teeth has spirit (Odin) as his father and nine powerful mermaids as his mother. The nine mothers represent the nine waves that carried him as he made his way into the here and now, onto the shore of this world. What is shown in other cultures as the nine branches of the world tree that the shaman ascends or the nine levels of Jacob's ladder were often represented in the mythology of the Germanic and Celtic tribes that settled the shores of the North Sea by the image of nine waves. The stages of a true shamanic journey are indeed often experienced as huge waves that carry the soul far away and back to shore again.

Thus, in the shape of a seal, this god surfed from the very depths of the spiritual universe into our world, into the here and now. His animal is thus a seal, and his plant is the nettle that makes us awake and present. It is this plant that can bring people back to the present whenever they are enchanted and drifting away from the here and now. Like a Zen master, it brings those affected back to solid ground with the blow of its stick. The stinging nettle, *wergulu*, offers deliverance to those suffering from enchantment by an unfriendly being or a false consciousness.

In modern phytotherapy, nettles are considered hematopoietic (blood-forming) and detoxifying; the seeds are invigorating and rejuvenating; and a tincture of the roots treats benign prostate inflammation.

Apple: It is not true, as is often claimed, that the barbarians in the north did not know the apple before the Romans came. Even the Neolithic farmers cultivated apples that were larger than the wild crab apples; the Romans only brought new cultivars. For forest peoples, as well as most Indo-Europeans, apples were a symbol of life and love. The vitamin-rich fruits held far into the cold season, and dried apple slices, still known in Alpine areas, cider, and cider vinegar helped ensure vitality over the winter months. As we learn from Germanic mythology, not even the gods could be without apples, which the goddess Idun had given them to stay healthy and young. The Celts, who called the world of the blessed Avalon ("Apple Country"), also knew the apples of eternal life. Apples and hazelnuts were cherished as food for the dead, and the spirit of the winter solstice, Santa Claus, brought apples and nuts as gifts of life. Since the pig was a sacred animal for all forest peoples, the suckling pig or roasted yule pig still gets an apple put in its mouth. The apple is to ensure that the animal may be born again.

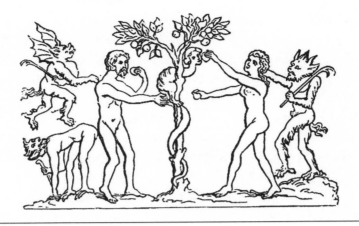

Medieval illustration of the devil seducing Eve under the apple tree

For the missionaries of the new faith, it must have been very difficult to turn the apple into a symbol of sin and death. Eve gave poor Adam this fruit to eat and so plunged them into misery. *"Malum e malo"* (the evil came through an apple), said the evangelizers. For the medieval monks, the apple was the symbol of sensual love and seduction, as well as female breasts.[22] A medieval image shows how the Christ child reaches toward the apple offered to him by the Mother of God. Symbolically, this action represents his taking the sins of the world upon himself. In the time when the Nine Herbs Charm was written down, things are no longer so clear. The Nine Herbs Blessing states:

> There the Apple accomplished it against poison
> that she [the loathsome serpent] would never dwell in the
> house.

In the meantime, the apple has been rehabilitated. "An apple a day keeps the doctor away" is still a popular adage among the English-speaking descendants of the old Anglo-Saxon states.

Chervil and fennel: The fragrant herbs chervil and fennel (*fille* and *finule*)[23] were not indigenous plants in England; they are typical monastery plants.

Chervil and fennel, two so powerful
herbs that were created by the powerful lord;
the holy one in heaven, as He hung;
he sent and placed them into the seven worlds
to help the rich and the poor alike.

The mighty Lord in heaven who was hanging there could be either Odin on Yggdrasil or Christ on the cross. The charm was probably intentionally ambiguous.

The Poisons

The Nine Herbs Charm ends with a list of the toxins that can be conquered:

Now these nine plants have power against nine powerful diseases
against nine poisons and against nine infections,
against the red poison, against the running poison,
against the white poison, against the pale blue poison,
against the yellow poison, against the green poison,
against the pale poison, against the dark blue poison,
against the bright poison, against the purple poison,
against worm-blister, against water-blister,
against thorn-blister, against thistle-blister,
against ice-blister, against poison-blister,
if any poison flying from the east
or any from the north should come,
or any from the west over the tribe of men.
Christ stood over the ancient, malevolent race;
I alone know the running rivers, and they enclose nine adders.
All weeds may now spring up as herbs,
Seas slide apart, all salt water, while I blow this poison from you.
Christ had power over all diseases. I alone know the flowing water,
and nine snakes fear it.

Now all the weeds like jumping from the herbs, the seas
were scattered, all the salt water,
if I blow this poison from you! (Pollington 2000, 217).

The Nine Herbs Charm (also called *Nine Worts Galdor*) is a magical song. While it does contain many pagan elements, it also has many Christian elements that blend in a syncretistic way. Philologists are of the opinion that this spell has not been preserved in its complete version and has been partly changed.

Hildegard of Bingen

Born in 1098 CE, Hildegard was a wise woman in the garb of a Benedictine nun. Although influenced by the dominant teachings of the classical antiquity, her medicine was a breakthrough: She knew not only the herbs of Dioscorides and the Bible but also mentioned native plants not previously mentioned in the cloister writings. In her eyes, these also partook of the divine luminosity, or the green power, that which she called *Viriditas*. She included the medicinal plants of the local herbalists in her medicine. She also did not hesitate to name them with the common German names of her times, in the language of the common people, such as *Wolfsgelegena* (arnica), *Huswurz* (houseleek), *Ringula* (marigold), *Hartenauwe* (Saint-John's-wort), *Lunckenwurtz* (lungwort), *Gunderebe* (ground ivy), *Cletta* (burdock), *Biboz* (mugwort), *Vehedistel* (Mary thistle), and so on. In this way, she joined again the healing art with Germanic and Celtic roots (Stille 2004, 33).

Hildegard was a seer. They say, as a five-year-old girl, she had pointed to a pregnant cow with her finger and said, "Look, what a beautiful little calf with a snow-white head." They thought she was just fantasizing, but, when the calf was born, it looked exactly like little Hildegard had described it. At the age of eight, Hildegard was sent to a convent, which was not uncommon for the times. Her clairvoyant ability carried her far beyond traditional monastery dogmas. She did not preach bloodless scholasticism. Like her pagan ancestors, she said yes, in almost poetic

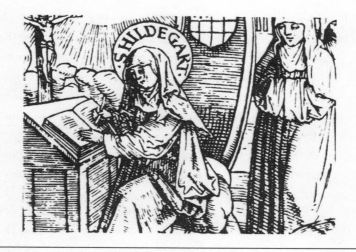

Hildegard of Bingen

words, to the sensual body and the act that leads to the procreation of new life: "In the heat of passion the love of the man behaves toward the woman's love as fire burning in the mountains which can be difficult to extinguish, in comparison to the wood fire of the woman that is easily put out. But the love of a woman stands in contrast to the raging fire of the man like the mild heat that emanates from the sun, and brings forth fruit" (Schipperges 1990, 43).

For Hildegard, infirmity meant too little fire of life, an excess of cold mucus, a lessening of green power *(Viriditas)*. For her, disease was not directly created by God; it is not a substantial entity but rather the result of something lacking. The nearness to God is lacking. Disease is an alienation from the divine source, an evil spell as it were. It is thus not primarily an imbalance of humors but arises due to self-inflicted separation from God.

Hildegard thought holistically: body, soul, nature, and the cosmos form a single unit. And if people, the microcosm, are lacking something, it can be retrieved from nature, the macrocosm, in particular from plants. Plants are remedies (Latin *remedium*), thus not only medicine but also mediators of divine salvation-giving powers.

217

With Hildegard, one encounters, again and again, popular, originally pagan, beliefs. For example, she writes about the magic power of the fern that contains the power of the sun and thus can drive off delusions and evil spirits: "Magic, demonic sorcery, diabolical words and other illusions make a wide detour around [dare not approach] the man who wears it on his person [. . .] And a woman when she gives birth to a child, should be surrounded by ferns and also the child in his cradle."

Further she wrote in the *Book of Plants (Liber medicinae simplicis):* For those suffering from gout, take fern, as long as it is green, cook it in water and bathe often in this water. Then the gout will recede." (Riethe 207, 388). It must be said that gout (Middle High German *giht*) was originally considered among the northern Europeans as a disease from spells or witchcraft. Almost the opposite of the fern, which "is a wisdom, and in the goodness of its nature, a symbol of goodness and holiness," is the poisonous belladonna. "In the countryside and in the place where it grows, diabolical influence abounds and aids the devil in his arts" (Riethe 2007, 38). Yet Hildegard used a few drops of this devil's plant with large, inflamed (in her words, durchsoden = thoroughly cooked) boils in an ointment of goose and deer fat to chase away the evil juices of the ulcers.

Belladonna *(Belladonna atropa)* was, by the way, one of the indigenous magical plants that grew in central Europe on limestone soils in the forest. This highly toxic fruit, *Wolfskirsche* (wolf's cherry) or *Wutbeere* (rage berry) as it is sometimes called in German, is said to have been part of witches' flying ointment and was associated with the god of ecstasy, Wotan. Like other tropane alkaloids, nightshade can catapult the soul into the lower astral world—into the devil's cauldron, so to speak, out of which one may not be able to get out (Raetsch 2005b, 80–81).

Hildegard used not only native plants but also, of course, the "Christian," exotic, expensive merchandise from the East for her remedies. Among them, were cinnamon, galangal, cloves, camphor, myrrh, muscle, lemon, and pepper. She made preparations and decoctions with vinegar or ale and, as is common in the Mediterranean cloister pharmacy, even wine. Following the Migration Period, wine grapes slowly but surely conquered much of the former Celtic and Germanic settlements. At the time of Hildegard, the edible chestnut was used as a panacea; even the smell was said to be curative. Fig and almond trees were no strangers in the Rhineland (central, western Germany), where they grew well because it was the climactic optimum and the temperatures were warmer than today.[24] Also, as a legacy of the healing of the Mediterranean countries, she used the *beom oleo,* or olive-tree oil, in addition to the usual animal fats in the preparation of ointments.

The Turning of the Wheel

Hildegard's medicine is in vogue nowadays, and not only with practitioners and doctors of natural medicine who are looking for their own cultural roots, but it is also diligently promoted by the Catholic Church. In this age of increasing environmental awareness, the Church is no longer the enemy of nature and is glad to have not just tree-felling religious fanatics on its list of monks and proselytizers but also saints such as Hildegard, Saint Francis of Assisi, or Mother Teresa. This is a heartening development.

Meanwhile, medicinal herbalism has even found protection under the wing of the Church. Father Sebastian Kneipp (1821–1897), who appears as a true shamanic personality in his biography, in addition to his water cure, also reinvigorated herbal medicine in a time of absolute materialism. He brought many forgotten healing herbs, such as horsetail, back into consciousness again. Similarly, the popular Swiss herbalist and priest Johann Kuenzle (1857–1945), in an age of questionable pharmaceutical products, made the "pharmacy of God" acceptable again. Both Kneipp and Kuenzle had to contend with strong resistance not only on the part of conventional medicine but also from their episcopal superiors. The gifted herbalist Maria Treben (1907–1991) was also a devout Christian and received her inspiration from the Mother of God. In earlier times, it would have been the Great Goddess who led her to the healing plants.

So times change, the wheel turns—or as the Taoist sage would say: Yin turns into Yang, Yang into Yin. Monastery gardens and faithful herbalists today have become a bulwark against a progressive pharmaceutical orthodoxy.

Regarding Hildegard medicine, a certain amount of caution should be exercised. Unlike the modern herbalist Maria Treben, whose statements are clear and comprehensible to us, we often do not know what the nun, who lived nearly a thousand years ago, meant exactly. She wrote in a difficult-to-decipher mixture of medieval Latin and Middle High German. It is not always clear what plant, what ingredient in the recipe, or what disease is meant. There are considerable problems of interpretation today, and what is practiced today as Hildegard medicine is based on uncertain and often quite creative interpretations.[25] What did Hildegard mean by "gout"? What is a "gouty migraine"? What is "sweating out the bone marrow"? Does she mean *Primula* as designated by Linnaeus (cowslip), or did she mean any other "first flowering" early spring flower? Although she had had much of her own experience in the proper use of medicinal plants, much has nevertheless been taken unchecked from the classic ancient writings. So Hildegard, yes, absolutely, but *cum grano salis*, with a grain of salt!

CHAPTER 7

Alcohol and Burning Pyres

When scholars study a thing,
they strive to kill it first, if it's alive;
then they have the parts and they've lost the whole,
for the link that's missing was the living soul.
GOETHE, *FAUST*, PART 1

The culture of the Middle Ages is the result of a successful synthesis. The ideas that came with the Christian missionaries and had seemed quite strange at first had by then been successfully integrated and incorporated into the worldview of the indigenous Germanic-Celtic forest peoples. As far as the medical system was concerned, there had been a reconciliation of the conflicting approaches. The nature-bound, indigenous, healing lore of the herbalists and the medicine of the cloister brothers and sisters had fused into a harmonious amalgam, or at least into an acceptable agreement and mutual understanding. This was reflected in the work and influence of the abbess, Hildegard of Bingen, who carried on in a similar spirit as clairvoyant wise women had always healed.

This balance was also reflected in the Gothic church architecture, which had begun during this time. The halls held aloft with high colonnades with their bold ribbed vaults and the light gently surging through the lancet windows almost gave the impression of forest silence. The cathedrals were, so to say, the rebirth in stone of the hallowed halls of the beech or oak forests that were sacred to the ancestors. The acoustics of the organ and polyphonic chorales, already introduced at that time, were close enough to the murmur of the gods in the sacred groves when the wind was blowing through the treetops. Ever more, the massive Romanesque churches, based on the Mediterranean model of damp, cool caves, were abandoned. In the hot Mediterranean where the sun can sting mercilessly, the gods had revealed themselves since ancient times in stone grottos, but in the north it was in the forest where one was close to God.

Professionalization

Alas, no sooner had the foreign influence been assimilated than the wind shifted again. A paradigm shift took place from the eleventh century onward. Again, the new cultural impulse came from the Middle East. One year after the birth of Hildegard of Bingen, the crusaders conquered Jerusalem and liberated the Holy City, including the Holy Grave.

Thereafter, contact with the Arab-Islamic world naturally grew in intensity. Shortly before these events, the learned North African doctor and drug trafficker Constantine the African (1017–1087 CE) appeared in the hospice in Salerno, which belonged to the Cloister Montecassino. As a baptized lay brother, the native Tunisian translated the Arabic writings of Avicenna, Rhazes, Ibn al-Baitar, and other Islamic scholars) as well as the lost (but preserved in the Islamic world) ancient Greek scriptures, into Latin.[1] Arabic writings were also translated in Moorish Spain at the University of Toledo. What came to light struck like lightning in the medieval world. Like hungry wolves, Western scholar monks pounced on the classical knowledge that had recently been made available again, particularly on Aristotle's and Persian-Arabic scholars' less lofty and less spiritual, but more objective, perspective on natural history.

Mineral remedies—alum, antimony, lead, iron sulfate, verdigris, lime, calcium carbonate, chalk, salt, copper ore, sodium carbonate, sulfur, sulfide, and other inorganic chemical substances—played a far greater role in Islamic medicine than in the West; perhaps this was so because the desert has less vegetation. In Arabic medicine, the plants themselves were not so much seen as independent, responsive beings one could talk to, but as

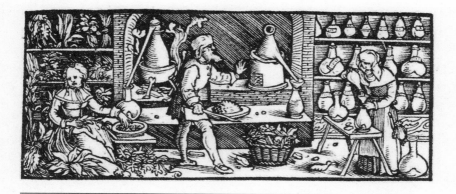

Alchemical processing of medicinal plants

carriers of material forces *(virtutes)*. These material forces can be extracted and transferred into elixirs, electuaries, pills, syrups, and other medicinal preparations (Stille 2004, 38). The aim of Arabic medical practitioners was to look for essences; they wanted to get rid of the rough fabric of impurities and slag *(faeces)*. It was based more on a materialistic perspective.

Arabic alchemy, dissolve and coagulate *(solve et coagula)*, came into fashion with the monks. They experimented, boiled, baked, calcined, distilled, filtered, and sublimated. It was the beginning of the laboratory and of modern pharmacy. Very important was distilled alcohol, the spirit of wine *(spiritus vini)*, the "fire water" *(aqua ardens)*. This alcohol *(spiritus)*, extracted as the essence of the crude plant mass, was practically seen as a panacea. It can especially alleviate the "cold" ailments and also serve as a solvent for precious exotic healing spices, such as cardamom, ginger, galangal, nutmeg, clove, and cinnamon. The monks and scholars were very enthused about all of this. Liqueurs, brandies, and herbal brandies became the monopoly of many monasteries. Uroscopy, bloodletting, cupping therapy, pulse taking, laxatives, purgatives, the making of electuaries (thick liquid medicine) and theriacs (pharmaceutical panaceas), Iatro astrology, and so on became part of medical science.

Yes, the wind had changed. The medical school of Salerno was revolutionary. An international scholarly elite gathered there. The founders' legend tells of four doctors, a Christian Orthodox Greek, a Jew, an Arab, and a Latin Christian who joined together in order to exchange views on the accumulated knowledge from India to Spain. In Salerno, anatomical experiments were done on pigs. Exceptional was also that women were admitted to the school, albeit only a few. Only one is actually recorded, namely medical doctor Trotula who hailed from a well-to-do family. She turned to gynecology, which had been left to primitive, illiterate midwives for centuries and wrote a scholarly work on the subject. Historians are not sure, though, if she was really a man who had given himself a fictitious name.

What took place in Salerno makes the hearts of many of today's enlightened contemporaries leap for joy. These medics were doing the job properly! What was developing there was encouraged and legally protected by emperor and pope. The Stauffer Emperor Frederick II issued a comprehensive set of laws (1240 CE), which led to the professionalization of physicians and pharmacists. No one was allowed to practice medicine who had not studied at a university for five years, taken three years of logic, and completed a one-year internship with an established physician. The future physician's knowledge of anatomy and the scriptures of the old masters, Hippocrates and Galen, had to be examined, by decree, by masters from Salerno (Schipperges 1990, 181).

The laws served to protect patients from charlatans and incompetent medical practitioners, who could neither understand humoral pathology nor draw logical conclusions. Pope John XXII and Paris Bishop Etienne joined the decree and also prohibited the practice of medicine by illiterates *(ignari)*, herbal healers *(herbarii)*, and old women *(mulieres vetulae)* (Chamberlain 2006, 44). With this, the rustic healers, leeches, wortcunners, midwives, and wise old women were decreed obsolete; they were considered illegal and henceforth liable to persecution. In their place appeared the Greek *iatros* ("medical practitioner"), the *fidicien* ("physician"; from Latin, "practitioner of natural science"), and the Latin *medicus* ("healer"), as well as the Latin *doctor* ("teacher"). As members of an independent profession, these physicians were no longer subject to the rules of celibacy but were permitted to marry and have families.

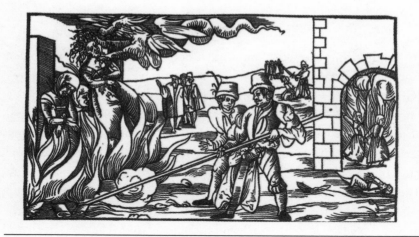

Burning witches

The new rules on professionalization also affected the mild-mannered monks. In various councils, such as the Council of Tours (1163 CE), they were forbidden to practice medicine. Priests, monks, and nuns should henceforth be restricted to their primary responsibilities, namely to see to the salvation of their flock. Monastic medicine came to an end. However, the monks were still allowed to produce medicines. And this they did; they busied themselves with the production and "examination" of various alcohols and distilled spirits, potions, powders, and the like.

Also during this time, apothecaries were established and regulated, and the practice of regular physicians was legally separated from that of surgeons. Now doctors alone were responsible for internal medicine and the prescription of pharmaceutical remedies (polypharmacy). The less prestigious, less educated barbers (surgeons) were responsible for blood-letting, pulling teeth, applying leeches, administering enemas, scraping out fistulas, sewing wounds, cupping therapy, and scarification.

The new regulations and laws had dire consequences for illiterate peasant healers, especially for the gifted women healers. Healing and herbalism, which had fallen within the range of female activity since time immemorial, had become a domain dominated by men.

Heretics

Just at this time, a heretical movement began to discomfort the Roman Catholic Church. The apostates called themselves Cathars, the "pure" (Greek *katharos* = pure), which became *Ketzer* (heretic) in German. They saw themselves as the only true Christians *(veri christiani)*. They practiced austerities and nonviolence and shamed the official Church and their secular clergy with their demonstrative virtuous conduct. They accused the Church of being too lax, unclean, unholy, and full of pagan practices. They rejected the idolatry of worshiping the cross, graven images, and saints; they rejected the doctrine of hell and purgatory: the material world in which we live, is in itself hell and Satan its master. They rejected baptism, marriage, and the Eucharist.

In addition, the Cathar worldview was strictly dualistic; that is, they divided the world into good and evil, light and darkness, spirit and matter, the kingdom of God and of Satan. In their view, the Catholic Church obviously belonged to the latter. Of course, this all went too far—the Church's reaction was to come down on the heretics, who had settled primarily in southern France, with full force. The pope called for a crusade against them. Under the leadership of the Dominicans, the Inquisition, a system of spying, torture, dispossession, and death by burning at the stake, was set up against them. The burning of the heretics could be biblically justified. Did Jesus not say, "If anyone does not remain in Me, he is like a branch that is thrown away and withers. Such branches are gathered up, thrown into the fire, and burned" (John 15:6)?

Spurred on by the Cathars, the Church tightened their ideological reins. All at once, Satan played a major role in theology. He was no longer the ordinary devil, the cloven-hooved, hairy, gaunt, nature spirit with horns that a clever farmer could outwit; he was also no longer the "poor devil" that a bishop could force to build a bridge. He was now "Lord of the World" and a veritable anti-god.

Even after the heretics were long eliminated, the Inquisition continued to exist as an institution. It was used against "witches," the last carriers of shamanism, which was very dangerous for the village healers and leech doctors, especially when they were more successful than the professional doctors, as was often the case. Successful healers got the full force of the law thrown at them. After all, only Satan could be responsible for their success!

Pestilence and Syphilis

In the fourteenth century, the medieval climate optimum came to an end. It gradually grew colder and the weather became unstable. Climatologists speak of the "Little Ice Age" between 1350 and 1800. The winters were longer; chestnuts, figs, almonds, and wine disappeared from northern Europe; grain acreage decreased; and there were crop failures, famine, and social unrest. Beggars and robbers made the roads unsafe. Flagellants traveled across the country, whipping themselves bloody in order to obtain God's grace.

Due to the wet and cold weather, rye, which thrives in a colder climate better than wheat does and was the most important grain for baking bread, was suddenly seized by the ergot fungus *(Claviceps purpurea)*. Because they were hungry, however, people did not stop baking bread, and the result was a pandemic ergot poisoning. Symptoms were convulsions, respiratory and circulatory disorders, and—because of the LSD-component of the fungus—crazed hallucinations. Because of circulatory disorders, fingers and toes

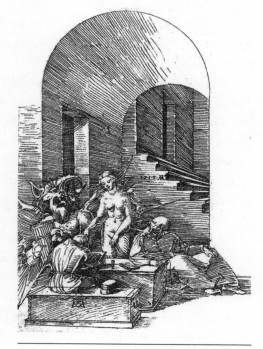

The Temptation of Saint Anthony
(Albrecht Duerer)

turned black and rotted off as if they had been burnt by fire. It seemed as if an army of demons had fallen upon mankind. The infestation was called St. Anthony's fire because only St. Anthony, the holy Egyptian hermit who himself had been attacked by hordes of demons and resisted them, could help.

The long, cold winters and insufficient food led to weak immune systems and susceptibility to various epidemics, including the plague. The pope and the emperor blamed the people themselves for their misery; their immoral and sinful life was responsible for God's punishment. They should buy indulgences. But above all, it was the fault of the witches, these covert heathens, who practiced harmful magic. And so witch persecution increased; the Inquisition had a new task. While the executed heretics had been both men and women, now the "witches" were mainly women, the heiresses of the old heathen seers, also traditionally called Walas, Voelvas and Veledas. By burning them at the stake, the cultural inheritance, the shamanic knowledge of healing and magic, were also burned, whose roots reached back to the Old Stone Age.

When the Black Death epidemic raged and wiped out one-third of Europe's population, the learned doctors were at their wits' end. Their visits to their patients were now called "death runs." In long leather garments that covered the whole body, with beak masks filled with aromatic herbs, with gauntlets and goggles meant to protect against infection by visual contact, they visited the sick. Bloodletting was the primary means of medical science because it was believed to guide the bad humors out of the body. Theriac, a broad-spectrum panacea made from expensive exotic spices, opiates, powdered toads, snake venom, and mithridate (a universal antidote also made of bizarre ingredients) should "master" the "pestilential poison." Perfumed smelling "apples" called pomander (small, hollow metal balls full of herbs) containing amber, civet, aloe, dittany, myrrh, and pimpernel were another medical remedy (Porter 2003, 127). Still other doctors prescribed brandy and other spirits for their patients. Houses were fumigated, and quarantines were enforced. This was how the Great Tradition reacted to the crisis.

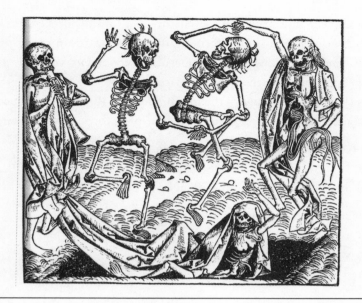

Dance of Death as imagined during the time of the plague
and famine (woodcut from the Nuremberg Chronicle, 1493)

For its part, the Church offered the frightened people the so-called pestilence saints, whose intercession should mitigate the scourge of God. The most important was Saint Roch, who had indeed himself suffered from the plague and had been healed. Saint Anne, the mother of the Mother of God, the grandmotherly being who had once replaced Mother Hulda (and was now the patroness of the miners just as the Paleolithic goddess had been responsible for the netherworld), should likewise be appealed to with consecrated "Saint Anne water" and pilgrimages to churches under her patronage. Saint Sebastian, who was studded with arrows, and the two divine physicians Cosmas and Damian were also part of what the Church officially had to offer. These were other answers from the Great Tradition.

In the Little Tradition of the common people, victims turned to local herbs and relied on revelations from the otherworld. Whenever people are at the extreme limit of what is tolerable and in the greatest danger, the veil that separates the everyday world from the supernatural world becomes very thin. In such times, nature and forest spirits come closer. Herbal women and simple farming folk now heard, in many places, angels, gnomes, talking birds, sea mermaids, moss dwarves, and various wee people who gave them good advice.

In the Giant Mountains, the mountain spirit Ruebezahl stepped out of the forest and told an exhausted and helpless forest farmer:

Cook saxifrage and valerian, so the plague will have an end.

In the Salzburg area, a bird called from a tree:

Eat juniper and burnet, then you die not so fast!

In St. Gallen, a mysterious voice said,

Burnet and masterwort are good for pestilence!

Dozens of such sayings have been recorded by folklorists. And if they are analyzed closely, they are always plants, especially the roots, that are not only rich in vitamins and have a vitalizing effect but also possess a strong immune-boosting component (Storl 2010a, 240). They include, first of all, saxifrage *(Pimpinella saxifraga)*, angelica *(Angelica sylvestris)*, masterwort *(Peucedanum ostruthium)*, juniper *(Juniperus communis)*, and the carline thistle (silver thistle, *Carlina acaulis*). Even ransoms, or bear's garlic *(Allium ursinum)*, tormentil *(Potentilla erecta)*, valerian *(Valeriana officinalis)*, and forest sanicula *(Sanicula europaea)* are frequently mentioned. According to modern phytotherapeutic criteria, these plants can be classified as more effective than the means of the Galenic academic doctors.

For the West Slavs, such as the Sorbs, it was similar. Here, too, voices were heard from the otherworld: "You shall need valerian, dorant [not clearly identified, possibly horehound, snapdragon, or some other plant], and frankincense." A young girl listens to a bird sing: "Valerian, valerian, valerian." It is said that all recovered who drank valerian afterward. If the plague threatened the Sorbs, they put out all fires, took an oak board and a thick spruce board, and rubbed them against each other until the spruce began to smolder and catch fire. With this fire, a so-called need-fire known since pagan times and which always signaled a new beginning, the plague then disappeared. Houses were also incensed against the plague—among others plants, juniper, elecampane root, oak leaves, birch bark, and even the hair of an uncastrated billy goat were used (Lehmann-Enders 2000, 34–35).

In 1492, yet another contagion was introduced when the ships of Columbus returned to Europe and brought syphilis. The European population had no natural immunity against this sexually transmitted, infectious disease. The victims rotted alive, and the nobility and the clerics were severely affected. Whole monasteries were depopulated; kings and princes succumbed. The common people, who had relatively strict customs and also lived a basically clean life, were less affected. All the stops of conventional medicine were pulled, but the Hippocratic-Galenic humoral teachings failed, and no cure was found. Even conventional herbs did not really help. Although the Caribbean indigenous peoples knew an effective cure with blood-purifying plants, such as guaiacum *(Guaiacum officinalis)* or sarsaparilla *(Smilax officinalis)*, combined with a special diet and frequent sweat baths, the Europeans had no understanding of such "savage practices." While it was previously believed that for every disease, there is a healing herb, the medical profession began to lose faith in the efficacy of herbal medicines.[2]

The modern medicine of the day found an answer in the so-called Saracen ointment which the crusaders discovered during their stay in the Middle East. This ointment consisted of mercury and other highly toxic mineral substances—and it seemed to help. Mercury was also administered internally in the form of calomel, or *Mercuris dulcis.* Even though the patient suffered severely and had adverse side effects due to mercury poisoning—salivating, drastic diarrhea, and later suppurating ulcers, kidney and intestinal inflammation, hepatitis, and hair and tooth loss[3]—mercury was considered a miracle drug, similar to penicillin, chemotherapy, and radiation in our age.

Doctors now prescribed, for those who could afford it, mercurial preparations for everything: asthma, colicky babies, gout, jaundice, madness, cancer, rickets, rhinitis, smallpox, and so on. To numb the pain that accompanied this therapy, laudanum, an opium preparation, was prescribed. Since opium paralyzes intestinal peristalsis and causes constipation, enemas and strong laxatives became necessary. (Bloodletting was still practiced because the "bad fluids" had to be flushed out.) This "heroic medicine," as it came to be called, was considered modern and scientific. The old herbal women could not keep up, and their "superstitious" knowledge was no longer in demand. On the contrary, it was ridiculed and increasingly punishable. The climax of the syphilis epidemic in the mid-seventeenth century was also the peak of witch persecution.[4]

In the eighteenth century, a clean sweep was made: it was the time of the Enlightenment. Only that which could be scientifically proven and based on accurate empirically supported observation and measurement and did not violate the laws of logic was considered real and substantial. Anything else was regarded as subjective, illusory, or simply superstitious. "Witches" no longer existed; if anything, they were henceforth declared poor, deranged old women. The witch hunt was passé. Anna Goeldin of Glarus was the last witch beheaded in Switzerland in 1782 for allegedly killing a child by conjuring pins into its milk. The very last execution of a witch in Europe took place in 1793 in Poznan (Poland).

And as little as it was believed in this new enlightened age that there are witches, wizards, elves, mermaids, or ghosts, no one believed in the effects of healing herbs and incantation. Medicine had become a rational science. Healing was now in the hands of men who were scientifically trained and rational. Even gynecology, obstetrics, and neonatology were now a matter for the doctors; midwives were only reluctantly tolerated as unskilled helpers. Chemical-pharmaceutical agents that can be dosed precisely replaced the herbs of the wise, old women. Sometime later, bourgeois women fought for the right to study and to practice the medical profession. This is good in itself, but basically they assumed a medical practice that is masculinized and in which all uncontrollable elements—vision, inspiration, intuition—are kept at a minimum.

In the countryside, far from enlightened city society, folk medicine lived on happily, with its herbal agents, healing incantations, and other so-called superstition. These rural folk used the same tried and true medicinal plants that their ancestors had always used. Monastic medicine had also left its mark. Not only were traditional teas, decoctions, powders, and ointments still made, but the old herb women who lived in virtually every village now also healed with herbal tinctures and spirits and made decoctions in wine, sweet electuaries, and ointments with olive oil. Again and again, herbal medicine revivalists, such as the brilliant doctor Christoph Wilhelm Hufeland and Father Sebastian Kneipp, who came from the simplest circumstances in Bavaria and whose family could not afford doctors, drew from the ancient traditions. Also herbalists, such as Maria Treben and Maurice Mességué, brought traditional knowledge into the modern age and traditional healing back to modern consciousness.

Arabic Influence in Medical Vocabulary

A new worldview requires a new vocabulary. The strong impression that Islamic medicine made on Western medicine from the twelfth century can be clearly seen if we bring the many concepts to mind that found their way into the language of scientific medicine and pharmacists.

Alchemy (Egyptian-Coptic *kami, chemi* = black, black earth): Arabian alchemy, material metamorphosis, the attempt to change ignoble, "sick" metals, step by step, into elixirs, or even gold, is the legacy of Ancient Egyptian culture. The transformation process that took place during certain constellations at exactly the right time included procedures such as distillation, crystallization, and

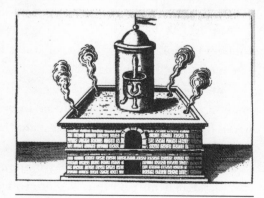

Athanor, an alchemical sand bath oven
(Museum Hermeticum, Frankfurt, 1678)

sublimation. In the course of time, exact weights and measuring methods were developed, and new materials were discovered, such as hydrochloric acid, sulfuric acid, nitric acid, ammonia, alkalis, many metal compounds, ether, phosphorus, Prussian blue, and so on.[5] Alcohol and minerals became part of medicine, of iatrochemistry. This new empirical direction of research fascinated the European clerical elite. It is the cradle of modern chemistry.

Alcohol (Arabic *al kuhl* = eye powder, antimony): The fine antimony powder was used as black eyeshadow and as a medical treatment for the eyes. The Spanish alchemists transferred the concept of the finest powder to the finest distilled spirits: *aqua vitae* (the water of life) and *aqua ardens* (distilled liquor), which represented the *quinta essentia* (quintessence) of the wine.[6] The famous Dominican and doctor, Arnold de Villanova, introduced "fire water," or "spiritus," as a medical panacea in the thirteenth century. After that time, alcoholic distillations were fervently produced in European cloisters, and not a few men of god became alcoholics.

Alembic (Arabic *al-inbīq* = distiller): The device that made it possible to distill alcohol and produce essential oils and perfumes.

Alkali (Arabic *quala* = roast): The word refers to roasted, saline beach plants out of whose ashes alkali (potash, sodium carbonate, etc.) can be gained.

Amalgam (Arabic *amalal-ğamā* a = work of fusion): This word, well-known due to mercury dental fillings today, refers to metal alloys with mercury. Mercury alloys played a major role in alchemical medicine.

Amulet (Arabic *hammāla* = a band to wear): An amulet is a pendant, which was spoken over with incantations or Koran verses to keep evil genies (djinns = bad spirits) away.

Aniline (Arabic *an-nil* = indigo plant; originally from Sanskrit nila = blue): Synthetic indigo was produced in the mid-nineteenth century by BASF (the multinational chemical-manufacturing company) from coal tar and used as a basis for many dyes, plastics, and drugs.

Antimony (Arabic *intimid* = stibnite): The Benedictine alchemist monk and alchemist Basilius Valentinus was very enthused about this silver-white lustrous metalloid. He heard that pigs eat it to purge themselves; then, he tried it on his fellow monks, who promptly died. Even

Paracelsus still believed that antimony is the strongest arcanum, if alchemically refined, and would transform an impure body into a pure one, such as with leprosy.

Artichoke (Arabic *al-haršūf* = goad, prod): This vegetable from the subfamily of thistles that the Moors imported to Europe was already used early on in Arabic medicine for liver and gall ailments. The root contains cynarine.

Benzine (a corruption of the Arabic *lubān gāw* = incense from Java; Catalan benjuyn; Middle Latin benzoe): Benzine resin was used as a healing means for chest ailments, catarrh, and abscesses. In the nineteenth century, the distillation of benzoin resulted in "gasoline," a word that came to be used for fuel for machines.

Bezoar (Persian *bādzahr* = antidote): This preventative and remedy for poisoning consists of the stomach stone of ruminants or hair balls from cat guts and was very popular with princes and cardinals in medieval Europe. They often wore them on pendants and dipped them into their beverages to neutralize possible poisons.

Bismuth (Arabic *itmid* = antimony): A chemical element with symbol Bi in the periodic table. The Arabs once also used this brittle white, silvery substance medicinally.

Boron, borax (Arabic *būraq* = borate sodium): The Egyptians already used this mineral for embalming. Medicinally, it acts as a disinfectant.

Camphor (Arabic *kāfūr,* from Sanskrit *karpūra*): In India, the fragrant white resin from the camphor tree is lit up, burning with a clear, white flame, and used when worshipping the gods. When the Muslims discovered it, they used it for washing and embalming of the dead and in medicine for nosebleeds, diarrhea, eye diseases, gout, and as an antiaphrodisiac. Hildegard was enthused about "Ganphora" that strengthens a feverish patient as "the sun brightens a cloudy day." Camphor, she said, "is so pure that witchcraft and delusions cannot manifest; instead they disappear in the face of its purity, as snow melts away in the face of the sun" (Riethe 2007, 383).

Cotton (Arabic *bitāna* = inner lining of garments): Loose mass of soft cotton fibers.

Elixir (Arabic *al-iksbī* = philosopher's stone, dry substance with magical properties; originally from the Greek *xēríon* = dry healing substance): It is one of the key words of alchemical medicine; it is the fifth essence, a life-supporting and life-extending substance. In Europe, one began to call herbal substances extracted in alcohol "elixirs."

Galangal (Arabic *halaṅǧān*): This plant from the ginger family grows in South Asia; it found its way to the Arab markets and pharmacies, has an antispasmodic effect on the digestive system, and is anti-inflammatory and stimulating. Hildegard of Bingen was highly enthused and prescribed the exotic root for everything from back pain, bad breath, hoarseness, and hearing disorders to spleen ailments.

Gauze (Arabic *qazz* = raw silk): Gauze is the thin, loosely woven fabric that is used for wound care.

Julep (Arabic *gulāb* = rose water, refreshing drink): In Europe, this drink of distilled water and syrup became a popular way to take medicine. We know the word as the refreshing mint julep in the hot south of the United States.

Kandis (Arabic *qand;* Punjabi khanda = *an angular stone*): Rock sugar, as well as crystalized sugar, was an expensive commodity that the Arabs brought from India and was used in many medicinal mixtures, such as syrup and electuaries. The modern word candy for confectionery goes back to it.

Massage, massage (Arabic *massa* = to touch, to feel; from the ancient Greek mássein = to knead): The treatment of touching or stroking out a disease is of course one of the oldest methods of therapy. However, this specific word was brought to the European languages by travelers to the East.

Mummy (Arabic *mūmiyā'ī* = earth pitch, bitumen, asphalt; from the Persian mum = wax): Embalmed body parts used as medicine (see page 238).

Myrrh (Arabic *murr*): The resin of the myrrh bush, which grows in southern Arabia, is regarded as precious incense. We know it from the story of the Three Wise Kings from the East, who bring the Christ child myrrh, frankincense, and gold. The ancient Egyptians used the resin along with soda to embalm corpses; the Arabs used alcoholic tinctures of it to make the gums firmer and to treat asthma, lung disease, worms, digestive ailments, and more. Hildegard saw the expensive imported good as a means against magic and satanic influences, but also as effective for fever and migraines.

Natron (Arabic *natrūn;* from the ancient Egyptian *ntr.j*): In British English, natron refers to the deposits of soda ash and sodium bicarbonate, which are chemically identical to soda and essential in preparing mummies. Today we know it as baking soda, as part of the effervescent powder used for neutralizing excess stomach acid. Arabs used it as an antiseptic and water softener.

Potassium (Arabic *al-qalya* = potash, ash salt): The element potassium, an alkali metal, is important in plant growth and living bodies to help maintain blood pressure and metabolism in the bones. The symbol for potassium in the periodic table is K, which refers to kalium, a word still used in British English and also comes from the Arabic al-qualya, meaning potash or "salt of ashes." Potash is essential in maintaining blood pressure, fluid balance, transmission of nerve impulses and the metabolism of the bones. Potassium was used for these purposes in Arab medicine.

Safran (Arabic *za'farān*): These orange pistils of a kind of crocus are a luxury (150,000 blossoms produce one kilogram of saffron); the plant was used by the Arabs for coloring and seasoning, but also for healing and as a cosmetic and an aphrodisiac.

Soda (Arabic *suuwād* = salt plant ash): Sodium carbonate, soda water.

Sugar (Arabic sukkar; as a loan word from Sanskrit sákara = grit, grains of sugar): The "white gold," especially that extracted from sugar cane, was recommended by Arab physicians as a remedy and was part of electuaries and syrup.

Syrup (Arabic *šarāb* = potion): Syrup is thickened sap with sugar, honey, or molasses. In Islamic medicine, remedies are often administered as syrups.

Talc (Arabic *talq* = talc, steatite): Powdered soapstone, used as talcum powder.

Mummy

In Arab-Islamic medicine, *mūmiyā* (bitumen, asphalt) was a highly valued, expensive remedy. It was processed into ointments and applied to treat broken bones, major bruises, skin diseases, inflammation, respiratory distress, gout, itching, and so on (Unger 2013, 208). Constantine the African made these exotic medicines in the exalted school of Salerno, which attracted the attention of European pharmacists and doctors.

After the Egyptians were defeated in battle against Muslim Arabs in the seventh and eighth centuries, the invaders opened the pharaohs' graves and claimed that the bitumen preservatives had penetrated the mummified dead bodies—if it were possible to extract it, one would surely have a panacea (Ludwig 1982, 250). Though they had concerns about whether the consumption of body parts would agree with their beliefs, they still sold the mummies to infidels who practically fought over them. Soon the supply of real mummies was depleted and replaced with less honorable bodies dried in the desert air, stored, and shipped with bitumen-impregnated cloth.

During the plague years in Europe, between the fifteenth and seventeenth centuries, medical authorities recommended powdered mummies as a remedy. When problems with the import arose, executed people were mummified with precise, legal regulations:

> One should take a raw, whole body of an unflawed person that has strangled on the gallows, or been executed on the torture wheel, or has run the gauntlet, and cut him into pieces, sprinkle with powdered Mumia [bitumen] and a little Aloe, then soak a few days in a distilled wine, hang up to dry, then pickle some more, then finally hang the pieces in the air. Let dry until it has the appearance of a cured meat and loses all stinking, and shows ultimately a nice, red tincture due to the wine or juniper brandy, demonstrating the art of the process (Ludwig 1982, 251).

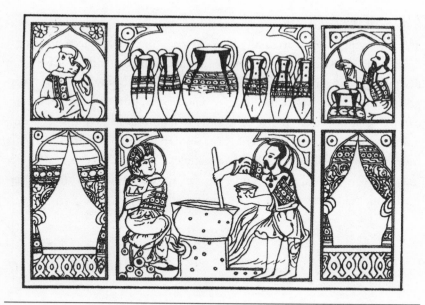

Preparing medicines in an ancient Persian apothecary

Mumia was available until the eighteenth century in Western pharmacies.

For Paracelsus, the term *mumia* assumed new meaning and importance. The great doctor used it metaphorically as a "force that draws diseased substances from the body, just as a magnet attracts iron filings." The *mumiae* of Paracelsus consisted of dried fat, blood, feces, and other organic substances of human or animal origin. The disease was transmitted to the *mumiae*, which was then wedged in a tree hole, buried in the ground, or given to a dog to eat. The concept for this practice was actually no different from that of folk medicine's "transmission" of illness: Fresh herbs that had the signature of the disease, such as lungwort for lung ailments or celandine for jaundice, were placed on the patient's body. When they dried out or wilted, they were replaced with fresh ones. These herbs would thus pull out the disease.

Plant Names from Arabic

The following words (originally from Arabic) for plants, spices, and preparations show what an impression the Arabic scholars made on European doctors, pharmacists, and scholars: aloe, barberry, borage, ebony, tarragon, galangal, harmal (wild rue), hashish, senna, ginger, jasmine, coffee, camphor, carob, calico (cotton), kermes (cochineal), kiff (cannabis resin), cumin, cubeb (pepper), turmeric, lime, loofah (sponge gourd), marzipan, myrrh, orange, saffron, salep ("fox testicles," boyhood herb), safflower (false saffron), sandalwood, senna, sesame, spinach, sultana, sumac, tamarind, teak, zedonary (bitter root), plum.

CHAPTER 8

Wise Women and Their Remedies

Heið they called, wherever she came to houses,
the Voelva with pleasing prophecies, she charmed staves,
Performed seið wherever she could,
Performed seið in ecstasy.
THE SEER'S PROPHECY (VOLUSPA, 22)

As we have already seen several times, the art of healing within folk culture (the Little Tradition) was mainly, but not exclusively, in women's hands. In some regions, medicine and herbalism were commonly passed back and forth between the genders; women passed it on to men, and in turn, their knowledge and experience were passed back on to women. Male and female healers were equally at home in the midst of nature, which surrounded house and yard, as they were in their cultural tradition. For all their lives, they had known the people and the animals with whom they had their dealings. They knew them personally and encountered them with that certain something, namely love. They also loved the native landscape and, as the Swiss writer Sergius Golowin writes, this love attracts the healing powers of the surrounding nature.

The medical professionals of the "higher culture" (the Great Tradition), who until recently were almost exclusively men, often lacked this heartfelt connection. The knowledge of the learned doctors and pharmacists is based on words and laboratories and less on inspiration and spiritual intuition. Paracelsus understood that: "It is not so that a doctor learns everything he knows at the universities; he must, from time to time, turn to the old women, the gypsies, the practitioners of the black arts, vagrants, and to all kinds of peasants and learn from them—because they have more knowledge of such things than all the universities do." And with regards to the fashion of the times, which were based mainly on Arab sources, he wrote, "They want medicine from overseas, though better medicine grows in the garden right in front of their houses" (Golowin 1993, 125).

Housewives and Grandmothers

In the traditional agricultural societies, the healing essence of the feminine was much more than simply a matter of taking care of the sick. In the traditional division of labor, whose origins date back to the Neolithic period, the women were responsible for the following areas.

Food and Drink

For the most part, the women prepared the food. They ground the grain, cooked the porridge, and baked the daily bread—the staple food. Bread, concentrated vitality, was sacred. It could serve as food offerings for the spirits and ancestors. In the presence of bread—also bees—cursing was forbidden. Bread and salt were thought to bring good luck, and in Germanic and Slavic households, it was offered to guests and newlyweds. In the Christian culture, God revealed himself in bread: "I am the bread of life," says the Savior. It builds community to eat bread together—a companion (Latin *cum* = with, *panis* = bread) is someone with whom one shares bread.

The housewife, the mistress of the home, kneaded the dough, shaped the loaves, and baked them in the oven. It was naturally she who performed the solemn custom of cutting the first ears of grain from the four corners of the field at the beginning of the harvest and made the first bread of the new harvest with it. In English, "lady" means "free woman." The word comes from the Anglo-Saxon *hlaef* (Proto-Germanic *hlaiba*

= loaf; related to Slavic *chleb*) and *dige* (dough-kneader). Thus, a lady is a bread-kneader.[1] In Sweden, however, the lady of the house is the *mat-moder,* the woman who cooks or roasts meat.

While turning the grain mill by hand, stirring the grain-porridge, or kneading the dough, the women hummed or whispered good charms and their good wishes and thoughts for the farm and community. Believed to bring blessings, the stirring and grinding had to be done, more or less, in a clockwise direction in accordance with the movement of the sun in the sky. The circle dances also always went, albeit with short backward movements, in this direction. But equal to how she could charm blessings into the bread, so could a disappointed or spiteful woman spoil the flour by milling it intentionally against the sun's path or while whispering curses. It could be a death spell, which in the Scottish dialect is called *widdershins* ("against the movement of the sun").

In addition to baking bread, putting away food for the winter—dried fruit and berries, parched, smoked, cured meat and fish, cheese, sauerkraut, and pickled vegetables—was an essential part of the female activities. Also brewing ale, called "liquid bread" and *kvass* (dry bread soaked in water until slightly fermented), as well as caring for smaller animals (chickens, house pets, orphaned sheep or calves) and the vegetable garden belonged to their realm.

How important food is to maintaining health hardly needs further explanation. In those days, all food came from the immediate surroundings. The specific methods of preparation, local eating and drinking habits, and the special foods within the cultural cycle of the seasons were part of the people's identity with their homeland and were nurtured mainly by the women. Today, in a global economy, in which one hardly knows where the food came from and international corporations such as fast-food chains do the cooking for many people, this old way of eating is unfortunately unimaginable.

Clothes

Clothing provides not only protection against the cold and the weather, but it is also part of the personality; it tells what and who a person is.

The manufacturing of clothing—from sewing, tending, and harvesting to the preparation of fiber plants such as hemp and, in particular, flax—was also traditionally women's work. They also knew the necessary growth charms sung or chanted to benefit fiber crops. They were passed on orally from mother to daughter. Often, the magical charms were rather crude and earthy, such as the following:

> Flax, flax do not be a runt,
> grow as high as my cunt,
> grow as high as my tit(s)
> and there stay and sit! [Meaning the plant should grow
> that tall.]

They danced flax dances with loosened hair, wore aprons as blue as flax flowers, and jumped as high over the midsummer bonfire as possible so that the flax would grow high (Baechtold-Staeubli and Hoffmann-Krayer 1987, Vol. 5, 1181). The spinning of the fibers—wool, linen, nettle—the weaving and dyeing, and the tailoring and sewing were women's work.[2]

Although there were tailors in the cities, the manufacturing of clothes was strictly a matter for women in the rural areas. Clothes not only warm and keep people dry, but they also give the soul protection. They protect those one loves, the children, the husband, in-laws, and maybe some friends. It is a magical protective skin. Again, it mattered what wishes and thoughts went into the weaving and sewing of each stitch of the needle. These procedures are archetypal—Native American women would sew the clothes and embroider magical, protective patterns onto them with dyed porcupine quills.

The spinning room was a female domain. Here, neither secular nor religious authorities had access. Here, ancient knowledge, often disguised in a fairy tale or a song, was passed on. Women's secrets and healing knowledge were exchanged. What may have been concealed throughout the rest of the year would inevitably come to light here in the darker half of the year while spinning and weaving. The clergy had harsh words

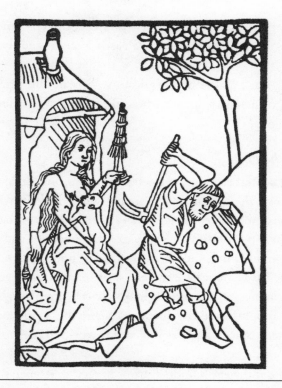

Adam toiling and Eve spinning, images of human occupations
(Basel, Switzerland, 1476)

for the spinning rooms according to this treatise from the seventeenth century: "The meetings in the spinning rooms are rarely without sin . . . they differ little from witches' meetings . . . they spoil all good manners and are a school for prostitutes . . . thus the authorities should go forward harshly against the spinning rooms" (Volkmann 2008, 34).

The textiles and plants for dyeing all came from the vicinity of the farm or village. The nature of the preparation and dyeing varied from place to place, and each area developed its own characteristics—even the colors were typical. In this manner, one could tell by people's clothes where they came from, their age, and their status or profession in life. Even today in Bavaria, unmarried women tie their apron in front on the left and married ones on the right when they wear the traditional costume, for example. A carpenter wears a certain costume, and chimney sweeps in most of Europe are easily recognized by their black costumes.

Clothing was a matter of one's destiny. Were not the primordial goddesses, the Norns, also spinners, who spun the fate of all beings, including that of the gods?

Keeper of the Fire

In an age of central heating and electric radiators, one can hardly imagine what the stove, the hearth, or the fire pit, which had always been at the center of the home, once meant. It was the warm heart of the community and at the same time the principal place of the housewife and family in the home. As yet, in Dutch and north German peasant houses, the mistress of the house has her seat here and can see from this spot everything that is going on in most of the rest of the abode. The fireplace, including the chimney, was considered the threshold where this world and the other-world connect. Smoke and fire linked this world to the world of spirits and ancestors.

Throughout the entire Indo-European region, women sacrificed bits of dough or butter into the flames, especially on holidays and other special occasions. This custom is still found in Hindu India, where it is done every day; the Slavs also still held firmly to the custom into modern times. Here in the hearth lived the house spirits (Old High German *stetigot,* Anglo *cofgodas,* Slavic *domovoi,* Latin *penates,* Norse *tompte* or *lokke*), which were interpreted by Christians as "poor souls" and revealed themselves through the knocking and crackling of the fire, for instance.

When the young bride moved into her new home, she was led by her husband, or in-laws, three times around the stove. In this way, the new or future mistress became acquainted with the home's familiar spirits. When a new house was built in Russia, an old woman brought embers from the fire of the old house, so as to provide continuity. In many places, it was a custom to carry the newborn child around the hearth after it was baptized—strictly speaking, here we are once again dealing with the sacred primordial elements of water and fire.

Wise Women and Their Remedies

Thus, we see that, when the housewife is brewing on the stove, the heart of the home, making herbal tea, or cooking or stirring an ointment, she is connected to the spiritual matrix of the home and the clan, and then the healing power is potentiated.

Herbalists

The housewives were the champions of healing herbs. Long before there were doctors, pharmacists, and hospitals, they were responsible for the care of the sick. They were heiresses of millennium-old tradition and experience. They knew where alongside the stream, in the hedge, or on the hill certain healing herbs were to be found. Their ancestors had already collected plants in the same places. They knew when and how to harvest and how to dry, store, and use them.

Conventional Guidelines
for Collecting Medicinal Plants

Here again is a brief summary of the general rules for collecting and applying the herbs.[3]

Seasons: Healing herbs for the year's use in the house and yard are collected during certain seasons, such as at midsummer (Saint-John's-wort) or at the time of the grain harvest in the hottest month, August. This makes sense because plants unfold their strongest healing powers by light and heat. Roots are better dug in late autumn or early in the spring before the plants sprout and the roots release their energy to the sprouts, leaves, and flowers.

Moon times: The rule to collect herbs during the time of the new moon, when the moon forms a small crescent, is ancient. At this time, the quality of medicinal plants is better. The herbalist Maurice Mességué, heir of an ancient Celtic herbal tradition from the Gascogne region says, "Herbs need a lot of solar power and less from the watery moon."

Time of day: In the morning, with the break of dawn and still wet with dew, the herbs will have the strength of the rising sun.

Holy days: In Catholic regions, it is customary to collect those herbs for which a certain saint is responsible on his or her name day. Saint John's Day is a particularly important one, as well as that of the days consecrated to Mary. The Holy Virgin appears in the place of the Great Goddess as the mistress of medicinal plants. Holy Thursday and Good Friday, when Jesus hung on the cross, and his tears, sweat, and blood soaked the earth, are the best days to collect early spring herbs.

Some herbalists still also carefully observe signs of good constellations between Venus, Jupiter, and the other "wandering stars" (planets). Herbal astrology, which assigns the plants to the seven visible "stars that move across the sky" (i.e., the planets, moon, Mercury, Venus, sun, Mars, Jupiter, and Saturn), dates back to ancient times and reached new heights during the Renaissance. This astrology of healing plants has been partially taken from traditional folk medicine.

Respect and gratitude: A nearly universal rule states that healing plants should not be cut with iron knives or dug with an iron spade. For as the Celts said, "Iron scares off the spirits. If iron is used, only the plant's body, but not its blessing will be harvested." The herbs are picked by hand, the earth is dug up, and the roots dug out with a stag antler, fire-hardened wood, and the like. But that is only for particular healing herbs; vegetables or herbs for everyday use can be cut with an ordinary knife or dug with a common iron spade.

Nothing is taken without giving something back. Good words or a small gift, such as some grain, bread, beer, or a copper coin are left in return for the plant. It is best to never take more than one needs, and to always leave enough of the plants growing so that they can continue to multiply. The golden rule is to leave at least half of the plant stand untouched.

Bundle of healing herbs: The herbs are hung in clusters in shady, airy places, under the attic, or in a particular herb-drying room, dried, and then put away in containers or jars. They are then used as needed.

Unique inspirations: Sometimes, in the case of a severe, sudden disease, the herbs present in the herb bundle are not enough. Then, the wise woman in the village or the grandmother, or nowadays the herbal practitioner, goes out to fetch an herb or root with special powers for that particular case. This is also known in other traditional cultures: If necessary, the patient is treated individually with specific herbs gathered just for him or her.

Even the night before they get the healing plant, the herbalists quiet their thoughts and go into deep meditation. They pay attention to their dreams. Sometimes, they get hints from the "angels" or deceased relatives; sometimes they also dream of the herb that can help. Then they go in the morning and pay attention to the signs along the way, to the animals who cross their path, to the songs of the birds. They go unwashed and unkempt—that is to say, unaffected by culture and in a natural state. In pagan times, they *(rhizotomoi)* would have gone naked as Sophocles writes about the root collector Medea: "She went naked to dig their roots." In Christian times, this practice was frowned upon, but the herbalists still went barefoot and with loosened hair. In this way, it was easier for them to receive the subtle messages from nature. Hairs are antennas with which delicate things are perceived; the soles of the feet as well—as has been rediscovered by reflexology—are extremely sensitive organs of perception. Often, after the conversion, the herbalist would pray to Mary or the Savior to obtain useful inspiration.

The herb or root is then blessed with charms to remind it of the healing powers it contains within itself. After digging the root or picking the herb, a small peace offering is left behind. The tea, salve, or poultice made out of the plant is unique and intended solely for this individual case. This remedy would not necessarily help in other similar cases. In this way, Maria Treben was able to heal a young woman who was ill with multiple sclerosis and make her healthy again using shepherd's purse; in another case, she was successful in using the calamus plant to treat colon cancer (Treben 2009, 28). These remedies came as inspirations to her during contemplation. In another sick person, at another time and in another place, these herbs would most likely not work.

The herbalist Father Sebastian Kneipp also managed to cure tetanus with silver weed—called "cramp herb" in a southern German dialect. Like Treben's cures, this one cannot be generalized in any way. It was probably—as any Native American medicine person would say—mainly the "healing power" or the medical charisma of the herbalist pastor himself that was responsible for his success.

Of course, mainstream physicians get up in arms against such "anecdotal" stories. Nevertheless, such cases arise more often than one might think. In the end, diseases are not necessarily predictable, mechanical processes. But, as the Shoshone medicine man Rolling Thunder said, "Each situation is new and unique, and every disease has different psychological, social, and karmic components, which cannot be lumped together."

Mothers

Among the forest peoples, women were also honored because they give birth to children. They give the ancestral spirits the opportunity to incarnate again and thus secure the future of clan and tribe. They nurture, guard, and teach the children at least until they are initiated and grown up. But this did not mean that women who did not have their own offspring enjoyed less respect; an unfathomable fate had merely doled out a different life's path for them. And just as the housewife cares for the little ones who have just arrived from the beyond and who rely on her protection and care, she also takes care of the infirm, sick, and elderly, who are on their way back to the otherworld. The housewife has the support of the extended family, without which nothing would be possible. In most Indo-European cultures, especially that of the forest peoples, a mother is associated through mythology with Mother Earth, for instance, Holda, Danu, Joerd, Hertha, Mati, Mokosch, and Zemes-Mate.

This reverence of the woman as mistress and mother has become alien to us. The woman has lost her stately seat at the hearth. Many of her activities, such as raising children, have been taken over by the government. Nursery school, day care, kindergarten, and after-school care are controlled by corporations, and mass-media programs tell the children the fairy tales (nowadays usually rather corny) they need for their development; the elderly come into retirement and nursing homes; the food is produced by large corporations, preserved and often even pre-cooked. In other words, compared to freshly cooked, maybe even freshly harvested and "home grown" living food, it is basically dead. Sexuality and fertility are also now successfully separated; one serves primarily hedonistic purposes, the other belongs to the field of reproductive medicine. Male sex life is completed with ejaculation; for women, coitus is only the beginning, followed by pregnancy, hormonal changes, and subsequent emotional changes, such as the natural good mood that "raises many pregnant women to the heavens" and allows her to dream the coming child into existence. (Her dreams are a guide for the ancestral soul that is returning to Earth).

Birth itself is experienced in traditional cultures as an important initiation for a woman. During natural birth, in the course of labor, the woman goes beyond pleasure and pain, beyond the limits of everyday consciousness, and enters the realm of the Great Goddess. Therefore, it was said in ancient times that Artemis, who otherwise lives in the wilderness with animals and shuns human civilization, will appear as a divine midwife and become visible to the soul's eye. In central Europe, it was always Hulda (Mother Goose), who stood by new mothers; in the Alpine regions, the *Saligefrau* (blessed woman) often appeared and helped the laboring mountain rustic's wife, charcoal burner's wife, or the milkmaid. Birth was and is a matter for women because the man had—even the head doctor of gynecology—no business there. The presence of the Goddess in this mystery when new life sees the light of day literally blows men away. In many cultures, there is therefore the couvade, a kind of men's sickbed into which the fathers retreat, completely exhausted. With birth, pleasant sensuality does not stop, because breastfeeding gives the infant as well as the mother bliss. We now know again how important breastfeeding is for a child's health and the development of a strong immune system.

The time of menstruation, the "monthly flower," is also part of female sexuality. Traditionally, these days were a time of reflection, of purification and renewal, of communion with the Goddess. Among most of the Native Americans, the woman withdrew for four days in the so-called moon hut. Even among the indigenous peoples in Europe, it used to be a special time with many taboos; gardening, baking, and brewing were banned, for example.

That which has long been an incontestable reality, as far back as historians can look, has now been put into question. The state-supported gender theory sees the roles of husband and wife or mother and father as arbitrary social constructions.

Herdsmen and Smiths

The grandmothers and housewives were not the only healers viewed by the representatives of the high culture as part of an inferior folk culture. Shepherds and herdsmen were also known to have special healing power. When the housewife was stumped, as the old farmer-philosopher Arthur Hermes told me, she went to seek advice from the shepherds.

The herdsmen were simple, natural people who already as children accompanied the herds into the mountains or in the lonely heath. Most of the slow, dreamy shepherd boys had never seen a school from the inside. Those who had attended only for a few short years so that they could barely read and write. The shepherds who lived close to nature were the exact opposite of the learned, studied doctors. Nevertheless, they were regarded as particularly gifted healers. They knew medicinal herbs and ointments with which they could make the animals entrusted to them healthy again after injuries or illness. And not only did they have practical knowledge based on experience, but in their solitude they were also frequently in the company of nature spirits, wild women, mountain ogres, and fairies.

Many tales and legends report thereof; for example, there is the legend of a virgin dressed in white who appears to a shepherd, gives him a cowslip flower, a "key flower," and tells him that he can use it to unlock the rock wall. Wonderful treasures are hidden in the rock, of which he could take as much as he wanted, but he should not forget to take the most important thing back with him, namely the flower. The shepherd tries it out. Indeed, the mountain opens, and gold, silver, and precious stones sparkle out at him. As if in a daze, he fills his pockets with the treasures, but forgets the cowslip, the most important thing, so a second access is impossible. The natural treasures of the otherworld—the gold of the sun (inspiration), the silver of the moon (intuition), and the precious stones of a crystal-clear mind—can be attained in the solitude of the wild.

How does the shepherd pass every day without friends to talk to, without reading material, without an iPhone, internet connection, or without an MP3 player? He plays the flute and he carves on his staff. And above all, he tends to and observes his animals, not objectively as a scientist, but he plunges in, merges spiritually with them, and goes on astral travels into their beings and bodies. In a trance, he smells the grasses and herbs through their noses; he imaginatively chews the cud with them and in this manner learns the characteristics of the plants that grow there. Not through the intellect, or the experimental procedure, does he learn herbalism but through the animals themselves who are his teachers. It is this profound, intuitive knowledge that makes him a respected healer in the village. Even with fertility magic he knows what to do because he has learned intuitively about it with his animal herds. That's why the farmers call him to "quicken" their cattle with his shepherd's staff (Storl 2009, 273). At times, the pastoral solitude in the heath or faraway mountain pasture lets his soul travel with the clouds; thus, he also has the ability to practice weather magic, a trait that is much appreciated by the farmers.

The blacksmith has also appeared as a healer since ancient times. The iron, which he smiths with the power of the fire and the hammer (and water), was regarded by the ancient peoples

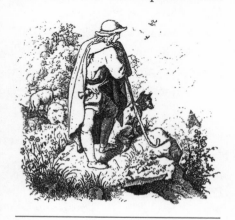

Shepherd (copper engraving by Ludwig Richter)

to be from a realm not of this world, not from Midgard, but from the otherworld. It falls as meteoric iron from the sky or is wrested from the depths of the earth. Only those who have a lot of power, such as the blacksmith who is the master of fire, can deal with it. Since the metals are from otherworldly dimensions, the Siberians consider smiths to be shamans. They possess magical heat (Eliade 1980, 29). It is interesting that the Shaman God Woden in the Anglo-Saxon *Lacnunga* (healing song) is referred to as a blacksmith. With the knife, "little iron, large wound," that he forged, he threatens the illness-bringing, magical arrow (little spear) (see pages 171–172).

Smiths were always seen as powerful magicians. They are dangerous: the sword that they forge can bring death, and the plow pulls off the skin of Mother Earth. In some societies, the smiths were banished from the village out of general precaution. But because forging could conquer the elements, it was believed that they could also even banish diseases and the devil. Children, for example, who suffered from "consuming" illness were brought before sunrise to the smithy and laid naked on the anvil. The blacksmith raised his hammer, as if he wanted to smite on hot iron, but stroked it very gently over the body instead. This was done three times, and the child was immediately healthy—perhaps out of sheer fright (Baechtold-Staeubli and Hoffmann-Krayer 1987, Vol. 9, 261)? Even the forge water was considered particularly healing and used to wash off scabies and rashes.

Like the smiths, a magical aura also surrounds the hunters, especially poachers. Through his contact with the animals and the spirits of the forest, the hunter is also, if to a lesser degree, in possession of healing powers.

Midwives

The midwife (French *sage-femme*, Slavic *baba*) has always been a woman with special status in her community. As midwife, she stood by the women in childbirth. This is and was more than just a technical task. She arranged the bedstraw in the birth room. She knew the birth herbs (mugwort, lemon balm, chamomile, ground ivy, and so on) and hemostatic agents such as ergot or groundsel *(Senecio fuchsii)*. She knew the charms and amulets that guard against the evil eye during the prenatal weeks and protect against the approach of bad spirits. After delivery, she cut a lock of hair from the child and tossed it as an offering—*pars pro toto*—to the elvish beings or the devil to ensure that they did not leave empty handed but left mother and child alone. She burned incense and made a pure atmosphere. She gave the child its first bath. She knew about postnatal care and how to stimulate milk production with herbal teas and beers with fennel, finial, cumin, or anise.

In ancient cultures, the midwife had an almost sacred status. For the Germanic people, she was the "the in-between woman" (Anglo-Saxon *myd wyf*), the mediator. After the birth, she put the newborn child on the floor to indicate that the child was not only of the biological mother but also a gift of Mother Earth. She walked around the newborn child clockwise and told it, in a clairvoyant state, its destiny. Then she picked it up and put it on the father's lap. (The German word for midwife is *Hebamme,* from the Old High German *hevan* = to lift, and *ana* = ancestor).

When the father took the baby on his lap, he acknowledged paternity and that he would take care of the child. Then the baby was sprinkled with the element of life, washed with water, and received its name. The dedication of a name and the consecration of water meant that this new-comer was now part of the community. It is this Germanic-Celtic water consecration that in the course of the conversion was finally adopted and institutionalized by the Church as infant "baptism." Obviously, it has little to do with the baptism of Jesus by John in the River Jordan. The child was considered a born-again ancestor, and sometimes the midwife even gave it the name this ancestor had carried in previous lives and would now carry again. A German word for grandchild is *Enkel* and means nothing less than "little ancestor" (Middle High German *eninklin;* Old High German *ano* = ancestor or grandfather, *klin* = diminutive suffix).

A baby that was not viable or was malformed or otherwise disfig-ured could be a changeling, or a fairy child.[4] Envious elves, dwarves, or mermaids had stolen the "real" child and foisted the ugly thing upon

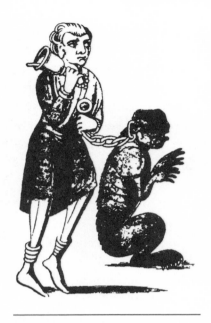

A charlatan exhibits a changeling
(Petzodt, *Kleines Lexicon,* page 177)

the mother. It was not lifted and embraced, but put out in the wilderness and exposed. Belief in changelings stretched from France to Russia. The right to continue the practice of setting unviable newborn children out in the wild was one of the conditions stipulated by the Icelandic Althing before the Icelanders would accept the introduction of Christianity. The missionaries had no choice but to agree (Hasenfratz 1992, 65).

From the beginning, the clerics observed the actions of the midwives with suspicion. Was there not quite a lot of paganism in play? Was it possible to carry out the birth so quickly and with so little pain? In the Bible, God said to woman: "I will greatly multiply your pain in childbirth, in pain you will bring forth children" (Genesis 3:16, *New American Standard Bible*). That was God's just punishment for Eve's original sin of being tempted by the serpent with the apple. Only Mary, as she was without sin, was granted a painless birth.

In the fifteenth century, midwives had to swear, by law, that no superstition or magical methods had played a part in the birth. They were told to sprinkle holy water and ask for the blessings in the name of the Father, the Son, and the Holy Spirit. During the peak of the witch hunts, it became ever more difficult for the midwives. What we can learn about them from those times does not come from the midwives but was written down by academic doctors and priests, who were not favorable to the illiterate women. They associated them with witchcraft, claiming, among other accusations, that the midwives would secretly kill children.

From the sixteenth century on, midwives in Europe had to be licensed and registered. Because of the persecution of witches, they

256

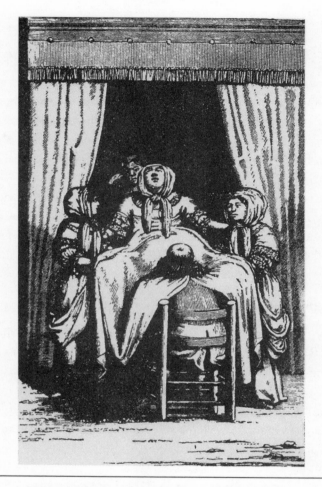

Male obstetrician treating under a sheet so as not to
embarrass the woman (woodcut, 1711)

had also been intimidated and ever fewer women entered the field
of midwifery. Innovative male doctors with knowledge of anatomy,
physiognomy, and surgery increasingly took over the business of childbirth, especially in the more affluent urban population. Instruments
such as the forceps were invented, and modern "chemical" means such
as chloroform gradually turned the natural occurrence of birth into a
technological process. Statistics from the time, kept since 1746, show,

however, that births assisted by midwives offered a far higher survival rate for the women and infants than those by physicians in hospitals (Achterberg 1991, 167). Mothers treated by doctors died three times as often as those cared for by midwives. Physicians examined pregnant women and newborns often without first washing their hands and with unsterilized instruments, giving the mothers puerperal fever. It wasn't until the middle of the nineteenth century that the observant physician Ignaz Semmelweis addressed the problem of medical hygiene (Humphries and Bystrianyk 2013, 73–74).

At the present time, scientific reproductive medicine only grudgingly admits midwives as helpers of the medical establishment. Extremely high insurance costs make it increasingly difficult for today's midwives to practice their profession.

Magical and Shamanic Women of the Forest Peoples

Since pre-Christian times in central Europe, the wise old woman, the *sagae,* as Tacitus calls her, had enjoyed respect and reverence. She was something of a shaman or worked at least similarly to a shaman, seer, herbalist, or midwife. In rural areas, she played a central role until the beginning of our modern era. The various activities of the wise women (as well as the visionaries), which we will consider here, overlap and are not mutually exclusive.

Witch

First, we want to say more about the wise old hag discussed earlier—the one who knew the nine herbs and how to let her soul fly through the chimney into the spirit world, the commonly called hedge sitter or fence rider (Old English *hægtesse*), who mediated between this world and the other. Seen through cultural anthropology, it can be assumed they still mastered the archaic shamanic technique of separating the soul from the body. At night, her soul could enter the body of her animal familiar as an owl, hare, fox, or cat. Thus, she could move through the village and countryside while her body lay at home in deep trance. She could check

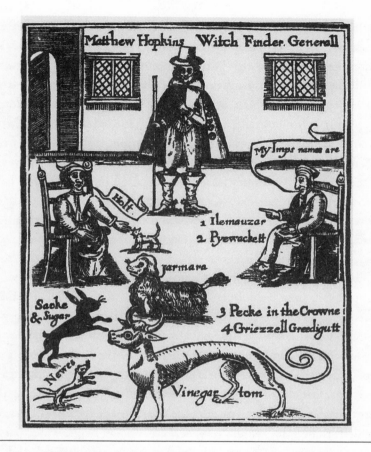

Witches name their animal familiars under interrogation
(in Mathew Hopkins's *The Discovery of Witches,* London, 1647)

on her neighbors through the eyes of her familiars; she was able to hear with their ears and smell with their noses.

The medieval scholars argued whether the witches could actually physically fly or whether it was just their demonic imagination. Definitely, people feared them and the Church made them subject to penitentials and inquisitions. The Abbot Regino of Pruem (846–915 CE) warned that "there are criminal women who, seduced by delusions and suggestions of demons, believe and confess that they spend the night with the heathen gods Diana and Herodias and innumerable other females, riding on certain animals all over the countryside, secretly and in haste in the dead silence of the night" (Habiger-Tuczay 1992, 120). Bishop Burchard of Worms wrote penitentials that served the priests as a guide for confession. In them, he lets the priest ask the confessors if they believe that a woman, while her husband sleeps and imagines his wife resting in his embrace, escapes through locked doors, flies through the air, and then, without any visible weapon, kills baptized people redeemed by Christ's blood. Even those who believed some women did these things (let alone those being accused of doing them) had to reckon with strict penance.

Presumably, these women knew about flying salves and flying herbs. Direct traditions of recipes do not exist. It was solely the priests, witch hunters, and early scientists who reported them and dealt with the salves. Giambattista della Porta, for example, describes a salve that an old woman is supposed to have used. In contrast to the Inquisition, della Porta considered witches' flights and the Witches' Sabbath on the Blocksberg (the Brocken) to be complete superstition. Through a crack in the door, he watched an old woman anoint herself with a salve and sink into a deep sleep. When she awoke, she told how she had flown over the sea and mountains. For della Porta, it was clear that it was all a subjective hallucination triggered by the toxic effect of the salve (Biedermann 1994, 355). Included in the salve were celery, aconite, poplar twigs, water parsnip, water iris, cinquefoil, nightshade (belladonna probably), oil, and bat's blood. A dangerous-sounding mix that should under no circumstances be imitated.[5]

Often, harmless analgesic ointments were found in the possession of the suspected person to serve as evidence *(corpus delicti)* for the offense. Witch hunting was, after all, a lucrative business because those found guilty had their possessions seized by the authorities.

Different types of magical women, heirs of heathen priestesses, were found for a long time in the villages of remote regions—as I know, from deep in the Alpine mountains—and can still be found today. Because they cannot be easily categorized, the following describes just a few of them.

Sorceress

The bad witch knows invocations and charms, has the power of curses, and can make voodoo dolls of her enemies. Perhaps she is also competent in sex magic, can cause infertility, or knows how to make someone lustful or love-crazy. A woman disappointed or jilted in love can hire a sorceress to make the man who has disappointed her impotent or her rival frigid. The spell is usually cast through "cord and knot magic"; that is, at certain moon phases, knots are tied in a string, while uttering spells: "By knot one, the spell is done; by knot two, it cometh true . . ."

Weather Witch

Weather magic was present in every archaic culture, and it played a role for the forest peoples as well. In the eleventh century, Burchard of Worms described a ritual to summon rain. If no rain fell for a long time, and the farmers needed it urgently, then the women gathered the little girls in the village. One of them was stripped naked, and, using the little finger of her right hand, she had to dig up a henbane plant and tie its root to the little toe of her right foot. Then the other children, with twigs in their hands, led the girl to the nearest creek. With the help of twigs, they sprinkled her with water and called out magical charms for rain. At the end of the ceremony, they went back to the village, whereby the naked girl had to walk back "like a crab and go backwards"—that is, she was not allowed to turn her back on the water (Gurjewitsch 1978, 379).

The Slavs also knew such rituals: a "rain girl," who was clothed only with green foliage, was doused with water. The Celts are said to have performed weather spells and preferred to use hemp agrimony *(Eupatorium cannabinum)* that grows in damp places. All this is reminiscent of rain rituals that anthropologists encounter throughout the world. Modern contemporaries are skeptical and see it as a pre-scientific attempt to exercise control, where no control is possible. The natives, for whom the world is a contiguous whole, on the other hand, claim that they can communicate with the cloud spirits.

In the witch trials, there was often talk of harmful weather spells by witches who maliciously summoned storms and hail. For example, there is the story of a witch-child, who conjured up a storm by whipping a puddle with branches. The clergy thought this would only be possible with the help of the devil—however, they themselves also made weather magic by letting the bells ring during thunderstorms. For a long time, the old country women still knew the charms and incense herbs that could avert an approaching thunderstorm that threatened the ripening cornfield. For example:

> Put on arnica, put on arnica,
> so the weather can depart!

Dried Saint-John's-wort was also burned as incense. In the Saxony-Anhalt region of Germany, when a storm raged for days, a voice from the clouds was heard to say:

> Is there not a single woman
> who knows about Saint John's Wort!

Village Sorceress or Shrew (Dutch, Low German toeveree, toeversche)

These are what the village magicians are called who could perform magic with red powder, ochre (iron oxide red), or blood. The German word for magic, Zauber (Old High German *Zoubar,* Anglo-Saxon *t afor,* Old Icelandic *taufr,* Middle Dutch *toever*), means just that, namely ochre, or red chalk. Since the Paleolithic times, at least since the Neanderthals, ochre was used magically to heal, rub on the dead, and paint. With white chalk, black charcoal, and red or yellow ochre, animal figures were drawn on the walls of the inner recesses of Paleolithic caves, the womb of the primordial goddess, to make the wild game fruitful and multiply. Similarly, the Druids dyed their magic wands red, and the Germanic priests used blood or ochre to enliven the runes they had scratched. Red, as we know, is the color of blood, which embodies the spirit of life; the blood sacrifice with which the gods are worshiped; woman's menstruation, which grants her fertility; and fire and embers. Red ochre was considered the blood of the earth. Indigenous people, such as the Australian Aborigines, say red ochre has the same vibration or quality as blood and can be used in its place.

Gydia and Gode (Gythia and Gothi)

The village witch, or *toeversche,* is heir to the old Germanic sacrificial priestess, the *gudia* (Gothic *gudja,* Anglo-Saxon *gydia*). She and her male companion, the *godi* or *gothi,* led the sacrificial ritual[6]—the *blót.* Participants in the blót ritual were dabbed with blood, or sprinkled with a branch that had been dipped in sacrificial blood. This was called *blédsian,* "to strengthen with blood or to bless." The English word "blessing" comes from the same root. As a sign of her trade, the female magician wears a ring and carries a staff or rod. She descends from a noble ancestral line.[7] In the fairy tale of Rapunzel, the *Gode* or *Gudja* reappears in the figure of Dame Gothel, the old sorceress in whose garden the Rapunzel vegetable (rampion, *Campanula rapunculus*) grows, which the pregnant women craved. Her husband is caught by the old woman in an attempt to steal the goodies for his pregnant wife. The witch is willing to let it be, but only with the promise that the child be entrusted to her when she is fourteen years old. Then, when the time has come, Dame Gothel takes the girl and locks her in a tower. Folklorists suggest the tower is reminiscent of puberty huts in which young women were initiated by priestesses into life as adult women.

Wickersche

Wickersche is another term for the soothsaying, fortune-telling, village wise person in the Lowland German dialect of northwestern Germany. The English word "witch" (Anglo-Saxon *wicca* or *wicce,* related to *witan* = wise) and the German word for consecrations, *weihen,* are related, as is the Middle High German *wich* (holy). In Iceland, the witch is the *vitki.* It is linguistically related to "wizard" as well as the Norman-French *wichard,* hence, the French first name *Giscard* ("the ingenious") or even the Old High German *wizago* (sage).

Galsterwoman

The *Galsterwoman* could perform *galster* and *vergalster* things; that is, she could sing charms (Old Nordic galdr; Anglo-Saxon *gealdor;* Old High German *galan*), invoke, conjure, beseech, and cast spells on someone or something. But the *galster* songs could also be songs and sayings of blessings and healing or even a call that dispels demons. The Indo-European root is **ghel,* "to yell, to scream."

The *Galster* songs or charms were different from our songs today. They did not rhyme at the end, a practice first introduced in the Middle Ages by minstrels influenced by Arab culture. The *Galster* songs were sung in alliteration and with magical tones (Old Norse *galdralag*), with modulated pitch, or in ancient storytelling tones ("way of ancient words"; German *Altmaerenton;* Old Norse *fornyrthislag*), and with specific breathing. Alliteration in general means that the same initial sounds are used in the stressed staves of the important words. The staves originally were related to the beech-wood staffs upon which reddened runes were carved. The sorceresses were generally known as possessors of such staffs. This is an example of an alliterative song from the *Edda* (Hollander 1962, 37):

> Runes wilt thou find and rightly read
> of wondrous weight,
> of mighty magic,
> which that dyed the dread god,
> which that made the holy hosts,
> and were etched by Odin
> (Havamal 142).

The word *galstern*, "magical tones," is reflected in the word "yell" (German *gellen*; Swedish *gaella* = ritual cries or war cry; Russian *galit'sja* = mock); in "nightingale" (from Old English *galan* = sing), the bird that sings enchanting songs in the evening; and in "celandine" *(Chelidonium),* which is attributed to the Greek *chelidon* (swallow). The swallow is the "screaming" bird.

Sinthgund and Sunna, who are known to us from the Merseburg Charm, were considered galster wives; Odin is known as *galster father;* and *Gjallerhorn* is the magic horn of Heimdall, the guardian of the Rainbow Bridge.

Leech Woman (Lachsnerin, Shamanic healer)

The leech doctor was the real healer of the common people. As we have already shown, the Middle High German word *lâchentoum* meant "remedies"; *lâchiron* (Old High German lâchen) means "to cure"; *lachi* (Anglo-Saxon *læce*, Middle English *leche*) is the "doctor"; the *lâchenaerinne* or her later name in German, *Lachsnerin,* was the healer in the villages. Her medicine (leechcraft) was deeply rooted in the traditional shamanic healing practice.

There were still female leech doctors for a long time in rural areas, remote mountain valleys, or the lonely heath. Until the nineteenth century, these women healed man and beast with archaic methods, with spells and plants, and with words and worts (roots). But soon enough, the clerical Church, the medical profession, and the government cracked down on them with laws and penalties. In Switzerland, new prohibitions against anyone practicing as a leech doctor were repeatedly adopted between the sixteenth and the eighteenth centuries. In 1533, during the early years of the Reformation, a decree by the "respectable Council of the City of Zurich" banned "in urban and rural areas all superstition, divination, leech practice, invoking the devil, magic, and the blessing of animals and people," under "the threat of stiff penalty." Ulrich Zwingli railed against the leech doctors, "who believe that they can show how to raise the dead by invoking the devil but are nothing but crooks." Johann von Muralt wrote in *Eydgenoessischen Lustgarten* (1715) about leech doctors, "who roam at night and in fog, and believe in such folly as that they can force the devil to do what they want. Or they practice witchcraft with their herbs, they use maidenhair or periwinkle for their love potions, poisons, magic, and leech doctor arts."

Knower of Poisonous Herbs, or Luepplerin

The *luepplerin* (Middle High German *luepplærinne*) knew the medicinal herbs, but especially the poisonous and magic herbs. She was considered a sorceress and poisoner. Astringent plant juice was known as *lueppe,* or *luppe;* the designated corresponding drug, salve, or magic formula was also called by this name. *Lueppe,* similar to the Greek pharmakon was, at the same time, a poison and a remedy. To *lueppen* someone (Anglo-Saxon *lubbian,* Middle Dutch *lubben*) meant to anoint someone with poison, poison someone, heal, or drive someone away. It depends, as Paracelsus said, on the dosage whether a plant is a simple healing herb or a poison.

The *luepplerin* knew about *luepp*-herbs, such as wolf's bane (aconite), lily of the valley, hellebore, belladonna, henbane, colchicum (autumn crocus), and so on. She had dangerous knowledge that was feared by the Church and state rulers. According to a court document from 1328, a person who interacts with a *Luepperin* is a heretic and should be judged. Elsewhere, from the fourteenth century, we read, "be it woman or man, who deals with magic and with *luppe,* and who know how to invoke the devil, should all be burned"—in other words, a death sentence (Rockinger 1883, 102). At this time, the pope forbade the craft of *lueppe.*

The word *lueppe* goes back to the Celtic word *lubi.* The Celts planted a *lubi-gortos* garden by their homes that contained not vegetables but effective medicinal herbs. From the word *lubi* or *lub-su,* the Celtic word for herb in general, *lussu,* originated (Hoefler 1911, 30).

Seidhkona (Seið-woman)

The mysterious magic of women is called *seið (sejd, seiðr).* The secret starts with the word. Some scholars claim it is related to "seething" (Old English *seothan* = boiling or cooking vigorously). Thus, it would refer to the "boiling" of cooking herbs, or the boiling of salt—salt was precious— and the prophesy read from the boiling cauldron. Perhaps the term also refers to the seething soul, the magical heat that shamans, berserkers, lamas, and ascetics possess. Other researchers believe *seið* could have to do with "rope" or *Seil* (Indo-European *$^*s$* , referring to a rope or, as a verb, "to bind"), binding spells and magical fetters, or even to "sing."

In any event, it was a woman's art. For men, it was considered shameful to practice *seið*. Freya, the *"seið*-bearer" was regarded as the champion of this knowledge. She taught this art to Odin, the shameless one. Loki mocks the shamanic god in his diatribes *(Lokasenna):*

> But though, say they on Sams Isle once
> wovest spells like a witch,
> in warlock's shape through the world didst fare:
> were these womanish ways, I ween (Hollander 1962, 95).

Visionaries

Clairvoyant, wise women played such an important role among the forest peoples that it astonished the Romans. In the Germanic-Celtic settlement area, they were known under the names Wala and Voelva and in southern and central Germany as *Walburg* or *Walburga,* which means "staff bearer" (Germanic *waluz* = stave, staff; from Indo-European **uel* = turn). They carried wands with which they were able to steer things magically. The Lombards knew the seer as *Gambara,* which also means "staff bearer" (Germanic *gand* = bar, *bera* = carrier). Other names for female seers were *Veleda, Heid,* or the Scandinavian *spákona* (from *spá* = see, peer; and *kona* = woman). The Veleda or Weleda goes back to the original Celtic *velet* or *fili,* which means "visionary" or "poet." These women were not priests, but prophets, or shamans, who prophesied while in an ecstatic state and so guided the destiny of their tribe. (Joan of Arc fits into this tradition, for instance.) On April 30th, the eve of the May Festival (May 1st), we still remember them when Walpurgis Night, or Witches' Eve, is celebrated. The patron saint of May 1st officially sanctioned by the Church is Saint Walburga, an English missionary and niece of Boniface, who could not stop the May Day celebrations.

These shaman women traveled about the land and were welcomed guests on the farmsteads as well as in the halls of the king. When they prophesied, they sat on a high seat or stool *(seidhallr)* on the roof of the house or on an ox hide on the crossroads, sang their *gladr* (magical songs) in magical tones, and subsequently journeyed into the world of the gods. Participants of these séances, who themselves were clairvoyant to the ethereal dimension, saw them covered in feathers and floating away as geese or swans. Freya herself appears in fairy tales and myths as a guardian of the geese; as a goose-maiden, she is the guardian of all souls. Particularly on special holy days, the shamans flew out as wild geese—on the Day of the Dead, the festival on November 1st, or the winter solstice, for instance. In many places, a goose, the totemic animal of flying Freya, is ritually slaughtered and seasoned with a bit of mugwort, the sacred shamanic herb. Reminiscent of shamanic flight is the ritual food of the Christmas or Saint Martin's goose; mugwort now serves merely as a "spice," its ritual context having been forgotten. The shamanic flights of these women were not simply psychedelic "trips" but served the kin community. In this way, they renewed the connections to the gods and spirit worlds, and brought blessings and healing back with them.

In the *Saga of Eric, the Red* a Voelva named Thorbjorn is described in detail and was called in to help Greenlandic farmers during a period of bad weather. They say she was wearing a full-length blue coat as her shaman costume, decorated to the hem with gems, a belt made from tinder polypore, a pouch with fire-making items, a leather bag with charms, a black lambskin cap lined with white cat fur, and a wand. She took a place on the high seat while a woman sang charms to invoke spirits. In her ecstasy, she prophesied the end of the bad weather spell, saw a happy marriage ahead for the woman who was singing, and answered the questions of all those present (Zingsem 1999, 266).

It is said of the Voelvas and Weledas that they were so powerful that even God, when he fell ill one day, descended to Earth so that the magical women could heal him. He was made to laugh and then felt better again. Of the mighty Thor, it is also told that he went to the prophetess Groa because a flint wedge was stuck in his head and was giving him headaches. She sang her magic charms, and the flint became loose. Enthusiastic about the effect, Thor told the singer that her husband would soon return. Groa was so happy that she forgot the rest of the healing song, so Thor still carries the wedge in his skull.

For the Christian missionaries and priests, these greatly honored wise women were an obstacle in their quest to convert people to the "one and only true faith." They were increasingly demonized. In 1326, the Icelandic Bishop Jon Halldórsson banned everything that had to do with magical practices, such as *seiđ*.

The Remedies of the Womenfolk

As we have already heard, herbal teas and decoctions were the main remedies of the indigenous forest peoples in central Europe. Wine decoctions, distilled spirits, tinctures, and herbal liqueurs only later became part of folk medicine under the influence of monastic and academic medicine. However, the healing plants were taken not only as infusions and decoctions but also in the form of beers and breads, or they were used externally as salves, poultices, and bandages.

Healing Ales

Paracelsus tells us, "Beer is not a bad drink, but a medicine . . . it enhances substance, it turns into blood. Therefore, it is also a nutriment and nutrition" (Kluge 2008, 71–92). He is probably right, because good (non-chemicalized) beer—consumed in moderation—keeps one healthy.

- Beer contains polyphenols, which are antioxidant and free radical scavengers with a cancer-inhibiting effect.
- Brewer's yeast is a good source of vitamin B.
- Because of lactate bacteria and yeast, beer has probiotic activity and improves the intestinal flora.
- Beer is relaxing and soothing. People who drink beer have a thirty percent lower chance of suffering from palsy.
- Beer cleans the arteries. Harvard Professor Walter Willett tells us, "Not drinking [beer] is a risk factor for heart attacks" (Willett 2005, cited in Kluge 2008, 82).
- Beer stimulates the metabolism so there is less constipation.

- Beer is a good diuretic; it stimulates the kidneys and reduces the risk of kidney stones.
- Because of the silica contained in it, it strengthens bones.

In folk medicine, beer has always been considered a good household remedy:

- A hot beer, not boiled, but heated up to a simmer—helps with colds, flu, and intestinal infection.
- Malt beer (a non-alcoholic beer) is good for pregnant and lactating women. It is strengthening and nourishing.
- Beer increases milk production because it contains the hormone prolactin.
- Applied externally, the beer grain residue cleanses and nourishes the skin.

Brewing, as well as baking, was traditionally women's work. The dowry that a young woman brought into her marriage included a brewing kettle. All sorts of herbs and other ingredients were added to the top-fermented ale (Proto-Germanic *aluth,* Baltic *alus,* Old Slavonic *olu,* Norse *oel*) the housewife brewed—except hops *(Humulus lupulus)*! Only the monks, who became more and more involved in the brewing business, flavored their beer since Carolingian times with the resinous, bitter female flowers of this dextrorotatory creeper from the hemp family. The hopped brew that the men of God called "beer" (from the Latin *bibere* = drink, *biber* = potion) kept longer and could be stored for longer periods. But that was not the only reason it appealed to them.

The monastery beer was also brewed to act against the incubi and succubi, underlying or overlying seductive demons who come in the form of provoking youths or flirtatious young women and rob the poor monks of their seed (semen). The seed is then used by the devil himself, because he has no innate creative power, to create cretins and monsters. Hopped beer was to curb the lust of the monks because sex and spirituality were seen as opposites. Although the beer seemed to be of only limited help because it increases general sexual pleasure, the monastic brothers drank it in vast quantities. Chroniclers tell us that each monk was allowed to take five liters of hopped ale per day (Kluge 2008, 21). Drinking such amounts causes hormonal disturbances—the phytoestrogens, which are similar to the female sex hormone, overwhelm the testosterone. In the hop-less ale the women brewed, that was not the case.

In northern countries, especially in England, people were initially not enthused about hopped ale. King Henry VI (1421–1471) forbade the cultivation of hops; Henry VIII said that hops are evil herbs that spoil the taste of the ale and harm people's health; and the botanist John Evelyn wrote, "Hops transmuted our wholesome ale into ale, which doubtless much alters its constitution. This one ingredient, by some suspected not unworthily, preserves the drink indeed, but repays the pleasure in tormenting diseases and a shorter life" (Grieve 1931).

Ordinary people, especially in Scandinavia, the Netherlands, Germany, England, and the Baltic states, held for a long time to the conventional gruit ale that contained many herbal ingredients and was often made with oats as brewer's grains.

As for daily, domestic brewing, women were gradually freed from this task as the brews that gave them, to a certain degree, control over the health and mentality of the household community now came increasingly into the hands of the high and mighty. The royal courts and gentlemen obtained their beer mainly from the cloisters, and, during the Middle Ages, the sovereigns and municipal leaders lent brewing rights to professional brewers and licensed premises, which were bound to strict regulations. It was thus taken out of the hands of the women. In 1516, Duke William of Bavaria enacted the *Reinheitsgebot*, "the German purity law," that permitted only water, malt, yeast, and hops as brewing ingredients. The law was said to prevent the use of impure and dangerous additives, such as henbane. According to Christian Raetsch, this was the first drug law. The common people found the law to be a repressive measure. At the present time, however, at least in Germany, one can be rather happy about it because the European Union is undermining the purity laws and allowing various, unwholesome chemical additives.

271

The pre-Christian forest peoples brewed various ales. In the first place, there was the everyday ale, containing very little alcohol and drunk by all, including older children. It was "liquid bread" and often more wholesome than the often impure water that was available. The main additive in this weak ale was the tart and spicy ground ivy (Glechoma hederacea). Common names, such as ale-hoof, tunhoof, or gill, betray the use of this creeping mint family plant for ale brewing. Other bitter or tannic, antimicrobial plants, such as yarrow, the leaves of ash or oak, heather, blueberries, pine tree shoots, and others, were also used in everyday ale.

In addition to the everyday beverage, people had ritual beers they drank at large festive events and sacrifices in honor of the ancestors, gods, or, later, saints. The Celts, who dedicated beer to the Great Goddess with the magical cauldron, the Grain Goddess and mistress of life and death, knew henbane beer. Henbane *(Hyoscyamus niger)* is a poisonous nightshade plant *(Solanaceae)* with strong psychedelic effects. Henbane beer was especially drunk during the festivals of the beautiful Sun God Belenos (Bhel) at the festival on the full moon of May, or at the summer solstice, and it catapulted the participants to numinous spheres. Henbane beer, *Bilsenbier* in German and named after the Sun God, is the original pilsner.[8] As a ritual drink, it was also adopted by the Germans and Slavs (Storl 2004b, 28–29). Further holiday and festival beers contained, accordingly, honey and certain herbs, which could make the drink "more inebriating": sweet gale *(Myrica gale)*, wild rosemary *(Ledum palustre)*, or possibly the neurotoxic darnel *(Lolium temulentum)*.

In folk medicine, medicinal ales, especially those brewed by the housewives, were important. By brewing daily ale, they had some control over the mood and well-being of the household. Here are some of the herbs that went into the ales, and their medicinal effect.

- angel hair or polypody *(Polypodum)*—hormonal, cholagogue
- ash leaves—diuretic, blood purifier
- avens—liver cleansing
- bedstraw—diuretic

- beechnuts—invigorates
- blueberry—antiseptic, astringent
- buckthorn—laxative, purgative
- caraway—digestive, emmenagogue
- cornflower—diuretic
- dandelion—encourages hepatic metabolism, diuretic
- elderflower—diaphoretic, strengthens the immune system
- juniper—diuretic
- marjoram (wild oregano)—stimulating, carminative
- meadowsweet—diuretic, analgesic
- mugwort—used in gynecological problems, promotes menstruation
- nettle—stimulates metabolism, cleansing
- parsley—stimulates menstruation
- rosehips—strengthen the immune system
- rowan—lymph cleansing
- Saint-John's-wort—antidepressant
- tansy—vermifuge, abortifacient
- thyme—antispasmodic
- wild ginger—encourages menstruation, abortifacient
- yarrow—increases appetite, strengthens the immune system

The herbs from the cloister gardens at the time of Saint Hildegard also found their way into the "medicinal beers" *(cerevisiae medicatae).* According to Hildegard of Bingen, beer is good for the humors. She did not like to add hops to beer; *Hoppo,* as she calls it, is not suited "because it increases melancholy in people, makes the mind of man sad, and with its dryness burdens the gut" (Riethe 2007, 397). Such herbs as horehound, a rather bitter cloister herb that increases bile and stimulates the appetite, garden sage as a disinfectant, and lemon balm to lighten the mood were added to the beer. Thistles or ground elder were boiled in beer to treat gout. Diarrhea can be stopped with oak leaves as an additive. Ulcers are healed with betony and cumin cooked in old beer. A "rising mother" (uterine displacement) was treated with southernwood boiled in beer. Enough recipes of this type can be discovered in scattered obscure writings to fill a book. Many found their way into rural medicine so that one can speak of a synthesis of folk medicine and cloister medicine.

Loaves, Bread, and Cookies

Bread has been, since humans started growing crops, a sacred life-sustaining staple. It was also suitable as a sacrifice for feeding the gods, spirits, and ancestors. In return, the gods and spirits passed their blessing on in the bread. The forest peoples of the heathen west knew of ceremonial breads that were shaped into the form of gods, animals, plants, or humans. When the consecration breads were consumed on sacred, ceremonial days, humans also consumed part of the blessing and healing power of the respective deity. The custom continued unbroken into Christian culture—the host, the bread of Holy Communion, which represents the body of God, is to be entirely understood in this sense. Soon, pretzels replaced the sun or spiral, which had been baked by the heathen women in honor of the resurgent spring sun.[9] Meant to represent the folded arms of the monks in prayer posture, pretzels were eaten during lent (with beer). Other medicinal loaves followed, into which healing herbs were often mixed as well as a prayer, charm, or small ritual, such as, for example, taking the breads to a sacred spring on Candlemas Day to bless them there.

Following the pagan example, an Easter loaf was flavored with tansy or sweetened with honey and baked in the form of a lamb, rabbit, or chicken; on November 1st, All Soul's Day bread was offered for the poor souls (the dead); and advent bread was popular on December 6th, Nicolas Day, on which breads were (and still are) shaped like Santa. Yule and Christmas breads were sweet breads full of nuts and dried fruit, such as the still very popular Dresdner Christ-Stollen (a long bread of one

kilo, representing the swaddling baby).
And just as bread was once identified
with the healing powers of the gods, so
they became identified with the saints
and their attributes.

Hubertus bread is said to help against
rabies and madness; Cornelius bread
works against epilepsy; Wendelin
bread against diseases of animals; and
St. Agatha bread against various ailments. Since the Middle Ages, for the
more affluent, Christmas gingerbread
was flavored with honey and expensive
exotic spices such as cinnamon, cloves,
cardamom, ginger, nutmeg, and pepper; the spices were believed to have a
healing effect. The German word for
gingerbread is *Lebkuchen*. *Leb* could
be traced back to the German word
for body, *Laib*, or to the Latin *libum*
(pancake); more likely, it goes back to
lueppe (Celtic *lubi*), which would refer

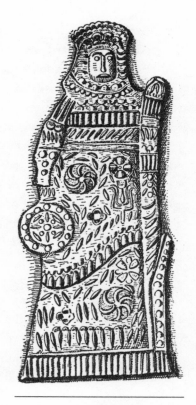

Holiday cookie

to the exotic herbs. Many of these breads are still baked in Europe on
the holidays; gingerbread men cookies are also a remnant of such festive baked goods.

Hildegard of Bingen knew the herbal cakes as "little breads." They
were made of wheat, bean flour, and egg yolks and baked in the oven,
or in hot ashes, or simply dried in the sun. A sort that should make the
heart strong and happy again had mullein in it, as well as meat or fish.
Another type of little bread, also with meat, contained ground ivy leaves
and is supposed to help people when they feel dull and feel their sense of
rationality is fading. Baking medicinal herbs into rolls or loaves is still a
way to provide phytotherapy.

Salves and Oils

Drugs do not necessarily need to be taken internally. The skin is an excellent absorber of fat-soluble medicinal agents. Salve making was one of the most important tasks of a housewife; it was, as today's herbalists still know, a "sacred matter," which is done in a state of meditative consciousness. Ultimately, it was not about active ingredients—of course, the people then did not yet know anything about that concept—but about stirring good healing magic into the salve. Every detail, every little detail, was important. The woman took note of when, where, and how the herbs were collected, the position of the moon, the kind of firewood used for cooking, and the atmosphere in the house. Good thoughts, carried by humming or soft singing and a stable stirring rhythm accompanied the work. As in the round dances, the general direction of the stirring was always clockwise. The stirring spoon was usually made of bad spell-repelling rowan or juniper wood. The best time to prepare salves was on Friday morning at sunrise, the day of Freya the goddess of women, the champion of *seiđ* art. The best lunar time for salve making was, just as it was with herb gathering, around the dark of the moon, when the moon was no bigger than a narrow sickle.

Of course, it mattered which fat was used as a carrier substance. For most Indo-European peoples, butter or clarified butter (ghee), the noblest gift of the sacred cow, was the preferred salve base.[10] In the Mediterranean, however, butter was little known. The Greeks and Romans, who insulted the northern barbarians by calling them "butter-eaters," cooked with olive oil and also used it in the production of salves. The fine, yellow May butter was considered the best butter by the forest peoples, because at this time of year the cows (or goats) ate the best vital greenery. The butter made during Saint John's time was also considered particularly strong for medicine. In southern Germany, it is said that the butter in which the elderflower fritters have been fried is curative.

In the Alemannic region, people liked to use the butter made on Saint Bartholomew's Day (August 24) because this saint had cooled and healed his broken body with butter. Hildegard of Bingen knows *Angosmêre* (butter salve) mainly as a healing ointment, especially for the head and eyes. In the Baltic region (Latvia), the butter made from the first milk after calving was considered a remedy for all kinds of evil. It worked best when a wooden spoon was used to smear the salve on the painful area, and then, without looking behind, the spoon was tossed over the shoulder (Kurtz 1937, 41).[11]

Lard was just as important a medium. Salves based on lard in the rural folk medicine are still preferred because this fat is the most similar to our own body fat and penetrates very well into the deeper layers of the skin. The great herbalist Maria Treben, like the rural population in general, cooked her various herbal salves—her famous marigold salve, for example—preferably in lard. Pigs are animals that are well adapted to a forest biotope. For forest peoples, pigs were an important protein source as well as sacred animals. For the Germanic people, Freyr's gold-bristled boar uses its strength to push the wheel of the new year back into motion after the sun-child is reborn at the winter solstice, on the sacred "mother's night" (Anglo-Saxon *modraniht*). Freyr's boar is still celebrated in the boar's head (with an apple in its mouth) or the Christmas ham served in England and Scandinavia at the yuletide banquet; it is also the piglet made of marzipan that symbolizes good luck for the new year.

For the Celts, roast pork was the best banquet and symbol of hospitality. A Celtic king had to spend some time as a swineherd, and Saint Patrick the patron saint of Ireland can boast of having done this as well. The wild sow was dedicated to the Great Goddess (Cerridwen, Demeter, Freya, and others), the Earth Goddess, and was an important animal in the matriarchal cultures. The Christian missionaries had trouble with this native worship of pigs, for they considered them impure and symbols of unchasteness and gluttony. Soon, however, a place was also found for pigs in the Christian cosmos with even their own patron saint, Saint Anthony.

The images a culture bears affect all areas of life, notably in healing and in the manufacture of medicines. Pig fat, this symbol of happiness, joy, and wealth (e.g., piggy bank), awakened expectations of salvation in the indigenous forest peoples.

Salve Preparation According to Maria Treben

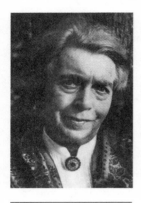

Finely chop two heaping handfuls of herbs. Heat 500 grams of pork lard in a deep frying pan. Stir in the herbs until they just patter. Remove the pan from the heat, cover, and let steep overnight. The next day, lightly reheat the mixture and then strain through a linen cloth. Pour the still-warm salve into sterilized jars. (Treben 2009, 8).

Maria Treben

Bear lard, as well as deer and badger fat were also used by the indigenous forest peoples as media for salves. Again, the symbolic meaning of animals played a fundamental role in what was expected of the salve: The bold, aggressive badger and the wise, knowledgeable herbalist "Bruin" (the bear) were once dedicated to the Earth Goddess, also the case among most Native Americans. Badger fat—similar to the still popular marmot fat—is said to help with tendonitis, gout, lupus, side stitch, tumors, and a number of other ailments. A salve made of bear fat was considered as strong as the bear itself and practically a panacea. Since the stroke of a bear's paw is deadly, hunters and poachers have used bear fat ointment to grease their firearms, hoping the magic will be transferred. And because the bear is hairy, the ointment can be used as hair growth pomade. Other animals had to serve for various salves and ointments, too. In the Middle Ages, buttered breast milk was even known. A salve made from mother's and daughter's milk was said to prevent eye ailments for a lifetime. Psychedelic flying ointment, mainly made with nightshade plants, such as belladonna, were prepared preferably with goose fat or bat fat for the best flying. The witches were claimed to cook the ointment naked at night—but who knows, that might have been a fantasy of the Inquisitors.

Today, there are ever fewer wild animals, and in industrial society where unhappy pigs and cattle are kept in large-scale factory-farming operations, conditions exist in which good, wholesome fats for such ointments cannot be produced any more. Not only are the fat and tallow of these unfortunate creatures penetrated with chemicals and antibiotics, but on an energetic level their suffering also affects the drug. How can it be otherwise? The same applies to the thousands of pharmaceutical products tested on animals as well. Over one hundred million vertebrate animals are still dying every year in such laboratories worldwide. How can true healing come from this? If one wants to make ancestral ointments, the fat of animals originating from organic farms that facilitate a happy and natural life should be used. And one should be grateful for their sacrifice as well.

More and more herbalists use olive oil and beeswax for health and ethical reasons, although these penetrate the skin less well than animal fat. Milking grease or Vaseline are popular as an ointment base, but these fats are made from petroleum. Other ingredients used today in alternative medicine as carriers include coconut oil, shea butter, cocoa butter, and other lipids that are available thanks to global trade.

Soap

The people north of the Alps discovered soap very early on in their history. The word seems to come from the West Germanic *sap* (juice, resin, dripping, sliding, slippery substance) and can be found as a loan word in the Latin *sapo* = soap (therefore, saponins are "foam-generating substances"). Pliny reported that the Germanic people made soap from tallow, ash, and plant juices, and for cultic reasons it was used to color the hair red (Pfeifer 2012, 1272). Soap is of course important for hygiene, which keeps the body clean and healthy. But not only that, it was also used as a remedy in itself. An old recipe from the Anglo-Saxon *Lacnunga* reads as follows:

> Take the nine herbs—mugwort, plantain, stune, attorlothe [these two plants cannot be definitely identified], chamomile, nettle,

apple, parsley, and fennel—and a piece of old soap. Crush the herbs into a powder; mix the soap and apple juice into it. Make a paste with water and ashes. Take fennel, cook it in the paste and mix it in the ointment. Sing the charm three times in the mouth, in both ears, and the wound of the patient before cleansing the wound.

In the medieval bathhouses—heirs of Stone Age sweat lodges—people used soap while bathing. But when the plague, cholera, and other diseases came, scholars and ecclesiastical authorities suspected that soap and water were harmful and mediated the disease, as they open the pores. The bathhouses, where the ongoings were quite unchristian anyway, were closed and washing was frowned upon. Instead, powdered underwear became the fashion. The distrust of washing with soap lasted until the early twentieth century. It was believed that it would make the bones soft; Arthur Hermes also never bathed because he thought it would wash away the "etheric body"; the body cleanses itself by itself, he said, if you live a morally clean life.

In folk medicine, there were many magical medicinal recipes with soap up until modern times. Especially effective for healing is, for example, a soap that has been used to wash a corpse. In Swabia, there is an ointment made of soap, lard, chalk, and vinegar, which was applied to swollen limbs.

Salt

Salt was valuable and one of the few trade goods of the Stone Age. It not only improves tastes and makes meat keep longer, but it is also important for the water balance of the body, the nervous system, and bone formation. It contains essential minerals and trace elements and maintains the electrolyte balance. But it is more than that. The mineral has the power to draw the soul into the body. Those who get no salt will have a soul that floats gradually into the otherworldly dimension. Therefore, in many places, it was the custom to put a little salt on the tongue or in the bathwater of the newborn so it would not leave Earth again. Lent pretzels

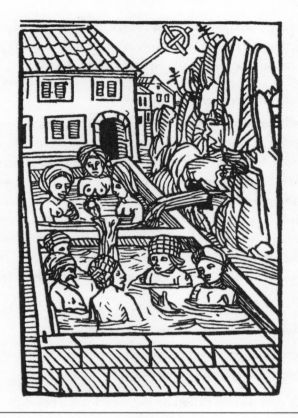

Medieval bathhouse

were sprinkled with salt so that the fasting person did not space out but remained anchored in everyday awareness.

On the other hand, it is said that witches eat no salt and the devil hates salt. Even Arthur Hermes, the farmer-mystic, avoided salt in his food; he claimed that salt binds too much on the material level. Food sacrifices for the dead are essentially not to be salted. This is also true in India, where the dead are given an unglazed clay pot filled with water from the Ganges and cooked rice for the long path to the *pitris* (ancestors). But the rice must not be salted, so as to not bind the soul.

It was a custom of mothers to sprinkle salt on lovesick daughters to bring them to their senses. To grind, boil, and blow salt was part of the art of Germanic *seið* women (Zingsem 1999, 219). Even into modern times, people in Latvia celebrated "salt blowers" *(sahl-puhschlotaji)*, who spoke to the salt and blew over it, and respected them as healers.

Compresses and Poultices

Herbal poultices, compresses, and bandages have always been effective and powerful remedies. Traditionally, hot wraps included chamomile, thyme, linseed, hay flowers, yarrow, or horsetail. Housewives and healers also knew cool compresses and bandages of sliced onions, cabbage, cheese, comfrey, fenugreek, clay, and so on. Skin-irritating, deep-working mustard and horseradish poultices were also used—usually with a thin cloth layer to protect the skin (Thueler 1995). It was especially herbalist Father Sebastian Kneipp who rediscovered the herbal wrap, like he did so many other traditional things that are valuable and effective in folk medicine.

Honey, Vinegar, Mud, and Urine

All sorts of substances found in the house and the barn could be part of the medicine chest. Here are some examples.

- Warm cow dung is placed on the back for sciatica. Mixed with old beer or vinegar, the dung is used for inflammation and ulcers.

- Cow urine helps wounds heal more quickly and repels skin fungus (of course, only from animals raised in a healthy manner).

- Honey has antimicrobial and antibiotic properties and nourishes the tissue. Honey helps for bed sores (decubitus) in bedridden people when nothing else does. Honey even soothes burns and psoriasis. Garlic milk with honey helps with pneumonia, and for a cough honey onion syrup, honey and radish syrup, honey and plantain syrup, or fennel honey milk is recommended. Honey water has a detoxing effect, improves digestion, and is supposed to be good for the kidneys as well.

- Vinegar, especially apple cider vinegar, has been rediscovered in alternative medicine as a panacea. Diluted with water (two teaspoons per glass) and sipped throughout the day, it stimulates the body's defenses. Vinegar water is said to help with joint pain; as a gargle, it has an antibacterial effect for sore throat and hoarseness. Vinegar water, drunk in sips, helps stomach pain and digestive disturbances (Hellmiss 1998). Father Kneipp used vinegar diluted with water "for weak natures" (cloth soaked in the mixture was used to rub the body down) or as a "wet shirt" for general strengthening.

- Clay packs were used to treat any kind of skin ailment.

- Cabbage leaves were used in many diverse ways. For the early Romans, Pliny wrote, cabbage was the panacea that guaranteed no doctors were needed for six hundred years and that only when they became decadent and soft did they turn to the wily Greek physicians and their expensive drugs. In folk medicine, grandmothers placed fresh, crushed cabbage leaves (preferably Savoy cabbage) on ulcers, poorly healing wounds, burns, neuralgia, gout, and tumors. Hot wraps helped with rheumatism and muscle pain. Internally, the juice of cabbage or sauerkraut helps with gastrointestinal problems.

Final Words: The Return of Ancestral Wisdom

And because the new things,
Build on the remains of the old,
Can an unclouded eye
Glancing backward, look forward.

FRIEDRICH WILHELM WEBER, DREIZEHNLINDEN
(*THIRTEEN LINDENS,* 1878)

Stone Age shamans, Indo-European charms, healing arts of old hags, root-diggers, and forest witches—what do they have to do with us? Is this not long-outdated history? Are we not infinitely more advanced with our scientific medical findings? The electronically networked knowledge of the world is a mouse click away. Who can deny such progress?

Despite all this, one can, as a cultural anthropologist, for example, have one's thoughts about it. Are we really so much smarter or wiser than the men of ancient civilizations? It seems that, in spite of the mountains of information readily available via Google or Yahoo!, we forget nearly as much as we believe we learn. Who knows about all the different herbs that grow right outside the front door, let alone their healing power? Who can telepathically talk to animals, slip into the consciousness of a plant, or experience nature spirits? We do not think that such a thing is possible anymore—if it ever was—but I have experienced it with the old mountain farmer Arthur Hermes, with tribal peoples in India and Nepal, and with Native American peoples. Who knows about the different heat qualities—as opposed to the mere quantity of calibrated heat—of various types of wood? Who can still milk a cow without a milking machine?

Some years ago, an elderly missionary came up to me at an ethnomedical conference that takes place every year in Munich.[12] He wanted to ask me a question. For decades, he had taught "the true faith" to the aboriginals in the Congo and communicated to them what a rational, modern worldview is. The syringe was one of the most effective means of conviction, he said with a smile. However, something left him no peace, and that was why he had come to the conference: An African boy had asked him if he could ask a plant which healing power it has, and could he get an answer from it?

"No one can do that!" The missionary had answered with certainty.

Nevertheless, the determined boy had replied: "But our *nganga* (medicine man) can!"

Over the years, this statement gave the priest no peace. Gradually, he even doubted his mission and wondered if what he was doing wasn't ultimately helping to destroy an indigenous culture.

One can also see progress as an ideology that promotes the progressive alienation from the things closest to us. To the degree that we are alienated from the earth under our feet, the smell of the forest and closeness of the animals, we move ever farther away from our own center, and from our many innate skills. Our fantastic technological support system is actually and ultimately made up of skills that we have within ourselves.

Telephone, mobile phone, and Skype not only replace our innate telepathic abilities, but they also turn them off and threaten to destroy them. Television and computers displace the inner vision that allows us to look into the deep dimensions of nature. Flights in heavy, metal, gas-guzzling airplanes let us forget the ability of the soul to fly. There are archaic techniques that allow the soul to leave the body temporarily and visit other people and regions that I could experience several times with Native peoples and elsewhere. Meanwhile, it has even gone so far that most people no longer believe that these innate skills even exist. Claudia Mueller-Ebeling, well-known ethnologist and art historian, wonders what impact the navigation satellite coordinate system GPS will have on spatial orientation skills of people in the long run. Will the time come when our instinctive sense of orientation and other inborn abilities are so stunted that one no longer believes that they even exist (Mueller-Ebeling 2010, 9)?

In one of my trips to see the Cheyenne medicine man Bill Tallbull, he shook his head and said, "We Indians always know where east, west, north, and south are. Each of these directions has their own character, their own power. How can it be that most whites who I meet have no idea where east or west is? How can they survive at all?"

Also, fewer and fewer people believe in the healing power of plants, the healing power of the word, or the innate healing ability of the body, the *vis medicatrix naturae*. They are convinced that the organism is similar to a complex cybernetic-controlled machine—the brain is a kind of information-processing computer, the heart is a pump, and the metabolism is some kind of process like in a test tube. The physiological processes—metabolism, hormone activity, enzyme reactions, and so on—can be pharmacologically guided and quantitatively, accurately, and experimentally confirmed by controlled experiments. Worn-out parts can be replaced like spare parts in a machine, or repaired. While all this may have its accuracy, it is a one-sided perspective and does not do justice to the essence of a living organism, a living body.

My friend and neighbor, Harald, a physician with a private practice, is convinced of this view. Once, when I happened to be passing by with a bunch of different healing herbs, he asked, "Well, Wolf, what do you have there?"

"Something that will replace the doctors," I said jokingly. He was not amused.

"Just you wait, when things get really serious, then only the hard facts count. Herbs are ineffective or toxic. With few exceptions, they have absolutely no meaning in medicine!"

That "ineffective or toxic" was an outright contradiction seemed to have escaped him. He simply did not believe in the potency of the plants. One of his colleagues, the renowned American physician Andrew Weil is of a different opinion. At a symposium in Munich, he expressed his belief: "If people would be taught about healing plants, they could treat sixty percent of their diseases and ailments by themselves—which would incidentally also be a great relief to the health care budget." I myself would go so far as to say—in the full knowledge that this is a heretical statement—that, with a substantial knowledge of phytotherapy, at least ninety percent of diseases, acute or chronic, are treatable.[13]

I have good reasons for saying that. For one, we now know—thanks to modern empirical, pharmacological research—much more about the complexity of medicinal plants. On the other hand—thanks to psychosomatic and psycho-neuro-immunological medicine—we are becoming increasingly aware of the mental and spiritual factors that are involved in health.

For shamans and healers of traditional peoples, spirit, soul, and body form an inseparable unit. They treat visible as well as invisible aspects of the human being with vocals, drums, incense, charms, stones, and herbs—with words and roots. This therapy moves the spirit and dissolves and loosens feelings that are blocked up in the body, and stimulates self-healing powers. In any case, psychological trauma and emotional shock, possibly even as far back as a birth trauma, filter down to the physical body and contribute to sickness. They can hardly be healed with pharmaceuticals alone.

Andrew Weil, MD, a Harvard graduate and professor of medicine at the University of Arizona, knows very much about states of altered consciousness and shamanism. In his book, *Spontaneous Healing* (Weil 2000), he deals with the effects of the spirit and the imagination on health and disease processes. Again and again, he writes, serious illnesses, such as cancer, go into spontaneous remission. This is by far not uncommon. The doctors who are treating the patient cannot explain it.

But is not wound healing in itself already a mystery? How do the cells know when the wound has finished healing and there is no need for them to multiply further? Who tells them that? In the human body, every second more than ten million defective cells are replaced; a permanent regenerative exchange is taking place in our bodies. It has been shown that even damaged DNA strands can repair themselves. What machine can do that? Could it be that the worldview of the technological medical establishment itself is actually a modern superstition?

Dr. Weil also finds it fascinating that warts can suddenly disappear through magical treatment: the grandmother speaks over them while circling them with a finger during a waxing moon and then "nicking" them into elderberry bark, or transmitting them onto a snail, which then slithers away with them. There is no rational explanation, yet these methods work again and again.

In the Slavic countries and in eastern Germany, it was customary to brush the hand of a still warm corpse three times over a sick body part, saying, "In the name of the Father, the Son, and the Holy Spirit, Amen." In this manner, even parts diagnosed with cancer would rapidly heal (Lehmann-Enders 2000, 65). Even to merely touch a just deceased person has brought about spontaneous healings. Clairvoyants say that the dead, especially in the first three days, have a strength that can change a loved one's deadlocked psychosomatic patterns. These are phenomena that go far beyond the limits of the scientific method. And yet experiments in quantum physics suggest that human consciousness exerts influence on the behavior of subatomic particles, electrons, and quarks. Experiments such as those of the physicist Paul Davis leave no other conclusion than that thoughts have an influence on this level; for example, they can even determine the direction of rotation of the electronic spin axes (Broers 2013, 37–38).

Dr. Weil also investigated the placebo effect. Obviously, unconditional faith is an important aspect of such methods of healing that are otherwise difficult to explain. We all know that a placebo is pseudo medication without pharmacologically active ingredients—pills made of sugar or starch, or injections with neutral saline. It can also even be sham surgery. The placebo effect has been repeatedly confirmed in randomized double-blind studies. For many patients, already the doctor's presence has a placebo effect. With the white coat, the diplomas on the wall, the often terrifying instruments, and the scientific Greco-Latin vocabulary barely comprehensible to the layman, expectations are aroused. "Fortunately, the natural self-healing ability of the body, the *vis medicatrix naturae,* helps us doctors out," my doctor friend Harald once confided to me.

Just as there are positive placebo effects, there are negative, so-called nocebo effects. Andrew Weil is convinced that the belief in the physician has a strong influence on the patient's healing potential. If the doctor does not believe that the treatment will be successful, or if internally, without saying so, is convinced that the patient cannot be helped, chances of recovery are negatively affected. A skeptical look or a careless word can thwart the recovery process. Andrew Weil calls this the "medical hex" (Weil 2000, 93). Some doctors fail to recognize that their words and gestures have strong suggestive power for their patients. They have forgotten that they are virtually exercising a priestly, reality-creating function.

An extreme form of negative placebo effect is practiced in many cultures by sorcerers and practitioners of black magic. For example, the voodoo death, in which a wax doll representing the victim is studded with needles while curses are spoken, can also be effective. This phenomenon was investigated in 1942 by Harvard ethnopsychologist Walter B. Cannon. He was able to confirm that among the indigenous Australians a completely healthy person—usually taboo breakers or criminals—can be put to death within three weeks if the old tribal magicians

(Kurdaitscha-men) point a bone at him or her while speaking spells (Cannon 1942, 169ff.).

In all of these cases, we see the effect of the mind on the body, the effect of the spirit on the processes that play out in physical space. What matters in these phenomena is *belief* in the original sense of the word. Belief is not what we mean when we comment dismissively, "As if!" Or, as Mark Twain once said cynically, "Faith is believing what you know ain't so." The word "belief" from the Germanic **ga-laub-jan* (to hold dear), the Middle High German *geloben*, or the Old English *gel fan* is related to "love" and "live." "Believe" meant, thus, "to be sure, to be convinced, to trust completely."

The Cheyenne medicine man George Elkshoulder was a strong, traditional healer. He sang, drummed, and incensed the disease demons from the bodies and souls of patients and treated them with his plant allies. When the U.S. government built a modern medical clinic with trained doctors and hospital staff on the reservation, he battled for its closure. "Why?" I asked. He replied, "They can't cure us because they don't love us—and only love can heal."

Our ancient herbal hags and wise women were masters not only of plant healing but also of psychology and matters of the soul. They could heal by using symbols—tales, magical charms, magic singing, rituals, and the power of love—thus removing obstacles in the souls and generating the faith in patients that they were healed and whole once again. They were able to break the bad spell of illness and replace it with the good spell of health. The gods and ancestors helped to bring this about.

The plant physiologist, biologist, and philosopher Rupert Sheldrake developed the theory, based on biological research, of morphogenetic fields that effectively extend through space and time. Custom and habit create these tangible fields. The more repetitions of the patterns take place, the stronger the field. This is also the case with time-tested remedies and healing rituals.

The Bernese librarian and author, Sergius Golowin, writes of ancient, often handwritten herbal books that have been family-owned for generations:

Such a book gains more strength the longer it is inherited within a family. In particular, the recipes that an old grandmother or grandfather had noted with clumsy handwriting how this or that had helped quickly and thoroughly, were especially healing. This is a clear indication of how much they recognized the importance of the power of belief in overcoming disease. Herbs that people only casually try have little effect. But those taken with the knowledge that the same cure had helped the ancestors are very effective due to the faith involved. The conclusion is then obvious: The medicine that made the ancestors healthy helps those, even in the present, who are convinced it will help (Golowin 1993, 68).

With the medicine of forest peoples, which goes as far back as the Stone Age, we have a powerful morphogenetic field that brings us into resonance with the distant ancestors and their gods. The healing plants they once knew still grow in our hedgerows, meadows, and forests; they grow between our front door and the garden gate. And beside these roots, we also have the language that connects us to and resonates with our ancestors. Even words are roots—cultural roots.

Traditional folk medicine is not part of a cultural heritage that has been long surpassed but a holistic view that includes the body, soul, spirit, cultural tradition, ancestral knowledge, and the nature surrounding us. Although much of it has, for the most part, become decadent and superstitious, there nevertheless remains a basic element of truth that is worth rediscovery. That which has been handed down to us through the tradition of folk medicine is not only worthy lore but also an art that requires intuition and spiritual vision—and it is our inheritance.

NOTES

Chapter 1

1. The literature regarding this theme is nearly inexhaustible. See the following books on the subject (details in the Reference List), most of which were written by medical professionals: Bigelsen (2011), Coleman (2003), McTaggart (2016), Mendelsohn (1979), Mendelsohn (1982), Moritz (2011), Trudeau (2004), and Weil (2000).

2. Galen's system, which has been refined and expanded over time, influenced medical science for the next 1,500 years.

3. An herbal (Latin *liber herbalis*) is a book used by apothecaries and physicians, listing the names of plants, their descriptions, and their medical virtues.

4. Theophrastus Bombastus von Hohenheim, who called himself Paracelsus, was a Swiss German physician, philosopher, astrologist, and alchemist. He revolutionized the medicine of his time by rejecting the teachings of Galen and the classical theory of the four humors. He advocated the use of alchemical preparations as well as the herbal medicine used by the rustics.

5. Alienation from the direct environment, from one's own roots, is a worldwide occurrence. Cultural imperialism has, for example, produced the urban African who would rather speak French than his or her Bantu mother tongue and for whom the Champs-Elysées and the Eiffel Tower are closer than the river or the baobab tree right in front of the door.

6. The word "book" in the Germanic languages can be traced to the word for "beech." In German, the word for "letter" is "beech stave" *(Buchstab)*. The word for "write" etymologically means "etch" (the runes); "read" means "ponder," or, rather, "decode the runes after they have been thrown."

7. Yggdrasil means the "carrier (or horse) of Yggr." Yggr is Odin in his terrifying form. And when the world, at the end of time, at the "twilight of the gods," falls apart, then it is the silent Vidar, the god who embodies the primordial forests, who will revive and rejuvenate the world. The basic idea is that renewal comes out of the forest wilderness.

8. The Irminsul was the world pillar of the Saxons. Like the "king post," the main upright beam that holds up the roof of a building, the Irminsul was believed to hold up the heavenly ceiling. The word irmin is thought to originate from megalithic culture and refers to a tall, upright megalith or stone pillar. In the year 772 CE, Charlemagne, in his attempt to eradicate heathen culture, had the Irminsul in Germany cut down.

9. More precise information about this church synod and the forbidden heathen customs can be found in the essay by Herman de Vries, "Heilige baeume, bilsenkraut und bildzeitung," in the 2000 book *Rituale des Heilens*, edited by Franz-Theo Gottwald and Christian Raetsch (Aarau, Switzerland: AT Verlag).

10. The desecration of the forest is not something that just belongs to the past. The need for wood no longer satisfies local requirements but the insatiable needs of a global market. The lungs of the earth are imprisoned in service to the god Mammon in all corners of the planet, from Siberia to the Amazons, with advanced technology (such as combine harvesters) that fell the trees with a velocity never seen before, so that even the world climate is endangered. In Germany, where the forests have basically become a wood business, one can barely find any trees that are over one hundred years old in the forests.

11. The Druids, even when they were competent in Greek and Latin, refused to put their knowledge down in writing. They considered the written word uninspired; only what the heart knows was true wisdom.

12. The idea that cultural areas are a geographic region that includes a multitude of different ethnicities is based on the work of anthropologists such as Leo Frobenius, Clark Wissler, Alfred Kroeber, and students of Franz Boas.

13. Matriarchal (Latin mater = mother, focus = hearth) cultures can be described as those in which inheritance follows the matriarchal line and the men move to their wives' family home upon marriage.

Chapter 2

1. Most people today understand the word "drug" to mean an inebriant. However, in herbal medicine and pharmacy, it means "dry goods," thus the dried medicinal plants. The etymology of the word goes back to the lower German *droog,* which means "dry."

2. The High Chinese Mandarin word for "tea" is *cha,* which was borrowed by Hindi to become *chai* and Russian to become *caj.*

3. More precise information about Cheyenne medicine gathering can be found in my book, *The Herbal Lore of Wise Women and Wortcunners* (2012).

4. Entheogen (Greek en = in, theos = god, genesthai = effect) describes plants and mushrooms that induce a spiritual, mystical experience and make religious visions possible.

5. According to most recent understanding, the Germanic peoples are the inheritors of the northern offshoot of megalithic culture. These "dolmen people" were "Indo-Europeanized" over the course of various Indo-European invasions, in particular the ones by the nomadic herders from the eastern steppes (2800–2200 BCE, corded-ware and battle-ax people). The corded-ware people, who introduced the indigenous European people to horses, were most likely the forefathers of the Slavs and the Baltic people. You can find more about this theme in my book *Pflanzen der Kelten* (2009)—unfortunately not yet available in English—on pages 32–60.

6. Voelva, the ecstatic visionary, sees Ymir, the primordial being, and the nine strung-together worlds of the world tree as a measurement of the various world ages and as the incarnation of the universe itself (Stroem and Biezais 1975, 243).

7. The not uncommon psychoanalytic interpretation—the blood as menstruation and the snow as sperm—is a reductionist view of this story.

8. Hollen and Hollinnen are the invisible masculine and feminine spirits.

9. In other geographic regions and cultural areas, psychoactive beer was not the sacred intoxicating substance. Because of a favorable climate, barley beer was able to dominate central and northern Europe after arriving there with Neolithic farmers. In the Mediterranean region, opium poppies and wine gave beer some competition. In Central Asia, hemp dominated; on the edge of the Indian Ocean, it was betel nut; in Siberia, fly agaric was preferred; and in South America, it was the coca leaf.

10. Hyperborean means "coming from the far north," where Boreas, the north wind, blows.

11. The Christian grail legends tell that the crystal goblet originally came from a jewel in Lucifer's crown, which had come off during his fall from heaven. The goblet contained wine—the blood of Christ—that had been drunk at the Last Supper. And when Jesus was crucified, young Joseph of Arimathea caught the blood flowing out of the Savior's body in the chalice. In order to protect the grail chalice from the Jewish priests, Joseph brought it, after wandering for many years, to Glastonbury, the most sacred location in the British Isles—the place the Celts identified with Avalon. Through this pious legend, the sacred vessel maintained its acceptance in Christianity and tied the new sacred teachings in with Celtic tradition. During the Middle Ages, the Legend of the Grail was expanded by the minnesingers and troubadours, and noble knights sought the grail. The Christian grail legends are

based not so much on the real world, but on an abstract spiritual otherworld.

12. "Mystery play" is a technical term used in comparative religious studies. They are theatrical performances that make the core values (the ethos) of a society explicit. Rooted in antiquity, these plays continued under Christian auspices as Christmas pageants or passion plays. Traditional American Westerns (movies) fulfill the criteria of the mystery play in that they show the victory of good against bad—high noon is often the climax of such a play.

13. For the Celts and the Germans, the breaking darkness was already the beginning of the next day—like the baby in the mother's womb, a new phase of time begins with the darkness and then breaks into the light.

14. It is probably indeed due to the influence of the Celts and Germanic people that the cross in its current form became the central symbol of the Church. The original "cross" or the stake on which Jesus was crucified, was the T-formed Tau Cross (St. Anthony's cross, the Egyptian cross). Only after the fourth century was the so-called High Cross, or Latin cross, worshiped.

15. In the Slavic region, the Harvest Goddess appears as Ziwena or Siva. The Baltic Harvest Goddess is called Žemyna or Jumja Mâte, and in the north she is known as the golden-haired Sif, the bride of the Thunder God, or as Fulla, Goddess of Plenty and Abundance.

Chapter 3

1. Excavations in Predmostí (Moravia) prove that Upper Paleolithic hunters of the Gravettien culture—those also responsible for many cave paintings and the well-known statue of "Venus of Willendorf"—already had dogs around 30,000 years ago. Analysis of carbon and nitrogen isotopes showed that the people survived mostly off mammoth meat, but that the dogs were fed with the less tasty reindeer meat.

2. The Cordillera ice sheet was found in the west and the Laurentian ice sheet in the east.

3. In our age of industrial, ready-made meals, sugary drinks, and chemical food, and the associated increase in obesity, diabetes, cancer, tooth decay, cardiovascular problems, and other diseases of civilization, some people have turned back to a so-called Paleo diet. The argument is that we have not genetically changed so much and that what the Stone Age ancestors ate for thousands of generations is the appropriate nutrition for us.

4. The term *frigida* has stirred up some controversy within the feminist movement. However, it has nothing to do with sexual frigidity, but simply means that this species of *Artemesia* grows well in the cold tundra of the far north.

5. Full and detailed information (in German) on the medicinal use of birch can be found here: www.smgp.ch/smgp/homeindex /faehigkeitsprogf/zertifikatsarbeiten/RuoffMarianne.pdf.

6. This consecration of healing plants, which has its roots in pre-Celtic European culture, has continued under the auspices of the Catholic Church and is dedicated to Mary. It is celebrated at Mary's Assumption on August 15th.

7. For those who are interested in the topic of the sweat lodge, Joseph Bruchac's book *The Native American Sweat Lodge: History and Legends* (1993) provides detailed, competent information.

8. For the Athabaskans in northern Canada, the sweat lodge is a moose.

9. The Eastern Woodland Indians covered the sweat lodge with elm or birch bark. On the Pacific coast, log houses served as sweat lodges but also as gathering places for men or sleeping places for unmarried bachelors (Hultkrantz 1996, 276).

10. The Lakota sweat lodge is an exception with the entrance directed toward the west.

11. For more information on the mugwort herb for women, see www
    .susunweed.com/herbal_ezine/May09/wisdomkeepers.htm and
    Brøndegaard (1985), "Artemisia in gynecological folk medicine."
    A discussion of homeopathic use is found in Vermeulen 2004 (pp.
    58–61).

12. The Danube and the Russian Don River also bear her name.

13. Within such ovens, which were very large and some still even are
    in Europe, a fire was made inside and then the burned-out ashes
    were pushed back to bake many breads at once.

14. Bishop Burchard of Worms (tenth to eleventh century) speaks
    of women who put their children into the oven to cure a fever or
    other diseases (Herrmann 2006, 93).

15. The religious scholar Mircea Eliade (1907–1986) created the
    word "shaman"—from a Siberian Tungus (Evenks) word—as it is
    known in the West. He defined shamanism as an "archaic ecstasy
    technique," a shaman as a "master of ecstasy."

Chapter 4

1. Matrilineal refers to the descent and inheritance through the
   female line. This "rule of descent" can be found in simple horti-
   cultural societies practicing, for the most part, shifting cultivation,
   such as the Iroquois, the Hopi, and some tribes in Papua New
   Guinea. The land belongs to the woman's clan because women, as
   bearers and carriers of life, are also responsible for the sowing and
   cultivation of food.

2. Meanwhile, soil surveys have shown that Neolithic farmers did
   not share their homes with their livestock, as was later the case
   with the Celts.

3. "Mother's sister"—or specifically *modrige,* as she was called in
   Old English (Proto-Germanic *m drijo;* German *Muhme*)—originally referred to a maternal aunt. In matrilineal plant societies,
   such as the Iroquois and presumably the Neolithic farmers,

mother, sisters, and daughters formed the core group of the settlement. Under such circumstances, an aunt plays an important role.

4. Pathogens infect animals and humans and are transferred between them. Today, this is especially problematic as we breed more and more multi-resistant bacteria in factory farms due to the use of antibiotics in industrial farming. We share twenty-six diseases with chickens and ducks, thirty-two with rats and mice (for example, the plague), thirty-five with horses, forty-two with pigs, forty-six with goats and sheep, and fifty to sixty-five with cattle and dogs (McNeill 1998, 70).

5. Botanists classify these plants that immigrated with the Neolithic farmers as "archaeophytes" as opposed to the "neophytes" that came from the New World and colonized the meadows, forests, and fields of Europe (and elsewhere after the discovery of America in 1492).

6. "Gowk" once described the cuckoo, the fool, the juggler, or a cuckolded husband.

7. There are still places in central Europe where ancient routes from the village lead directly to the cemetery and end there. They are known as paths of the dead (Dutch doodwegen), and folk superstition tells of ghost trains that move on special days (Devereux 1994, 130).

8. The plantain has many names that indicate its medicinal properties: Danish *laegebald;* Swedish *laekeblad, laekesblaeder;* Anglo-Saxon *laecewyrt;* English *leechwort.* In German dialects, plantain still is called *Laegenblatt, Lugi,* and *Lugenebletter.* In Tirol, it is called *Lugenbladeless;* elsewhere in Austria, eastern Germany, and German Bohemia, it was called Luegenblatt. In English, it is also called waybread and ribwort-plantain. It is used in the popular children's game by picking a leaf and then counting the hanging threads (of the leaf's veins): that was how many lies you had already told on that day, how many children you would have, how many other girls the boy had kissed, and so on.

Chapter 5

1. *Kurgan,* Slavic for "grave mound," because they buried their dead in hills.

2. Šiva, Slavic goddess of life and of the grain.

3. Saule, Baltic Sun Goddess, "Lady Sun."

4. In this sense, the Indo-European healer is similar to the Native American medicine man or medicine woman. For them, "medicine" is not a physical, pharmacological substance but simply a means of spiritual power (medicine power).

5. Then, the elf invites the Lord Oloff to a dance, who refuses, however, and the daughter of the elven king says (Herder 1778, 79):

   "And, if you, Mr. Oloff, will not dance with me,
   Then pestilence and sickness shall follow you!"
   She struck him a blow across his heart:
   "Woe is me, my fear and pain is great!"
   Then she lifted him pale upon his horse:
   "Ride home and greet your treasured bride!"

6. The weevil (German *Wiebel,* Old High German *wibil,* Lithuanian *vabalas*) is a beetle that moves quickly "back and forth" and brings diseases.

7. The Vedic Indians believed, for example, that a person not only physically reincarnated when born on Earth, but that the person's real name also incarnated as part of his or her being.

8. Ethnobotanists identify the plant as balsam herb, costmary *(Tanacetum balsamita),* or costus root *(Saussurea* spp.); this plant was introduced to Europe in the Middle Ages. It has sharp, bitter, and sweet characteristics, was used as a fumigant, vermifuge, ameliorating substance, aphrodisiac, emmenagogue, and for chest pain, liver complaints, jaundice, digestive problems, and skin diseases (De Vries 1989, 345). Kúshta is probably not a specific herb, but more generally the god of aromatic plants (Findly 2008, 5). The

Rigveda (see footnote 19, this chapter) refers to Kúshta as growing high in the Himalayas where eagles are born, and as the Moon God Soma's brother.

9. The Germanic Alcis or Alkene that Tacitus (*Agricola and Germania* 43, 3) equates with Castor and Pollux are also manifestations of these philanthropic twin deities. In Anglo-Saxon mythology, Hengist and Horsa are the two chieftains who conquered Britain around 445 CE. In Latvia, the horse head–like gable beams can also be interpreted as crossed rye haulms and symbolize the Harvest God, Jumis.

10. In Old Norse, the healer is *læknir*, in Old High German, *lachnar*. An English word for a physician is still *leech*.

11. The Germanic medicine man—as the cultural historian Hanns Ferdinand Doebler speculates—probably carried a mask and a belt; like the Lapps, he may have used a drum to summon the spirits, dipped his fingers in the red sacrificial blood of the animal, and, then, with his thumb, the "Odin Finger," marked the wound (Doebler 1975, 311). Other anthropologists identify the leech finger or doctor finger (Norse *læknisfingr*) with the ring finger of the left hand; that goes back to the adoption of classical antiquity, which states that this *digitus medicalis* is connected by a nerve or a vein directly to the heart.

12. For more information, see www.galdorcraeft.de.

13. Sarasvati, the virginal White Goddess and the Swan, the goddess of new beginnings, of spring and birch, is the companion of the Creator Brahma. She is the primordial word. She names all of the beings that Brahma creates in his meditation. Like her Celtic counterpart, Brigit, she brings everything to flow, the natural waters, the flow of thought, and the speech flow of inspired poets or healers.

14. Fol (Vol, Pfol) is probably not, as is often read, another name for Baldur, but for Fro (Freyr). Vol is always mentioned along with

Vulla; Vol and Vulla are none other than Freyr and Freya, the fertility gods of the Vanir clan. Balderes in this case means "Lord," and not Baldur. Odin is the rider of the horse (Mettke 1979, 85). Baldur is the Scandinavian name probably inherited from the masculine Celtic Sun God (Bel, Belenos) during the Iron Age because, originally among the Nordic indigenous peoples, the sun was feminine; it was the dear "Lady Sun."

15. Sinthgunt, the "Night Walker," is probably a Moon Goddess, and Sunna the Sun Goddess (Stroem and Biezais 1975, 92).

16. Mahra, the Virgin Mary, is barely concealed as none other than the beloved Fate Laima, the mistress of the sweat bath. Mahra "carries water in diamond bowls" to pour on the hot stones: "The beloved Mahra heats the bath-house, for which the sons of gods are waiting" (Biezais 1994, 171).

17. Among the West Slavs, the Sorben, it is said that, if one uses elder wood to make fire, then the "lamenting one" *(Boza losc)* comes in the midnight hour and screams, *Be da wam! Be da wam!* ("Woe to you! Woe to you!").

18. This book of leechcraft was written by the scholar Bald in the ninth century, when Alfred the Great was ruler of England.

19. Rigveda 10.97, In Praise of the Healing Plants (Michel 2008 306ff.; Zysk, 1996: 99–100).

20. Mistletoe is still associated with fertility in common folk medicine. Herbalist Maria Treben prescribes that women drink mistletoe drops with yarrow and chamomile tea to treat the unfulfilled wish for children.

21. Vaseneyi Samhit 12.98.

22. Diancecht was long remembered. On a parchment from the eighth or ninth century (*Stiftsbibliothek St. Gallen*, manuscript from 1395), a probable Irish-Scottish monk wrote: "I trust in the ointment that Diancecht gave his people, that would heal all that it touches."

23. "I tell you: My shoe buckles are more learned than your Galen and Avicenna, and my beard has experienced more than all your High Schools" (Paracelsus, *Paragranum*).

24. According to Rudolf Steiner, plants are primarily extroverted beings; they can grow into exuberant forms and shapes and express themselves in the most outrageous colors. If human organisms were to do the same, they would be ill, to say the least: When our body flushes red, it indicates a blood condition; when we turn yellow, we suffer from jaundice; when our skin turns orange, we might have cellulitis; or, when our body has bulges or protuberances, we tend to be in bad shape. Thus, what are normal processes in the plant world tend to be pathological in the human being. Plant signatures, thus, become a key to finding the corresponding medicine: Red plant parts, such as red grapes or cayenne peppers, have a positive effect on the circulatory system; madder root is blood thinning; and red staghorn-sumac berries are blood staunching. The yellow juice of the greater celandine (tetterwort) or yellow-flowering plants, such as the dandelion, help with jaundice. Orange peels can be used to treat cellulitis, and hemiparasitic plants like the mistletoe growing on trees are used as therapy for tumors.

25. *Whirl* also comes from this Indo-European word.

Chapter 6

1. The Church Synod of Laodicea (366 CE) and later the Synod of Ratisbon (877 CE) forbade priests the study or application of medicine.

2. This celebration is the origin of the largest peasant feast, namely the autumn fair, *Kerwa* or *Kilbe*—different versions of the German *Kirchweihmesse* (ceremony of blessing a church) where a lot of dancing, feasting, flirting, and drinking takes place.

3. The historical Nicolas, Bishop of Myra (third to fourth century), had a tree felled that was dedicated to the goddess Diana. He is also supposed to have performed many miracles, such as the

resurrection of the dead or calming a storm. From his grave, a spring is supposed to have flowed with anointing oil.

4. Meanwhile, after over a thousand years, these plants have adapted through natural selection to the cooler climate. Only in the Allgaeu, in southeastern Germany, in my garden on the mountain, they do not survive some winters.

5. The monastery plan of St. Gallen, written 819–826 CE, is the earliest representation of a medieval monastery in central Europe.

6. The famous Way of Saint James (Camino de Santiago de Compostela) is dedicated to him, a patron of pilgrims.

7. In Norway, the possession of cowslip has been transferred onto Mary and is called Marienoeglebaand, "Mary's keychain."

8. Rye, which is susceptible to the ergot fungus responsible for the disease, grows better than wheat in the damp, cold climate of the north. The disease, St. Anthony's fire, was, therefore, a threat to agriculture-based peoples of the northern woodlands. The first recorded outbreak was in Xanten in 857 CE.

9. Warning, not recommended for imitation! The juice is corrosive and may, if it gets in the eye, trigger conjunctivitis.

10. The name has been preserved in Swiss German as *Züschtig* for Tuesday.

11. The three Beths, who visit the houses and farms of the people to bless them toward the end of the Twelve Days of Christmas from December 24th to January 5th, were replaced in the course of conversion not only with the three holy virgins but also with the three kings from the East—Caspar, Melchior, and Balthasar. These carolers come to each house on January 6th (Three Kings Day) and put their initials (C + M + B) with chalk on every entryway— which is meant as a protection for the house dwellers.

12. Lucian is said to have forced a bear that had mauled an ox to pull the plow. If, in the lives of saints, such as that of Saint Gall, compulsory labor of bears is mentioned, the heathen Alemannic

berserkers, who had to bow to the greater power of the saint, are linked.

13. So at least the legend goes. Unfortunately, there are several "Veils of Veronica" that have emerged and, on closer scientific examination, reveal fabric and weaving techniques of the Middle Ages (Pabst 2013, 213).

14. *Lacnunga* CXXV B, Charm against a sudden stitch. The sudden stitch could be an elf shot, a witch's shot, or a stroke in the modern sense.

15. The shields were brightly painted with the images of helping totem animals and helping spirits. Why linden wood? To understand the purpose of this action, one must know that the shields used in ordinary battle were covered with the inner bark, the bast fiber, of linden wood.

16. According to Wikipedia: Nine Herbs Charm.

17. According to Raven Kaldera, *Northern Shamanism* (2004).

18. According to R. K. Gordon, *Anglo-Saxon Poetry* (1962).

19. From the *Old English Dictionary.*

20. According to Raven Kaldera, *Northern Shamanism* (2004).

21. Bosworth-Toller, *Anglo-Saxon Dictionary* (1898).

22. The "apple" of Eve was probably a pomegranate *(Punica granatum)*, which comes from West Asia and was dedicated to the Great Goddess; in Greece, it was consecrated to the Underworld Goddess Persephone. Since the pomegranate did not grow in the north, the missionaries carried on the symbolism with the local apple.

23. Occasionally, *fille* is translated as sweet cicely *(Myrrhis odorata)* or as wild thyme *(Thymus serpyllum).*

24. In the so-called High Medieval Warm Period (circa 900–1300 CE), the annual average temperature was two degrees higher than today, and the tree line in the Alps rose to 6,500 feet (2,000 meters). Mediterranean plants spread out to the north, and the

growing season became longer as the warmer temperatures shifted northward (Behringer 2009, 103ff.).

25. For more detailed information on this issue, see Hildegard von *Bingen's Physica: The Complete English Translation of Her Classic Work on Health and Healing,* or Irmgard Mueller's *Die pflanzlichen Heilmittel bei Hildegard von Bingen*, 2008.

Chapter 7

1. Among these writings preserved in the Islamic realm were those of Pythagoras, Hippocrates, Aristotle, Dioscorides, and Galen.

2. The belief that there is a healing plant for every disease is universal. The Christians have no doubt to date. In the didactic poems of the school of Salerno, the *Regimen Sanitatis Salernitanum,* one can read the famous saying, "Why does a man die if a medicinal plant *(Salvia)* grows in his garden?" The answer comes in the next verse: "Because for the poison of death there is no cure."

3. Severe salivating and profuse sweating were seen as very positive by the doctors; they claimed that the bad humors left the body this way.

4. A detailed discourse on the cultural effect of syphilis and the end of herbalism can be found in my 2010a book, *Healing Lyme Disease Naturally.*

5. Justus von Liebig, the great chemist, points out that alchemy was far more than just trying to make money: "it was never anything other than chemistry" (Liebig 1840, 36).

6. Quintessence: the "fifth essence" in addition to the four elements of earth, water, air, and fire. Christ was considered the spiritual quintessence of man.

Chapter 8

1. Lord, however, was originally *hlaford* and older yet, *hlafweard,* meaning the "bread warden" or "guardian of the loaf."

2. In some regions, though, weaving was the men's occupation.

3. More on this subject can be found in my book, *The Herbal Lore of Wise Women and Wortcunners* (2012).

4. These babies probably suffered from hydrocephalus, cretinism, or some other cruel act of nature. To care for such children is a luxury that only a modern affluent society can afford.

5. Those who are interested in psychoactive plants should consult *The Encyclopedia of Psychoactive Plants* by Christian Raetsch (2005).

6. Interesting in this context is that the name of the great poet Johann Wolfgang von Goethe can be traced back to Gode, the heathen priest who led the blessings.

7. Gode or Gydia incidentally has the same origin as the word "God" (Germanic *god, gud*). God has nothing to do with "good," as one would like to believe, but comes from the Indo-European **gheu,* "to pour." "God" is the lofty being for whom the libation is poured or more likely the lofty being who pours his blessings out. That would be consistent with the Slavic *Bog* (God) or the Indian *Bhagvan,* which also means "the giving one," or "the provider."

8. Since henbane contains, among other things, the narcotics scopolamine and hyoscyamine, henbane beers should be addressed with great respect. The indigenous people drank this beer as a community ritual. Without ritual control and exact dosage, these beers can be a ticket to the astral world with no return. Stories from the Thirty Years' War tell of mercenaries who tipped off the bench with their beer mugs still in their hand, and never got up again (Storl 2004b, 31–32).

9. "Pretzel" comes from the medieval Latin *bracciatella* (small arms) or *precari* (prayer).

10. The Alemannic name for butter is *Anke* (Old High German *ancho*); the ancient Celts had a similar name. *Schmer* (Norse

smoer; "smear" is related) is the Northern Germanic name. The word "butter" comes from the Latin, which borrowed the word *bútyron* (dairy cheese) from the Greek *bous* (cow) and *tyros* (cheese).

11. In general, many butter spells have been known since heathen times; they sacrificed the precious substance to friendly house spirits and the sun (Norway) and gave it as a harvest sacrifice. Germanic peoples once "oiled" wooden idols with butter and later the crucifix.

12. See www.institut-infomed.de.

13. That would be, without a doubt, an economic catastrophe for the pharmaceutical industry that, according to a report by the German Business News (18.04.15), earned a trillion dollars in 2014 (http://wiw.adpo.org/die-pharma-mafia-der-flexner-report/).

BIBLIOGRAPHY

Achterberg, Jeanne. 1991. *Woman as Healer.* Boulder, CO: Shambhala.

Aigremont, Dr. 1910. *Volksesoterik und Pflanzenwelt.* Halle, Germany: Hallescher Verlag.

Baechtold-Staeubli, Hanns, and Eduard Hoffmann-Krayer. 1987. *Handwoerterbuch des deutschen Aberglaubens.* 11 vols. Berlin: De Gruyter.

Beckmann, Dieter, and Barbara Beckmann. 1997. *Das geheime Wissen der Kraeuterhexen.* Munich: DTV.

Behringer, Wolfgang. 2009. *A Cultural History of Climate.* Waco, TX: Polity.

Biedermann, Hans. 1994. *Dictionary of Symbolism.* New York: Plume (Penguin).

Biezais, Haralds. 1994. "Die soziale Grundlage synkretistischer Prozesse." *In Tradition und Translation,* edited by Christoph Elsas. Berlin: De Gruyter.

Bigelsen, Harvey. 2011. *Doctors Are More Harmful Than Germs.* Berkeley, CA: North Atlantic Books.

Birkhan, Helmut. 2012. *Pflanzen im Mittelalter.* Vienna: Boehlau.

Blake, William. 1977. *The Complete Poems.* London: Penguin.

Blofeld, John. 1997. *Chinese Art of Tea.* Boulder, CO: Shambhala.

Bosworth-Toller, Joseph. 1898. *Anglo-Saxon Dictionary.* Oxford: At the Clarendon Press.

Botheroyd, Sylvia, and Paul F. Botheroyd. 1995. *Lexikon der keltischen Mythologie.* Munich: Eugen Diederichs.

Braun, Lucien. 1993. *Paracelsus.* Munich: Heyne.

Broers, Dieter. 2013. *Gedanken erschaffen Realitaet.* Munich: Heyne.

Brøndegaard, Vagn J. 1985. *Ethnobotanik: Pflanzen im Brauchtum, in der Geschichte und Volksmedizin.* Berlin: Verlag Mensch und Leben.

Brosse, Jaques. 1990. *Mythologie der Baeume.* Olten, Switzerland: Walter.

Bruchac, Joseph. 1993. *The Native American Sweat Lodge: History and Legends.* Berkeley, CA: Crossing Press.

Cannon, Walter B. 1942. "Voodoo Death." *American Anthropologist* 44(2):169–181.

Chamberlain, Mary. 2006. *Old Wives' Tales.* Stroud, Gloucestershire: Tempus.

Coleman, Vernon. 2003. *How to Stop Your Doctor Killing You.* European Medical Journal. Kindle edition.

Demitsch, Wassily. 1889. "Russische Volksheilmittel aus dem Pflanzenreiche." In Vol. I of *Historische Studien aus dem Pharmakologischen Institut der Kaiserlichen Universität Dorpat,* edited by Rudolf Kobert. Halle: Verlag Tausch & Grosse.

Descola, Philippe. 2014. *Beyond Nature and Culture.* Chicago: University of Chicago Press.

Devereux, Paul. 1994. *Shamanism and the Mystery Lines.* Woodbury, MN: Llewellyn Pub.

De Vries, Herman. 1989. *Natural Relations.* Nuremburg: Verlag fuer moderne Kunst.

Diamond, Jared. 1997. *Guns, Germs and Steel.* New York: W. W. Norton & Co.

Doebler, Hannsferdinand. 1975. *Die Germanen.* Barcelona: Prisma.

Duerr, Hans-Peter. 1990. *Sedna oder die Liebe zum Leben.* Frankfurt am Main: Suhrkamp.

Eliade, Mircea. 1980. *Schmiede und Alchemisten.* Stuttgart: Klett-Cotta.

Erichsen-Brown, Charlotte. 1989. Medical and Other Uses of North American Plants. Mineola, NY: Dover.

Findly, Ellison Banks. 2008. *Plant Lives: Borderline Beings in Indian Tradition.* Delhi: Motilal Banarsidass.

Gardner, Laurence. 2000. *Realm of the Ring Lords.* Dubai: MediaQuest.

Golowin, Sergius. 1993. *Paracelsus.* Munich: Goldmann.

Gordon, R. K. 1962. *Anglo-Saxon Poetry.* London, Dent: Everyman's Library.

Grienke, Ulrike, Margit Zoell, Ursula Peinter, and Judith M. Rollinger. 2014. "European Medicinal Polypores—A Modern View on Traditional Uses." *Journal of Ethnopharmacology* 15:564–583.

Grieve, Maud. 1931. *A Modern Herbal.* London: Jonathan Cape.

Griffith, Ralph T. H. 1895. *Hymns of the Atharva Veda.* www.sacred -texts.com.

Grimm, Jacob. 2012. *Teutonic Mythology.* Translated by James Steven Stallybrass. London: George Bell & Sons. Kindle edition.

Gruschke, Andreas, Andreas Schoerner, and Astrid Zimmermann. 2001. *Tee: Susser Tau des Himmels.* Munich: DTV.

Grzega, Joachim. 2008. "Hi, Hail, Hello: Greetings in English Language History." *In Speech Acts in the History of English,* edited by Andreas Jucker, 165–193. Amsterdam: John Benjamin.

Gurjewitsch, Aaron J. 1978. *Weltbild des mittelalterlichen Menschen.* Dresden: VEB Verlag der Kunst.

Habiger-Tuczay, Christa. 1992. *Magie und Magier im Mittelalter.* Munich: Diederichs.

Hasenfratz, Hans-Peter. 1992. *Die religioese Welt der Germanen.* Freiburg: Herder.

Heise, Thomas. 1996. *Chinas Medizin bei uns.* Berlin: VWB.

Hellmiss, Margot. 1998. *Natural Healing with Cider Vinegar.* New York: Sterling Pub. Co.

Hempel, Werner. 2009. *Die Pflanzenwelt Sachsens von der Spaeteiszeit bis zur Gegenwart.* Jena, Germany: Weissdorn-Verlag.

Herder, Gottfried. 1778. "Erlkoenig." *In Des Knaben Wunderhorn.*

Herrmann, Paul. 2006. *Deutsche Mythologie.* Augsburg, Germany: Weltbild.

Hoefler, Max. 1911. "Volksmedizinische Botanik der Kelten" *Archiv fuer Geschichte der Medizin* 5(1/2):1–35.

Hollander, Lee M. 1962. *The Poetic Edda.* Austin: University of Texas Press.

Hultkranz, Åke. 1996. *Shamanic Healing and Ritual Drama.* New York: Crossroad.

Humphries, Susanne, and Roman Bystrianyk. 2013. *Dissolving Illusions: Diseases, Vaccines, and the Forgotten History.* CreateSpace Independent Publishing Platform.

Kaldera, Raven. www.northernshamanism.org/herbalism.html.

Kay, Margarita A. 1996. *Healing with Plants in the American and Mexican West.* Tucson: University of Arizona Press.

Keller, Hiltgart. 1979. *Reclams Lexikon der Heiligen und der biblischen Gestalten.* Stuttgart: Philipp Reclam.

Kluge, Heidelore. 2008. *Die Heilkraft des Bieres.* Munich: Herbig.

Korn, Wolfgang, and Flemming Bau. 2006. *Unsere Geschichte.* Stuttgart: Theiss.

Kurtz, Edith. 1937. *Heilzauber der Letten in Wort und Tat.* Riga: Verlag der AG "Ernst Plates."

Lehmann-Enders, Christel. 2000. *Was die schwarze Kuh scheisst das nimm ...: Vom Aberglauben, Heilen und Besprechen im Spreewald.* Luebben, Germany: Heimat-Verlag Luebben.

Liebig, Justus. 1840. *Organic Chemistry in Its Applications to Agriculture and Physiology.* Translated by Lyon Playfair. London: Bradbury and Evans. Reprint, Amazon Digital Services LLC, 2014. Kindle edition.

Lissner, Ivar. 1957. *The Living Past: 7000 Years of Civilization.* London: G. B. Putnam's Sons (Penguin).

Loux, Francoise. 1978. *Le jeune enfant et son corps dans la medicine traditionelle.* Paris: Flammarion.

Ludwig, Otto. 1982. *Im Thueringer Kraeutergarten.* Guetersloh: Prisma Verlag.

Lurker, Manfred. 1991. *Woerterbuch der Symbolik.* Stuttgart: Koerner.

Madejsky, Margret. 2008. *Lexikon der Frauenheilkraeuter.* Baden und Muenchen: AT-Verlag.

Mannhardt, Wilhelm. 1875. *Wald und Feldkulte.* Berlin: Gebrueder Borntraeger.

Marzell, Heinrich. 2002. *Geschichte und Volkskunde der deutschen Heilpflanzen.* St. Goar: Reichl Verlag.

_____. 1979. *Wörterbuch der deutschen Pflanzennamen.* Vols. I–IV. Leipzig: S. Hirzel.

McKee, Paul. "Spanish-English Medical Plant Names for Southwest United States and Mexico." Last modified December 12, 2007. www.intk.org/plants/Swl.htm.

McNeill, William H. 1998. *Plagues and Peoples.* Garden City, NY: Anchor Books.

McTaggart, Lynne. 2013. *What Doctors Don't Tell You.* London: Avon.

Bibliography

Mehta, Gita. 1998. *Snakes and Ladders.* London: Vintage.

Mendelsohn, Robert S. 1979. *Confessions of a Medical Heretic.* New York: Warner Books.

_____. 1982. *Mal(e) Practice.* Chicago: Contemporary Books.

Mettke, Heinz, ed. 1979. *Aelteste deutsche Dichtung und Prosa.* Leipzig: Philipp Reclam.

Michel, Peter (Publ.). 2008. *Rig-Veda—das heilige Wissen Indiens.* Wiesbaden: Matrix.

Michener, James A. 1965. *The Source.* New York: Random House.

Moerman, Daniel E. 1999. *Native American Ethnobotany.* Portland, Oregon: Timber Press.

Mone, Franz Joseph. 1823. *Das Heidenthum im noerdlichen Europa.* Leipzig: C. W. Leske.

Moritz, Andreas. 2011. *Vaccine-nation: Poisoning the Population, One Shot at a Time.* Ener-Chi Press.

Mueller, Irmgard. 2008. *Die pflanzlichen Heilmittel bei Hildegard von Bingen.* Freiburg: Herder.

Mueller-Ebeling, Claudia. 2010. *Ahnen, Geister und Schamanen.* Aarau und Muenchen: AT Verlag.

Mueller, Irmgard. 2008. *Die pflanzlichen Heilmittel bei Hildegard von Bingen.* Freiburg: Herder.

Ody, Penelope. 2011. *The Chinese Medicine Bible: The Definitive Guide to Holistic Healing.* New York: Sterling.

Pabst, Maria Anna. 2013. *Die Wunderwelt der Pollen.* Aarau und Muenchen: AT Verlag.

Pfeifer, Wolfgang. 2012. *Etymologisches Woerterbuch des Deutschen.* Koblenz: Edition Kramer.

Pfleiderer, Beatrix. 2009. *Die Kraft der Verbundenheit.* Klein Jasedow: Drachen Verlag.

Ploberger, Florian. 2011. *Das grosse Buch der westlichen Kraeuter aus Sicht der traditionellen chinesischen Medizin.* Schiedlberg: BACOPA.

Pollington, Stephen. 2000. *Leechcraft: Early English Charms, Plantlore and Healing.* Anglo-Saxon Books.

Porter, Roy. 2003. *Blood and Guts: A Short History of Medicine.* New York: W.W. Norton and Co.

Probst, Ernst. 1999. *Deutschland in der Steinzeit.* Munich: Orbis.

Raetsch, Christian. 2005a. *Der heilige Hain.* Baden und Muenchen: AT Verlag.

———. 2005b. *The Encyclopedia of Psychoactive Plants.* South Paris, ME: Park Street Press.

Redfield, Robert. 1953. *The Primitive World and Its Transformations.* New York: Macmillan.

Reichholf, Josef H. 2008. *Warumm die Menschen sesshaft wurden.* Frankfurt am Main: S. Fischer.

Riethe, Peter. 2007. *Hildegard von Bingen: Das Buch von den Pflanzen.* Salzburg: Otto Mueller Verlag.

Rockinger, Ludwig von. 1883. *Berichte zur Untersuchung von Handschriften des sogen.* Schwabenspiegels, 14./15. Century. Vienna: Wiener Akademie.

Rosenbohm, Alexandra. 1991. "Der Fliegenpilz in Nordasien." In *Der Fliegenpilz,* edited by Wolfgang Bauer, Edzard Klapp, and Alexandra Rosenbohm. Cologne: Wienand.

Ruoff, Marianne. "Beeren und Blumen im Baerenland." Unpublished manuscript, last modified 2014.

Scheffer, Mechthild, and Wolf-Dieter Storl. 2012. *Die Seelenpflanzen des Edward Bach.* Bielefeld: Aurum in J. Kamphausen.

Schipperges, Heinrich. 1990. *Der Garten der Gesundheit.* Munich: DTV.

Schlesier, Karl H. 2013. *The Wolves of Heaven: Cheyenne Shamanism, Ceremonies, and Prehistoric Origins.* CreateSpace Independent Publishing Platform.

Schmitz, Rudolf. 1998. Vol. 1, *Geschichte der Pharmazie.* Eschborn: Govi-Verlag.

Schubert, Rudolf, and Guenther Wagner. 2000. *Botanisches Woerterbuch.* Stuttgart: Eugen Ulmer.

Seyr, Birgit. 2009. *Mit Pflanzen verhueten.* Ampass, Oesterreich: Pflanzenwerkstatt.

Stille, Guenther. 2004. *Kraeuter, Geister, Rezepturen.* Stuttgart: Konrad Theiss.

_____. 2004b. *Goetterpflanze Bilsenkraut.* Solothurn, Switzerland: Nachtschatten Verlag.

_____. 2005. "Wuermlein klein ohne Haut und Bein—schamanische und ethno-botanische Aspekte der indigenen Heilkunde Nordeuropas." In *Der grosse Institut fuer Ethnomedizin.*

_____. 2006. *Wandernde Planzen.* Aarau, Switzerland: AT Verlag.

_____. 2009. *Pflanzen der Kelten.* Aarau, Switzerland: AT Verlag.

_____. 2010a. *Healing Lyme Disease Naturally.* Berkeley, CA: North Atlantic Books.

_____. 2010b. *Mit Pflanzen verbunden.* Munich: Heine.

_____. 2010c. *Das Herz und seine heilenden Pflanzen.* Aarau, Switzerland: AT Verlag.

_____. 2011. *Kraeuterkunde.* Bielefeld, Germany: Aurum Verlag.

_____. 2012. *The Herbal Lore of Wise Women and Wortcunners: The Healing Power of Medicinal Plants.* Berkeley, CA: North Atlantic Books.

_____. 2014a. *Planzendevas.* Aarau, Switzerland: AT Verlag.

Strassmann, René A. 1994. *Baumheilkunde.* Aarau, Switzerland: AT Verlag.

Stroem, Åke V., and Haralds Biezais. 1975. *Germanische und Baltische Religion.* Stuttgart: W. Kohlhammer.

Tacitus, Publius Cornelius. 2010. *Agricola and Germania.* London: Penguin Classics.

Thueler, Maya. 1995. *Wohltuende Wickel.* Worb, Switzerland: Maya Thueler Verlag.

Treben, Maria. 2009. *Health Through God's Pharmacy.* Innsbruck: Ennsthaler Pub.

Trudeau, Kevin. 2004. *Natural Cures.* Elk Grove Village, IL: Alliance Pub. Group.

Unger, Andreas. 2013. *Von Algebra bis Zucker.* Stuttgart: Reclam.

Van Schie, Christiane. 2010. *Im Schoss der Erdmutter.* Klein Jasedow, Germany: Drachen Verlag.

Vermeulen, Frans. 2004. *Homoeopathische Substanzen—Vom Element zum Arzneimittelbild.* Stuttgart: Sonntag.

Volkmann, Helga. 2008. *Purpurfaeden und Zauberschiffchen.* Goettingen, Germany: Vandenhoek & Ruprecht.

Weil, Andrew. 2000. *Spontaneous Healing.* New York: Ballantine Books.

Willett, Walter. 2005. *Eat, Drink and Be Healthy.* New York: Free Press.

Wolters, Bruno. 2000. *Zur Entwicklung der altsteinzeitlichen Phytotherapie im westlichen Eurasien und der Indianischen Medizin in Sibirien und Nordamerika.* Duesseldorf: Duesseldorfer Institut fuer amerikanische Voelkerkunde.

_____. 1999. "Die aeltesten Arzneipflanzen." *Deutsche Apotheker Zeitung,* no. 39.

Zingsem, Vera. 1999. *Goettinnen Grosser Kulturen.* Munich: DTV.

Zuk, Marlene. 2008. *Riddled with Life.* Fort Washington, PA: Harvest Books.

Zysk, Kenneth G. 1996. *Medicine in the Veda.* Delhi: Motilal Banarsidass Publishers.

INDEX

A

Abenaki, 80
Achillea millefolium. See Yarrow
A. ptarmica. See Marsh yarrow
Aconitum napellus. See Monkshood
Acorus calamus. See Sweet flag
Adam and Eve, 16, 214, 245, 256, 304
Aegopodium podagraria. See
    Goutweed
Aesir, 97, 193
Agatha, Saint, 275
Agni, 133–34
Agrostemma githago. See Corn
    cockle
Ainu, 72
Ajuga reptans. See Creeping bugle
Albertus Magnus, 92
Alchemy, 223, 233–34, 305
Alcohol, 223, 234
Alembic, 234
Ales. *See* Beer
Algonquin, 22, 69, 73, 80, 81
Alkali, 234
Allantoin, 147
Allium ursinum. See Bear's garlic
Aloe, 240
Amalgam, 234
Amanita muscaria. See Fly agaric
Amator (bishop), 17
Amulets, 234
Anagallis arvensis. See Pimpernel
Ancestors, wrath of, 131–32
Andromeda polifolia. See Bog
    rosemary
Angelica (*Angelica* spp.), 68, 85,
    106, 230

Aniline, 234
Anna Perenna, 88, 116
Annapurna, 88
Anne, Saint, 88, 229
Anthemis nobilis. See Roman
    chamomile
Anthony, Saint, 190, 227, 228
Antimony, 234–35
Anu, 88
Aphanes arvensis. See Field
    parsley-piert
Apollo, 47, 89, 131
Apollonia, Saint, 195–96
Apophytes, 113–14
Apple, 213–14
Arabic influence, 222–23, 233–40
Arapaho, 68
Arctium lappa. See Burdock
A. minus. See Burdock
Arctostaphylos uva-ursi. See
    Bearberry
Aristotle, 222, 305
Arnica (*Arnica montana*), 193
Arnold de Villanova, 234
Artemis, 89, 251
Artemisia absinthium. See
    Wormwood
A. dracunculus. See Tarragon
A. frigida. See Fringed sage
A. ludoviciana. See Steppe
    sagebrush
A. tridentata. See Steppe sagebrush
A. vulgaris. See Mugwort
Artichoke, 235
Arum (*Arum maculatum*), 169

Arundhati, 135
Asclepius, 5, 6
Asgard, 103
Ashvins, 134–35
Athanor, 233
Atharva Veda, 121, 133, 142–43,
    148, 149, 159, 160, 161
Atterlothe, 208–9
Audumbla, 37
Autumn crocus, 164–65, 266
Avicenna, 222
Ayurveda, 2, 3, 10–11

B

Baba Yaga, 13
Bach, Edward, 48, 170
Baking soda, 237
Baldur, 185, 210
Balsam herb, 299
Bantu, 33–34
Barbara, Saint, 196–97
Barbara vulgaris. See Winter
    rocket
Barberry, 240
Barnyard grass, 208
Bartholomew, Saint, 276
BASF, 234
Bearberry, 68, 78, 193
Bear root, 193
Bear's garlic, 230
Bee balm, 85
Beech, 291
Beer, 42–44, 269–74, 294
Beetles, 157–59
Bel (Belenos), 185, 210, 301
Belief, power of, 288–89
Belladonna (*Belladonna atropa*),
    193, 218, 266
Bellis perennis. See Daisy, common

Beltane, 54
Benedict, Saint, 195, 197–99
Benzene, 235
Bergamot, 85
Bernhard, Saint, 195
Betony, 209
Betula spp. *See* Birch
Bezoar, 235
Bhishàjs, 136–38
Big cordgrass, 137
Birch, 69–74, 85, 231
Birch bracket mushroom, 71
Birch polypore, 71
Bismuth, 235
Bistort, 79, 165, 209
Bitter clover, 75
Bitumen, 236, 238
Black Death, 228
Blackfoot, 77
Black nightshade, 113
Blacksmiths, as healers, 253–54
Blackthorn, 187–88
Blake, William, 140–41
Blessed thistle, 199
Blofeld, John, 31
Blois, William, 174
Bloodletting, 7, 223, 228, 232
Blueberries, 273
Blue weed, 188, 209
Boas, Franz, 293
Bock, Hieronymus, 153
Bogbean, 75
Bog myrtle, 85
Bog rosemary, 67
Boniface, Saint, 17–18, 174, 182
Borage, 240
Borax, 235
Boron, 235
Botheroyd, Sylvia and Paul, 47

Brahmins, 147, 197
Bran, 46
Brandies, 223, 228
Bread, 274–75
Brewing, 42–44, 270
Brigit, 70, 155, 300
Brihaspati, 160–61
Brunfels, Otto, 80, 119
Buckthorn, 78, 273
Bugle, common, 200
Burchard of Worms (bishop), 175, 260, 261, 297
Burdock, 114, 165
Burial mounds, 116–17
Burnet, 230
Burnet-bloodroot, 201
Butter, 276–77, 306–7
Butter-and-eggs, 112
Butterbur, 202

C
Cabbage, 283
Caesar, Julius, 15, 17, 19
Caillech, 39
Calamus, 85
Calico, 240
Calomel, 231
Caltha palustris. See Marsh marigold
Camellia (*Camellia sinensis*), 28
Camphor, 235, 240
Candlemas, 54, 274
Cannabis, 82
Cannon, Walter B., 288
Capsella bursa-pastoris. See Shepherd's purse
Caraway, 273
Cardamine hirsuta. See Hairy bittercress

Carline thistle (*Carlina acaulis*), 198, 199, 230
Carob, 240
Carrot, wild, 114
Cathars, 226
Catherine, Saint, 196–97, 200
Catholic Church
  herbalism and, 175, 194–95, 203–4, 219–20
  heretics and, 226–27
  Inquisition, 98, 226–27, 228
  monastic medicine, 6, 180, 223, 225, 233
  pagan customs and, 203–16
  women and, 175
Cauldrons, 42, 44–48
Cave art, 93, 94
Celandine, 165
Centaurea cyanus. See Cornflower
Ceres, 44
Cerridwen, 44, 46, 184
Chaga, 72, 170
Chamomile, 27, 67, 110, 111, 118, 146, 182, 192, 194, 203, 209–10, 254, 279, 282
Changelings, 255–56
Charaka, 162
Charlemagne, 18, 47, 48, 179, 180, 198, 199, 292
Chelidonium maius. See Celandine
Chenopodiaceae. See Goosefoot
Cherry, 85
Chervil, 214–15
Cheyenne, 31, 32, 40, 41, 60, 68, 82, 83, 85, 109, 149, 161, 170, 293
Chicory, 114, 188–89, 211
Chimaphila umbellata. See Wintergreen
Chippewa, 77

Christianity, spread of, 173–74
Chrysanthemum leucanthemum.
   See Oxeye daisy
C. parthenium. See Feverfew
Church architecture, Gothic,
   221–22
Cichorium intybus. See Chicory
Claviceps purpurea. See Ergot
   poisoning
Clematis, 170
Climatic Optimum, 99
Clinker polypore, 72
Cloister gardens, 178–80
Clothing, manufacturing of,
   243–46
Clubmoss, common, 75–76, 193,
   205
Cnicus benedictus. See Blessed
   thistle
Cockoo-pint, 169
Coffee, 240
Colchicum autumnale. See
   Autumn crocus
Colic-wort, 112
Columbus, 90, 231
Comfrey, 165, 282
Compresses, 282
Confucius, 30
Consolida regalis. See Field
   larkspur
Constantine the African, 222
Cookies, 274–75
Corn cockle, 111
Cornelius, Saint, 275
Cornflower, 111, 273
Corn Mother, 110
Corn poppy, 112
Cosmas, Saint, 135, 229
Costmary, 299

Costus root, 299
Cotton, 235, 240
Council of Agde, 175
Council of Tours, 225
Cowslip, 189–90, 303
Cow-wheat, 112
Crab apple, 211
Cree, 72
Creeping bugle, 200
Croll, Oswald, 169
Cross, as symbol, 53–57, 177
Crowberry, 78
Cubeb, 240
Cumin, 240
Cupping therapy, 223
Curses, 130–31
Cynarine, 235

D

Dagda, 46
Daily cycle, 48, 50–53
Daisy, common, 203
Dakota, 64, 68
Damian, Saint, 135, 229
Dandelion, 165, 273
Daphne, 193
Darbha grass, 137–38
Daucus carota. See Carrot, wild
Davis, Paul, 287
Dea Ana, 46, 88, 116
Della Porta, Giambattista, 169, 260
Demons, 128–29
*Desmostachya bipinnata. See
   Kusha* grass
Devil's claw, 76
Dhatr, 136
Diana, 88, 259
Diancecht, 46, 163, 301
Dioscorides, 5, 180, 216, 305

Dipsacus sylvestris. See Teasel

Disease

  causes of, 5, 34, 126–32

  chants for dispelling, 147–50

  sedentary lifestyle and, 107–9

  in the Stone Age, 65

  transferring, onto trees and

    animals, 150–53, 157–59

Docks, 114

Doebler, Hanns Ferdinand, 300

Dominicans, 185, 226

Donar, 17

Doshas, 11

Druids, 15, 147, 197, 262, 292

Drunemeton, 15

Dryopteris filix-mas. See Male fern

Duerr, Hans-Peter, 93

Dung, 282

Durga, 186

Dwarf birch, 78

Dwarf elder, 178

Dwarf mallow, 114

E

Earth smoke, 112

Easter water, 20

Ebony, 240

Echinochloa crus-galli. See
  Barnyard grass

Echium vulgare. See Blue weed

Egyptian medicine, Ancient, 10

Elder, 76–77, 85, 92, 151–52,
  153–57, 180–81, 274

Elecampane, 146, 231

Electuaries, 223

Eliade, Mircea, 93, 297

Elixirs, 236

Elkshoulder, George, 289

Emetics, 91–93

Enlightenment, 12, 98, 232

Epilobium angustifolium. See
  Willowherb

Equisetum arvense. See Field
  horsetail

E. hyemale. See Rough horsetail

Ergot poisoning, 190, 227–28, 303

Ethnomedicine, 9

Etienne (bishop of Paris), 224

Euphrasia officinalis. See Eyebright

Eve, 16, 214, 245, 256, 304

Evelyn, John, 271

Evening, significance of, 52

Eyebright, 165–66

F

False Face Society, 22

Farmers

  first, 21, 100–103

  sedentary lifestyle and, 107–9

Fennel, 214–15

Fenugreek, 169, 282

Feverfew, 203

Fiacre, Saint, 199

Field cow-wheat, 112

Field horsetail, 26, 77–78

Field larkspur, 112

Field parsley-piert, 112

Field pennycress, 208

Figwort, 166, 199

Filipendula ulmaria. See
  Meadowsweet

Fir clubmoss, 76, 205

Fire and water, 36–37, 42, 47

Fireweed, 74, 78, 190

Fly agaric, 67, 72–74, 294

Fomes fomentarius. See Tinder
  polypore

Food preparation, 242–43

Forest culture, 12–13, 15–19, 21–23
Forest sanicula, 230
Four, symbolism of, 50
Frederick II (Holy Roman emperor), 224
Freya, 98, 144, 175, 182, 183, 189, 192, 201, 267, 268, 276, 301
Freyr, 73, 144, 181, 277, 300–301
Fringed sage, 68, 85, 88
Frobenius, Leo, 293
Fuchs, Leonhart, 202
Fuller, Buckminster, 8
Fumitory (*Fumaria officinalis*), 112

G
Galangal, 236, 240
Galen, 5, 6, 7, 11, 27, 180, 224, 291, 305
Galium verum. See Lady's bedstraw
Gall, Saint, 176, 303
Galsterwomen, 264–65
Garden of Eden, 5
Garlic, 146, 193
Gautama Siddhartha, 137
Gauze, 236
Geranium robertianum. See Herb Robert/Rupert
Gerard, Saint, 195, 199–200
German chamomile, 210
Gertrude, Saint, 177
Geum rivale. See Water avens
G. urbanum. See Wood avens
Ginger, 240, 273
Gitxsan, 72
Glechoma hederacea. See Ground ivy
Gnomes, 128, 129
Gode, 263, 306
Gods. *See also individual gods*

healing, 132–36
wrath of, 131–32
Goeldin, Anna, 232
Goethe, Johann Wolfgang von, 221, 306
Goldenrod, 166
Golowin, Sergius, 241, 242, 289–90
Goosefoot, 114
Goutweed, 200
Grain Wolf, 110
Greater celadine, 191
Greater figwort, 199
Great Tradition and Little Tradition, 19–21, 162, 241–42
Gregory the Great (pope), 174, 176
Gregory von Tours (bishop), 175
Grieve, Maude, 210, 211
Groa, 268
Gromwell, 109
Groundhog Day, 54
Ground ivy, 181–82, 193, 272
Ground pine, 75
Guaiacum (*Guaiacum officinalis*), 231
Gydia, 263

H
Hairy bittercress, 208
Halldórsson, Jon (bishop), 269
Harmal, 240
Harvest Queen, 110
Hashish, 240
Hawthorn, 169
Healing plants. *See also individual plants*
animals using, 59–60
apophytes, 113–14
arable weeds, 110–13
circumpolar, 67–71, 75–81

collection guidelines for, 247–50
discovery of, 59
essence of, 159–62
power of, 25, 285–86
pre-historic use of, 60–62, 66–67
roots of, 170–71
saints and, 194–203
signatures of, 162–70
Hearth, role of, 103, 246–47
Hedge mustard, 112
Heimdall, 212
Hellebore, 266
Hemp, 82, 294
Hempel, Werner, 99
Henbane, 196, 266, 272, 306
Hennepin, Father, 81
Henry VI (king of England), 271
Henry VIII (king of England), 271
Heracleum. See Meadow
  hogweed
Herbal teas
  in China, 28–31
  of indigenous forest people,
    26–27
  making, 26–27, 30
  in other cultures, 31–35
Herb Barbara, 197
Herb Bennet, 199
Herb-paris, 202
Herb Peter, 189
Herb Robert/Rupert, 166, 190
Herdsmen, as healers, 252–53
Heretics, 226–27
Hermes, Arthur, 104, 252, 280, 281,
  284
Herodias, 259
Herodotus, 82
Hibiscus, 178
Hierochloe odorata. See Sweetgrass

Hildegard of Bingen, 7, 89, 111,
  118, 167, 180, 216–19, 220, 221,
  235, 236, 237, 273, 275, 276,
  305
Hippocrates, 5, 6, 11, 162, 175, 180,
  224, 305
Holbein, Hans, the Younger, 106
Holle, Mother, 45, 46, 52, 88, 116,
  117, 152–55, 158, 180, 207
Holocene Thermal Maximum
  (HTM), 99
Holy Grail, 47, 294
Holy thistle, 167
Honey, 282
Hopewell, 81
Hops, 270–71, 273
Horehound, 273
Horseshoes, 204
Horsetail, 26, 77–78, 166, 282
Houseleek, 193
Hubertus, Saint, 104, 275
Hufeland, Christoph, 233
Hulda, Mother, 45, 46, 52, 229, 251
Humoral pathology, 11–12, 174
Huna, 2
Huperzia selago. See Fir clubmoss
Hvergelmir, 37
Hyoscyamus niger. See Henbane
Hypericum perforatum. See Saint-
  John's-wort

I

Iatro astrology, 223
Ibn al-Baitar, 222
Imbolc, 54
Impatiens glandulifera. See Indian
  jewelweed
Indian jewelweed, 170
Indian tobacco, 91

Indra, 131–32, 141, 193
Inonotus obliquus. See Chaga
Inquisition, 98, 185, 226–27, 228
Inuits, 69
Irminsul, 18, 20, 292
Iroquois, 22, 69, 81, 92
Islamic medicine, 222–23, 233–40

J
James the Elder, Saint, 184
Jasmine, 240
Jesus, 5, 55, 144, 148, 152, 177, 181,
    182, 183, 188, 189, 191, 200,
    214, 226, 236, 248, 294, 295, 305
Jewel pills, 33
Joan of Arc, 267
John the Baptist, 177, 182, 185
John XXII (pope), 224
Joseph of Arimathea, 294
Judas, 155, 181
Julep, 236
Juniper (*Juniperus communis*),
    39–42, 78–79, 85, 191, 230, 231,
    273
J. virginiana. See Red cedar
Jupiter, 193

K
Kandis, 236
Kapha, 11
Kermes, 240
Key flower, 189
Key of heaven, 189
Khanty, 72
Kiff, 240
Kneipp, Sebastian, 78, 219, 233,
    250, 282
Knotted figwort, 199
Knotweed, 79, 114

Korean medicine, 2
Kroeber, Alfred, 293
Kuan Yin-Tse, 3
Kuenzle, Johann, 219
Kusha grass, 137

L
Lacnunga, 139, 144, 205–6, 209,
    254, 279
Ladybugs, 157–59
Lady's bedstraw, 182–83
Laima, 16
Lakota, 82
Lakshmi, 139
Lammas, 54–55
Lancelot du Lac, 139
Lard, 277
Larkspur, 112
Laudanum, 232
Lawrence, Saint, 200
Laxatives, 91–93, 223
Ledum palustre. See Marsh
    Labrador tea
Leech doctors, 138–40, 265
Lehmann-Enders, Christel, 173
Leschij, 13
Lesser celandine, 166, 199
Levisticum offinale. See Lovage
Liftinae, Boniface, 175
Ligusticum meum. See Bear root
Lily of the valley, 266
Lime, 240
Linaria vulgaris. See Toadflax
Linden, 166–67, 183
Linear Pottery culture, 100, 101
Linseed, 282
Liqueurs, 223
Lithospermum. See Stoneseed
Little Ice Age, 227

Little Tradition and Great
    Tradition, 19–21, 162, 241–42
Lobelia inflata. See Puke weed
Loki, 16, 192, 267
Lomi, 2
Loofah, 240
Lords-and-ladies, 169
Lovage, 178
Lucanus, Marcus Annaeus, 17
Lucian, Saint, 201, 303
Luepplerin, 266
Lugh, 184
Lughnasadh, 54–55
Lungwort, 167
Lupercalia, 54
Lycopodium clavatum. See
    Clubmoss, common
L. selago. See Fir clubmoss

M

Macer Floridus, 180
Maiden hair fern, 146
Male fern, 146, 209
Mallow, 114
Malus sylvestris. See Crab apple
Malva neglecta. See Dwarf mallow
M. sylvestris. See Mallow
Manabozho, 71
Marcellus Empiricus, 19, 92
Margaret, Saint, 196–97, 202–3
Marian thistle, 167
Marjoram, 273
Marsh Labrador tea, 79
Marsh marigold, 79–80
Marsh yarrow, 200
Martin, Saint, 17, 176
Mary (mother of Jesus), 78, 125,
    181, 183, 184, 186, 191, 201,
    248, 256, 296, 301, 303

Marzipan, 240
Massage, 2, 236
Masterwort, 230
Matricaria chamomilla. See
    Chamomile
M. discoidea. See Chamomile
M. recutita. See Chamomile
Mayweed, 209
Meadow hogweed, 193, 194
Meadow saffron, 164
Meadow saxifrage, 168
Meadowsweet, 167, 273
Médard, Saint, 145
Medicine Buddha, 33
Medicine Crow, Joseph, 59
Melampyrum arvense. See Field
    cow-wheat
Menominee, 92
Menstruation, 251–52
Menyanthes trifoliata. See Bogbean
Mercuris dulcis. See Calomel
Mercury, 231–32, 234
Merlin, 15
Mességué, Maurice, 191, 233, 247
Miach, 163
Michener, James A., 5
Micmac, 72
Midday, significance of, 51–52
Midgard, 102
Midnight, significance of, 52–53
Midwives
    effectiveness of, 258
    methods of, 20, 88
    persecution of, 224, 256–57
    role of, 254–55
    status of, 254, 255
    toleration of, 232
Milfoil, 191–92
Milk thistle, 167

Mineral remedies, 222–23
Mint, 85, 146
Mistletoe, 160, 301
Modern medicine
  alternatives to, 2–3
  skepticism toward, 1–3
Molitor, Ulricus, 45
Monarda fistulosa. See Bee balm
Monastic medicine, 6, 180, 223,
  225, 233
Monkshood, 193, 196, 198
Morning, significance of, 50–51
Morphogenetic fields, 289–90
Morrigan, 187
Mothers, role of, 250–51
Mountain ash, 193
Moxibustion, 87, 89
Mueller, Wilhelm, 1
Mueller-Ebeling, Claudia, 285
Mugwort, 40, 66, 78, 84, 85, 87–89,
  167, 207, 209, 273, 297
Mullein, 114, 183–84
Mummies (mumia), 236, 238–39
Myrica gale. See Bog myrtle
Myrrh, 236–37, 240
Myth, role of, 8–9

N
Naked lady, 164
Nasturtium (*Nasturtium*
  officinale), 208
Natron, 237
Nature spirits, 13, 63
Neanderthals, 60, 61
Nemeton, 15
Nemetonia, 15
Nerthus, 116
Nettle, 67, 80–81, 85, 114, 185,
  211–13, 273

Nicolas, Saint, 177, 274, 302
Nightmares, 129
Nine Herbs Charm, 88, 97, 117,
  141, 207–16
Nocebo effect, 288
Noon, significance of, 51–52
Nuada, 163

O
Oak, 17–18, 231, 274
Oats, 85
Odin, 15–16, 37, 73, 97–98, 141,
  144, 147, 151, 181, 193, 204,
  206, 207, 265, 267, 292, 301
Oetzi, 69, 71
Oils, 276–79
Ojibwa, 70, 71
Okanagan, 71, 77
Omaha, 68
Opium, 232
Orange, 240
Ostera, 20, 177
Ostyaks, 72
Our Lady's keys, 189
Ovens, 44, 90–91
Ovid, 44
Oxeye daisy, 203

P
Palm Sunday, 54, 187
Papaver rhoeas. See Corn poppy
Paracelsus, 1, 7, 129, 163, 185, 235,
  239, 242, 266, 269, 291
Paris quadrifolia. See Herb-paris
Parsley, 178, 273
Pashupati, 87
Pathways of the dead, 115, 117
Pawnee, 68
Perkunas, 16, 193

Index

Persephone, 117
Pestilence saints, 229
Petasites hybridus. See Butterbur
Peter, Saint, 17, 144, 181, 189
Petroselinum crispum. See Parsley
Peucedanum ostruthium. See
   Masterwort
Pfleiderer, Beatrix, 59
Physicians
   effect of, 288
   professionalization of, 222–25
   shamans vs., 95–96
Pimpernel, 106, 113, 201
Pimpinella saxifraga. See Saxifrage
Pine, 85
Pipal, 160
Pipsissewa, 81
Piptoporus betulinus. See Birch
   polypore
Pitta, 11
Placebo effect, 288–89
Plague, 90, 106, 108, 228–31, 238
Plantain (*Plantago major*), 114–19,
   208, 298
Pliny, 19, 205, 279, 283
Plum, 240
Poisons, 266
Poludnitsa, 51
Polygonaceae. See Docks
Polygonum bistorta. See Bistort
P. spp. *See* Knotweed
Polypody (*Polypodum*), 272
Pomander, 228
Potassium, 237
Potawatomi, 77
Potentilla anserina. See Silverweed
P. erecta. See Tormentil
Poultices, 282
Prairie sage, 66

Pranayama, 2
Professionalization, 222–25
Progress, as alienating ideology,
   284–86
Prosperina, 117
Puke weed, 91
Pulmonaria officinalis. See Lungwort
Pulse taking, 223
Purgatives, 91–93, 223
Pyrethrum, 178
Pyrola umbellata. See Winter green
Pythagoras, 305

Q
Qi-gong, 2

R
Raetsch, Christian, 73, 209, 271
Ragwort, 184–85
Ransoms, 230
Ranunculus ficaria. See Lesser
   celandine
Red, symbolism of, 262–63
Red cedar, 87
Redfield, Robert, 21
Regino of Pruem (abbot), 259
Reichholf, Josef H., 45
Reiki, 2
Rhazes, 222
Rhododendron palustre. See Marsh
   Labrador tea
R. tomentosum. See Marsh
   Labrador tea
Richter, Ludwig, 14
Rigveda, 121, 159, 161, 170, 300,
   301
Robert, Saint, 190
Robert geranium, 190
Roch, Saint, 201–2, 229

327

Roman chamomile, 200, 210
Roots, 170–71
Rose hips, 169, 273
Rosemary, wild, 193
Rough horsetail, 26, 77–78
Rouquouyennes, 86
Rowan, 273
Rudra, 131
Rue, 178
Ruebezahl, 13, 14, 230
Rumex. See Docks
Rupert, Saint, 190
Rusalka, 13
Ruta graveolens. See Rue
Rye, 227, 303

S
Safflower, 240
Saffron, 237, 240
Sage, 178
Saint Anthony's fire, 190, 228, 303
Saint James wort, 184
Saint-John's-wort, 27, 40, 167–68, 185, 247, 262, 273
Saints. *See also individual saints*
    bread and, 275
    festivals of, 177
    healing plants and, 194–203
    pestilence, 229
Salep, 240
Salerno, medical school of, 223–24
Salt, 280–82
Salves, 276–79
Salvia spp. *See* Sage
Sambucus canadensis. See Elder
S. ebulus. See Dwarf elder
S. nigra. See Elder
Samhain, 55
Sandalwood, 240

Sanicle (*Sanicula europaea*), 200, 230
Saponoria officinalis. See Soapwort
Saracen ointment, 231
Sarasvati, 70
Sarsaparilla, 231
Satan, 226–27
Saussurea spp. *See* Costus root
Saxifrage (*Saxifraga* spp.), 168, 230
Schmitz, Rudolf, 139
Scrophularia nodosa. See Figwort
Sebastian, Saint, 229
Sedentary lifestyle, 107–9
Self-heal, 85
Seminole, 91
Semper pervivum. See Houseleek
Senecio jacobaea. See Tansy ragwort
Senna, 240
Sen No Rikyu, 25
Sesame, 240
Shamanism, 2, 72–73, 93–98, 168, 297
Shavegrass, 166
Sheldrake, Rupert, 289
Shennong, 28–29
Shepherds, as healers, 252–53
Shepherd's purse, 113
Shiatsu, 2
Shiva, 87, 186
Shoshone, 109
Shou-Hsing, 4
Signatures and signs, 162–70
Silver thistle, 199
Silverweed, 114
Silybum marianum. See Milk thistle
Sisymbrium officinale. See Hedge mustard

Sloe, 187–88
Smilax officinalis. See Sarsaparilla
Smiths, as healers, 253–54
Soap, 279–80
Soapwort, 114
Soda, 237
Solanum nigrum. See Black
  nightshade
Solidago virgaurea. See Goldenrod
Soma, 136, 160, 161
Sonchus oleraceus. See Sow thistle
Sorceresses, 261, 262–63, 266
Sow thistle, 111
Speedwell, 203
Spells, evil, 126–27
Spinach, 240
Springs, sacred, 46–47
Spruce, 85, 151
Spurge, 193
Stachys officinalis. See Betony
Stag, as symbol, 104–5
Stag's horn clubmoss, 75
Steam baths, 82, 90
Steiner, Rudolf, 164, 302
Stephen, Saint, 148
Steppe nomads, culture of, 122–25
Steppe sagebrush, 87
Stinging nettle. *See* Nettle
Stone Age medicine, 60–61, 63–67,
  91
Stoneseed, 109
Storkbill, 190
Strabo, 19
Strabo, Walafrid, 173, 179
Strassmann, René, 153
Stune, 208
Sugar, 237
Sultana, 240
Sumac, 240

Surya, 134
Sushruta, 162
Swallowwort, 191
Swantowit, 73
Sweat lodges, 82–86, 90, 296
Sweet flag, 67
Sweet gale, 85, 193
Sweetgrass, 87
Symphytum officinale. See
  Comfrey
Synod of Ancyra, 175
Synod of Laodicea, 175, 302
Synod of Liftinae, 18, 182
Synod of Ratisbon, 302
Syphilis, 90, 231–32
Syrups, 237

T
Tacitus, Publius Cornelius, 15, 16,
  19, 116, 258
Tai chi, 2
Takmán, 133, 149
Talc, 237
Taliesin, 44
Tallbull, Bill, 285
Tamarind, 240
Tanacetum balsamita. See
  Costmary
Tansy (*Tanacetum vulgare*), 146,
  209, 273
Tansy ragwort, 110
Tarragon, 67, 85, 240
Teak, 240
Teasel, 168
Tegernsee Charm, 143
Tertullian, 175
Teutonic Order, 18
Theodosius I (Roman emperor),
  173

Theriacs, 27, 223, 228
Thlapsi arvense. See Field pennycress
Thor, 17, 141, 193, 268
Thoth, 10
Thoughts, influence of, 287–89
Three, symbolism of, 48–49
Thuja plicata. See Red cedar
Thujone, 146
Thunder beard, 193
Thyme, 273, 282
Tibetan medicine, 2, 3, 32–33
Tilia spp. *See* Linden
Tinder polypore, 71–72
Toadflax, 112, 200
Tormentil, 199, 230
Traditional Chinese Medicine (TCM), 2–3, 11, 28–31, 87, 89
Traditional European Medicine (TEM)
    myth and, 8–9
    origin of, 3–7
    popularity of, 7
    woodland culture and, 12–13, 15–19
Treben, Maria, 191, 219, 220, 233, 249, 278
Trees, transferring sickness onto, 150–53
Trotula, 224
Turmeric, 240
Twain, Mark, 289
Tyr, 193–94

U
University of Toledo, 222
Urine, 282
Uroscopy, 223

Urtica dioica. See Nettle
Utgard, 102

V
Valentinus, Basilius, 234
Valerian (*Valeriana officinalis*), 230
Vata, 11
Vayu, 134
Vedas, 37, 70, 121, 129, 133, 135, 136, 142, 147, 148, 161
Verbascum thapsus. See Mullein
Vermifuges, 146–47
Veronica (*Veronica officinalis*), 203
Veronica, Saint, 203
Vidar, 292
Villi, 37
Vincetoxicum hirundinaria. See White swallowwort
Vinegar, 282–83
Viper's bugloss, 209
Vishnu, 139
Visionaries, 267–68
Voelvas, 267–68, 294
Von Muralt, Johann, 265

W
Walburga, Saint, 267
Walnut, 146, 169
Water and fire, 36–37, 42, 47
Water avens, 81
Water pepper, 79
Weather magic, 261–62
Weber, Friedrich Wilhelm, 283
Weil, Andrew, 286, 287, 288
Weledas, 267–68
Wendelin, Saint, 275
White Goddess, 45, 54, 70, 187, 300
White swallowwort, 200
Wickersche, 263

Wiegele, Miriam, 152
Wild people, 105–7
Willett, Walter, 269
William of Bavaria (duke), 271
Willowherb, 74, 78, 190
Winnebago, 92
Winter green, 81, 85
Winter rocket, 197
Wissler, Clark, 293
Witches
    abilities of, 258–60
    brooms of, 70
    cauldrons of, 44–45
    as mediators between worlds,
        104, 105
    persecution of, 98, 185, 225,
        226–27, 228, 232, 259–60
    weather and, 261–62
    wood and, 104
Woden. *See* Odin
Wolf berry, 193
Wolfsbane, 193, 266
Wolf's claw, 75
Wolters, Bruno, 77, 85
Women. *See also* Midwives;
    Witches
    Catholic Church and, 175
    farmers, 100–101
    herbal knowledge of, 103–4, 247
    magical and shamanic, 258–69
    as mothers, 250–52
    remedies of, 269–83
    at Salerno, 224

traditional division of labor and,
    242–47
Wood avens, 199
Woodland culture, 12–13, 15–19,
    21–23
Woodland figwort, 166
Words, power of, 130–31
Worms
    as cause of disease, 92, 96,
        129–30, 140–41
    colors of, 145
    destroying, 140–59
    intestinal, 146–47
Wormwood, 85, 146
Wortcunners, 170–71
Wotan. *See* Odin

X
Xhosa, 60

Y
Yajur Veda, 159
Yarrow, 67, 85, 106, 191–92, 193,
    197, 273, 282
Yggrdrasil, 16, 292
Ymir, 37, 294
Yoga, 2

Z
Zedonary, 240
Zeus, 193
Zwingli, Ulrich, 265

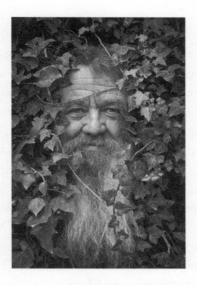

ABOUT THE AUTHOR

Born in 1942 in Saxony, Germany, with a green thumb and the gift of writing, cultural anthropologist and ethnobotanist Wolf Dieter Storl, who emigrated with his parents to the United States in 1954, has had a special connection to nature since childhood. His specific area of research is shamanism and healing in traditional societies, focusing on the role of plants in all aspects of life, including sacred symbolism, magic, medicine, foods, and poisons. He has pursued this interest in many parts of the world.

After finishing his PhD in anthropology (magna cum laude) on a Fulbright scholarship in 1974 in Berne, Switzerland, he taught anthropology and sociology in Grants Pass, Oregon. During this time, he also offered an extremely popular organic-gardening course, as he was one of the pioneers of the organic/biodynamic gardening movement. While preparing for his doctoral exams in Switzerland, he also lived in an experimental community and helped tend a five-acre organic garden. There, he had the good fortune to learn from master gardener Manfred Stauffer, who specialized in composting organic matter.

Storl is also an avid traveler and has observed nature around the entire globe, spending time with people who are very connected to the nature that surrounds them. From 1982 to 1983, he spent a year as an official visiting scholar at the Benares Hindu University in Varanasi, India. After returning to the United States in 1984, he spent much time with traditional medicine persons of the Cheyenne and taught courses at Sheridan College in Sheridan, Wyoming. He has traveled and conducted research in South Asia, India, Mexico, the Canary Islands, South Africa, and much of Europe, pursuing ethnobotanical and ethnomedicinal interests. He has written some twenty-five books and many articles, which have been translated into various languages, including Czech, Danish, Dutch, English, French, Italian, Japanese, Latvian, Polish, Portuguese, Spanish, and Russian. Storl is a frequent guest on German, Swiss, and Austrian television and has also appeared on the BBC.

After another visit in India and Nepal in 1986, Storl and his wife moved to Germany, where he is both a freelance writer and lecturer. They live on an old estate with a large garden in the foothills of the Alps.

Storl's books are unique in that he does not treat nature with cold objectivism. He is able to delve into nature's depths and supports his experience with ancient lore from all over the world that has been, for the most part, left on the wayside in the wake of objective science. He theorizes that science is not always as objective as it claims to be. He invites his readers on a journey into a world of nature that is completely alive and has its own rhyme and reason. Myths and lore from many cultures also have a prominent place in his writings, as he claims that the images portrayed in this way often tell us more about the true nature of things than dry facts can.

TITLES BY WOLF D. STORL

available from North Atlantic Books

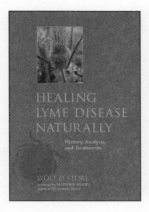

*Healing Lyme
Disease Naturally*
978-1-55643-873-8

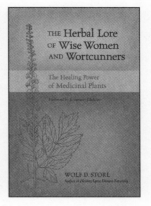

*The Herbal Lore of Wise
Women and Wortcunners*
978-1-58394-358-8

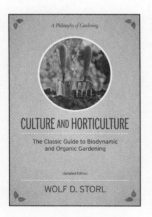

Culture and Horticulture
978-1-58394-550-6

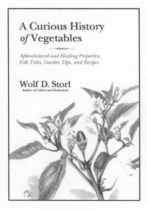

*A Curious History
of Vegetables*
978-1-62317-039-4

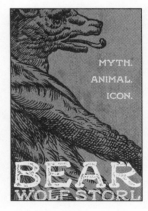

Bear
978-1-62317-163-6
Available January 2018

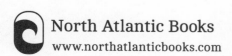

North Atlantic Books
www.northatlanticbooks.com

North Atlantic Books is an independent, nonprofit publisher committed to a bold exploration of the relationships between mind, body, spirit, and nature.